WHEN PEOPLE COME FIRST

CRITICAL STUDIES IN
GLOBAL HEALTH

EDITED BY
JOÃO BIEHL &
ADRIANA PETRYNA

PRINCETON UNIVERSITY PRESS

PRINCETON AND OXFORD

Copyright © 2013 by Princeton University Press

Published by Princeton University Press, 41 William Street, Princeton, New Jersey 08540

In the United Kingdom: Princeton University Press, 6 Oxford Street, Woodstock, Oxfordshire OX20 1TW

press.princeton.edu

Cover art by Vik Muniz, *Atlas (Carlão)*, 2008, digital C-print, 229.9 × 180.3 cm, © Vik Muniz/Licensed by VAGA, New York, NY
Cover design by warrakloureiro

All Rights Reserved

Library of Congress Cataloging-in-Publication Data

When people come first : critical studies in global health / edited by Joao Biehl and Adriana Petryna.
    pages cm
    Summary: "When People Come First critically assesses the expanding field of global health. It brings together an international and interdisciplinary group of scholars to ad-dress the medical, social, political, and economic dimensions of the global health enterprise through vivid case studies and bold conceptual work. The book demonstrates the crucial role of ethnography as an empirical lantern in global health, arguing for a more compre-hensive, people-centered approach. Topics include the limits of technological quick fixes in disease control, the moral economy of global health science, the unexpected effects of massive treatment rollouts in resource-poor contexts, and how right-to-health activism coalesces with the increased influence of the pharmaceutical industry on health care. The contributors explore the altered landscapes left behind after programs scale up, break down, or move on. We learn that disease is really never just one thing, technology delivery does not equate with care, and biology and technology interact in ways we cannot always predict. The most effective solutions may well be found in people themselves, who consis-tently exceed the projections of experts and the medical-scientific, political, and humani-tarian frameworks in which they are cast. When People Come First sets a new research agenda in global health and social theory and challenges us to rethink the relationships between care, rights, health, and economic futures"— Provided by publisher.
    Includes bibliographical references and index.
    ISBN 978-0-691-15738-2 (hardback) — ISBN 978-0-691-15739-9 (paperback)
    1. World health. 2. Public health—International cooperation. I. Biehl, João Guilherme. II. Petryna, Adriana, date.
    RA441.W44 2013
    362.1—dc23
                        2012049338

British Library Cataloging-in-Publication Data is available

This book has been composed in Sabon and Helvetica Neue

Printed on acid-free paper. ∞

Printed in the United States of America

10 9 8 7 6 5 4 3 2 1

Contents

WHEN
PEOPLE
COME
FIRST

Critical Global Health

JOÃO BIEHL AND ADRIANA PETRYNA

A Visit with the Patient

Janira lies in bed at home while her mother, Carmen, visits the public defender's office in Porto Alegre, Brazil. Carmen is filing a lawsuit to obtain
the medicine that her daughter urgently needs to treat severe pulmonary
hypertension. A heart attack the year before led to a loss of mobility,
and Janira has not been able to resume work. Her doctor has prescribed
six medicines; five are provided through Brazil's universal health system,
while the sixth, a high-cost vasodilator, is not. The doctor advised the low-
income family to seek free legal assistance at the public defender's office.

Carmen hands the doctor's prescription to Paula Pinto de Souza, the
public defender responsible for her case. "Is it here that I get the medicine?" she asks.

Paula welcomes Carmen "to the juridical hospital," but she explains
that getting the medicine will not be so simple. In her role as a legal advocate for the poor and chronically ill, Paula's job is to ameliorate suffering and to restore the rights of her clients. "The person," she explains,
"comes here sick. Her right to health has been profoundly injured by
public power. Even if the medicine might not bring them life, the claim is
also for their dignity." That, at least, is Paula's goal.

Given the severity of Janira's condition, Paula will ask the district judge to issue a court injunction compelling the state to provide Janira's treatment right away. She cautions Carmen not to get her hopes up too high, however, as state attorneys will most likely appeal the lawsuit. "It might take years to reach a verdict," she says. And this is not unusual. It is in fact typical of the right-to-health lawsuits that now inundate the Brazilian judiciary. And the problem does not end there. Carmen complains that she has already gone to the state pharmacy several times to obtain the five other medicines that Janira needs, and that should be publicly available, "but they are always out of stock."

Carmen, whose husband died of cancer, is retired and lives on a small pension. Her home is a one-room shack on the outskirts of the city, which she shares with her daughter and two granddaughters. A monthly course of the vasodilator Janira needs costs about US$1,000. Carmen has been purchasing the medicine in small amounts with borrowed cash, indebting herself to members of her extended family. She makes a little extra money performing Afro-Brazilian rituals in her home and occasionally receives a food basket from her religious organization. When we visited the shack, we noticed an offering to the *orixás* filled with packaged sweets.[1] "I do this so that all patients who need medicines win their lawsuits," Carmen explains.

What Janira really needs is a heart transplant, and all the medicines she takes are meant to keep her healthy enough to undergo the surgery. Janira's brother, who lives in another shack on the same lot with his own family, routinely checks the status of her case at a nearby Internet station. Within days of the public defender's filing, the district judge issues an injunction for the medicine to be delivered to Janira. Two months later it has still not arrived.

At a time of great medical progress, Janira is barely clinging to life. Her family is locked in a daily struggle for survival on several fronts, for in order to preserve Janira's life they must not only battle her disease but also resist political and economic death and social oblivion. Theirs is only one story, but it accurately reflects the way in which broad-based questions of access to technology and social justice are often contested in today's rapidly changing public health context. Anthropological fieldwork or home visits, such as the one we have described, can vividly capture and draw attention to these efforts and to the real persons whose imperiled lives they impact. For anthropologists, these peopled accounts—stories that are so often hidden from view, obscured by more abstract and bureaucratic considerations of public policy—are the very fabric of alternative social theorizing. By looking closely at life stories and at the ups and downs of individuals and communities as they grapple with inequality, struggle to access technology, and confront novel state-market formations, we begin to apprehend larger systems. We are able to see them in the making or in the process of dissolution, and we understand more intimately the local realities, so often unspoken, that result when people are seen or governed in a particular way, or not at all.

In the course of the twentieth century, innovations in public health and medicine helped to increase life expectancy at birth by almost thirty years in the United States and other rich countries. Meanwhile, mortality rates remained high and life expectancies short in poor countries (Cutler, Deaton, and Lleras-Muney 2006). Advances in medical technology continue to give cause for hope, as does the substantial increase in financial resources now available to address some of the world's most pressing health challenges. New state policies, public-private partnerships, and multidisciplinary research collaborations are reshaping the field that has come to be known as Global Health and, in the process, putting older paradigms into question and transforming realities on the ground. In key developing democracies—such as Brazil, India, and South Africa—we see activists and patients engaging in struggles over access to high-quality care and, at a more fundamental level, debating the meaning and implications of health conceived as a right rather than a privilege (Biehl et al. 2012; Fassin 2007).

Magic-bullet approaches—the delivery of health technologies (usually new drugs or devices) that target one specific disease without regard to the myriad societal, political, and economic factors that influence outcomes—have been the norm in international health interventions for decades. There are, however, significant practical and epistemological downsides to this approach, which is now being challenged. Social scientists and health-policy advocates caution that a narrow focus on the triad of technology delivery, patient compliance, and the basic science of disease, as important as they are, is insufficient. Also, unintended consequences may be unleashed by even the most carefully designed interventions (DelVecchio Good, Good, and Grayman 2010; Larson 2011).

The global health community has overemphasized individual risk factors that ignore how health risks are shaped by law, politics, and practices ranging from industrial and agricultural policies to discrimination, violence, and lack of access to justice. We need to better attend to breakdowns in public health systems and to the many political and social determinants of health (such as education, water, sanitation, vector control, air pollution, and accident prevention) that make people vulnerable to disease and injury in the first place (Amon and Kasambala 2009; Cueto 2007; Farmer 2004; Freedman 2005; Hahn and Inhorn 2008; Singer and Hodge 2010; Utzinger et al. 2002). Given the extreme inequalities that are so intricately woven into the current international order as well as into the social and political fabrics of countries and regions (Reinhardt, Hussey, and Anderson 2004; Deaton 2008), we need integrated approaches that recognize the profound interdependence of health, economic development, good governance, and human rights. Any sustainable development has to reach and improve the conditions of the poorest and most vulnerable groups carrying the highest burdens of ill health.

Moreover, as is evident in Janira's case, disease is never just one thing, technology delivery does not translate into patient care, and biology and technology interact in ways we cannot always predict. So, we ask: What really happens when new treatments are introduced into epidemiologically diverse and variable social worlds? How is care organized by providers, by state and nonstate institutions? By what trajectories and means do the people who desperately need care access it (or fail to access it)? And how can the stories of real people dealing with insecurities of all kinds find their way into and improve current practices in global health?

When People Come First brings together an international group that includes anthropologists, historians, and an epidemiologist and human-rights scholar to produce an ethnographic critique of the contemporary global health enterprise. While global health initiatives and programs are booming in the United States and have begun also to displace earlier framings of the field (such as "tropical medicine" or "international health") in Western Europe and Latin America, critical analyses of the social, political, and economic processes associated with this quickly evolving field are still few and far between. The contributors to this volume are engaged in both empirical and theoretical investigations of global health-related initiatives and epistemologies, and are concerned with the actual impacts of these initiatives on care, health systems, and governance. The book emphasizes ethnography as a crucial methodological tool for achieving better comprehension of health services at all levels of analysis and advocates anthropological case studies and crosscultural analysis as foundational to a much-needed critical global health perspective.

Our case studies explore the agonistic relationships among people, medical technologies, markets, and public institutions and reflect on the limits of the evidence-making practices, models of care delivery, and moral calculus that underpin large-scale health interventions. Contributors attend to the variable intended and unintended effects of these interventions on those in need, and they challenge the certainties of planners and implementers while probing the limits and possibilities of the social theories informing their works. Cases draw from fieldnotes, interviews, life histories, and database and document analyses, and they are constructed in dialogue with rich bodies of applied and theoretical work carried out in specific countries and regions. While each case has something important and original to say about a particular facet of global health today, the cases also play off each other to produce a critical cumulative effect that is greater than the sum of its parts.

When People Come First offers innovative ways of thinking about older debates in light of emerging realities, and it sets a new agenda for research in global health, one aimed at a more comprehensive framework for understanding the human, technical, and political issues involved. The title of the book expresses our shared respect for the dignity and singularity of the people with whom we work, and our close attention to the ways in which their own struggles and visions of themselves and others create holes in dominant theories and interventions. People constantly exceed the projections of experts. The medicoscientific, political, and humanitarian frameworks in which they are temporarily cast cannot contain them. Their plights and travails demand intense listening and continuous attention. We must hold social theory accountable for the full range of human conditions, for all the polyvocal and contradictory realities that we encounter in the field, and that are too often obscured by the lens of established thought. *When People Come First* is thus as much a critical study of global health as it is a field guide for a global health humanities that can challenge perceptual deficits of all kinds, open new avenues of thought, and inform the continuous efforts of multiple stakeholders to create a health sufficient to liberate human potentials and futures, wherever they are thwarted.

The Field of Global Health

In the twentieth century, international health initiatives were by and large implemented by states, subject to the coordination of specialized bodies such as the World Health Organization (WHO). In this paradigm, the main source of authority was the state, which took the lead in setting priorities and allocating resources. The politics of international health care were, as a result, subject to the usual constraints of diplomacy (Fidler 2007; Brown, Cueto, and Fee 2006), while the WHO and related bodies played a coordinating role, often using the discourse of human rights to orient and instigate efforts. These dynamics would be somewhat altered in the context of the United Nations' Millennium Development Goals (MDGs), which recognized health as an essential value and as a key pillar of development (United Nations 2000). New forms of cooperation and intervention were established to reach the targets of reducing maternal and child mortality and expanding access to treatment for infectious diseases, for example. In the process, the interests and practices of the private sector began to play a larger role in global public health. Humanitarian schemes and health system building have made common cause with the technical and financial know-how of the private sector (Cueto, this volume). A complex mix of partnerships linking state and nonstate actors—the latter including philanthropic agencies, nongovernmental organizations (NGOs), and the pharmaceutical industries—has arisen and is shaping health interventions worldwide under the rubrics of humanitarianism, development, and security (Fassin 2012; Lakoff and Collier 2008; Birn 2005b).

We now see a multiplicity of actors, all vying for resources and influence in the political field of global health, each seeking to remain a relevant and powerful player. Ranging from the Gates Foundation to pharmaceutical company drug donation programs and PEPFAR (the [US] President's Emergency Plan for AIDS Relief), to research initiatives, South-South cooperation and myriad rights-based pilot projects, these diverse interests are setting new norms for institutional response, sometimes providing the public health resources that states and markets cannot or have failed to furnish. Locally, such multiple and fragmentary global health interventions consolidate what Susan Reynolds Whyte and her colleagues call, in this volume, "projectified" landscapes of care (see also DelVecchio Good, Good, and Grayman 2010). While enabling much-needed access to AIDS treatment, for example, the amalgamation of public-private interventions can also endow states with new (and sometimes abusive) powers. The "projectification of care" is thus a key venue in which the scope and roles of government are redefined, micropolitics diversified, and entrepreneurial prospects of all kinds explored (Ecks and Harper, this volume).

There is considerable confusion about how these new players and initiatives fit together in a global health architecture, and how they inform the ongoing debate about whether such architecture can and should be constructed and, if so, by whom and in whose interest (Cohen 2006; Garrett 2007; Frenk 2010; Keusch et al. 2010). In practice the concerns of donors, not recipients, tend to predominate (Schieber et al. 2007; Easterly 2006; Epstein 2007; Ferguson 2006; Ramiah and Reich 2005; Farmer 2011). Often, donors insist on funding disease-specific and technologically oriented vertical programs at the expense of the public sector (Pfeiffer, this volume). Thus, in settings as diverse as neoliberal Mozambique and urban America, state-of-the art facilities for HIV/AIDS testing, treatment, and clinical research coexist with dilapidated public hospitals. Coinfections, which are not built into the calculus of disability-adjusted life years (DALYs), are yet another indication that global health interventions that limit their target to one disease can miss the mark. Such is the case with malaria. No one contracts it or recovers from it in a vacuum, and its biological and immunological uncertainties beg for a more nuanced science (Packard 2007).

Whatever differences in interest and ideology may divide corporate, activist, and state public health agendas, the imperatives of "saving lives" and "increasing access" seem to reconcile these differences and fold them into an ethos of collective responsibility in the face of "crisis." Global health players can become impervious to critique as they identify emergencies, cite dire statistics, and act on their essential duty of promoting health in the name of "humanitarian reason" or as an instrument of economic development, diplomacy, or national security (Fassin 2011; Adams, Novotny, and Leslie 2008; Buss and Ferreira 2010). We are left, however, with an "open-source anarchy" around global health problems—a policy space in which new strategies, rules, distributive schemes, and the practical ethics of health care are being assembled, experimented with, and improvised by a wide array of deeply unequal stakeholders (Fidler 2008:410; Pogge 2010).

Treatment access is one of the central tenets of global health activism and a professed goal of interventions. Biological and medical sciences have greatly contributed to today's therapeutic armamentarium, and the metrics of epidemiology and pharmacology have productively shaped the design and implementation of interventions. Amid fluctuations in funding, the field of global health has been consistently driven by scientifically based schemes of evaluation revolving around natural experiments, randomized controlled trials (RCTs), and statistical significance (Hammer and Berman 1995; Anand and Hansen 1997; Duflo and Kremer 2008; Imbens 2010). In this dominant regime of veridiction and falsification (Foucault 2008), evidence-based medicine has migrated to the realm of health interventions and has quickly positioned itself as the default language for both public- and private-sector actors concerned with identifying problems and measuring outcomes (Deaton 2010; Cartwright 2011).

Indeed, "RCTs have been given a free pass in the name of rigor," development economist Angus Deaton argues. "But there are no magic bullets and there are no gold standards" (2012).[2] With the hegemony of this theoretical and technical fix, the kinds of data we collect and our capacity to apprehend heterogeneity are compromised. Moreover, biosocial approaches to disease and health that could help to specify dynamic causal connections and local politics are relegated to the low-authority category of "soft science" (Adams, this volume; see Krieger 2011).

The advent of for-profit institutions as purveyors of services (be it the fulfillment of specialized functions or an entire intervention) has demanded the incorporation of systematic economic assessment techniques, of which the cost-benefit analysis and the audit are the most salient. In this new landscape of global health saturated with NGOs and special-interest groups, there is a movement toward making interventions cost-effective and scalable. Thus, interventions themselves become producers and consumers of marketable and comparable information. Entrepreneurship over capitalizable data has taken hold.

Needless to say, such approaches perpetuate a limited understanding of narrowly conceptualized problems and support a rhetoric that offers only temporary control over isolated aspects of a given disease—a rhetoric that is aligned with the demands of funding organizations for immediate technical solutions (Amon, this volume). This preoccupation with scientific and economic issues results in less attention to on-the-ground social dynamics of programs and in assumptions that a particular model will work in an array of countries and situations, despite the fact that each is home to distinct institutions, practices, and rationalities, not to mention persistent inequalities and stubborn deficits in local infrastructures (Moran-Thomas, this volume).

Global health, according to business scholar Michael E. Porter, mirrors the limitations of health care delivery in the United States and "is stuck in an access and volume mindset, rather than focusing on the value delivered to patients" (Porter 2010; Porter 2009; Porter and Teisberg 2006). That is, narrow measurements of efficacy concentrate exclusively on the vertical intervention level and can assess only discrete preventative steps, drugs, or services. Porter and his colleagues call for a goal shift away from increasing access to treatments and toward delivering value for patients (Kim et al. 2010; Denzter 2009).[3] The former goal assumes a consumer-patient capable of seeking out and paying for appropriate treatment as long as it is available; the latter puts greater responsibility on health systems and providers for actively reaching the patient in need and attending to the full cycle of care and health outcomes for his or her medical condition. The focus must be on the results obtained by the patients (measured in survival rates and in the degree and sustainability of recovery) and *not* on a program's success (measured, for example, by its compliance with standardized guidelines or by the number of drugs distributed).

A more holistic understanding of health is called for, and diverse disciplines (including anthropology) must be engaged as we seek to understand the complexities of the context and content of interventions as well as the trial and error, the endless tinkering, of real people in specific circumstances trying to figure out what works for them (Cartwright and Hardie 2012). Such multiscale empirical knowledge is crucial to the development of a patient-centered care delivery framework. This alternative knowledge can and should challenge the reductionist epistemic frameworks that tend to inform donors' priorities and funding decisions as well as global health evaluation schemes (Epstein 2007; Stepan 2011; Feierman et al. 2010).

Anthropologist-physician Paul Farmer is one of the most prominent proponents of a community-based approach that blends technological intervention with a focus on making health systems work (2004, 2011). Farmer and Partners In Health, the organization he cofounded, understand diseases as loci where biology, environment, and medicine have gone awry, and their notion of intervention accordingly tackles the structural conditions that perpetuate disease at the local level.[4] In the interest of making the best care available to the poorest, Farmer and his colleagues reject economic orthodoxies such as demands for structural adjustments to eliminate health and education expenditures in the name of development, cost-effective benchmarks that limit the provision of wraparound services, and human rights discourses that privilege political over socioeconomic rights (Farmer 2008; Bourdieu 1998; Pfeiffer and Chapman 2010). In Partners In Health's social justice approach, accounting for individual patient trajectories and staying with patients throughout the progression of their disease and rehabilitation (the work of local *accompagnateurs*) is as important as tackling the economic and social factors that impact families and mitigating the decay of clinical infrastructures. In this vision, the health care system is seen no longer as a drain on the economy, but as an enabler of social and economic development. While Farmer's project is by no means accepted as a gold standard, it has, alongside other initiatives of this kind, created dents in the prevailing rationalities that guide global health interventions, and has redefined the perceived boundaries of feasibility.

Indeed, multiple approaches, moral principles, methodological techniques, and epistemologies cohabit within the broad framework of global health. Many would agree that global health "is more a bunch of problems than a discipline" (Kleinman 2010:1518). While the field still debates fundamental questions of self-definition and values, it has nonetheless become a significant political, economic, technological, and social nexus for a variety of actors and interests that engender projects that "are complex, diverse, temporally unstable, contingent, and often contested or resisted at different social scales" (Janes and Corbett 2009:169; Nichter 2008; Rylko-Bauer, Whiteford, and Farmer 2009). So far few, if any, institutions have been put in place to conceptualize, evaluate, or monitor the immediate and broader impact of this expanding field.

There are profound discrepancies between how global health policies and campaigns are envisaged to work and the concrete ways in which they are actually implemented or received by target populations that are routinely facing multiple morbidities and economic insecurity (Han, this volume; Livingston 2012; Manderson and Smith-Morris 2010). So, how are we to measure the value that interventions have for people, their health, and their subjective well-being, and how do interventions affect health systems over time? And how can people and their advocates resocialize ill health and mobilize for a comprehensive right to health?

When People Come First grapples with the transnational and local realities that are emerging through and in the shadow of large-scale health and development interventions that come and go in a climate of ever-expanding global medicine. Amid broken public institutions and deepening rifts, the targets of global health interventions often implode the units through which they are conceptualized. In the meantime, the externalities created by interventions are real, impacting institutional capacities and social relations—a multivalent impact that people trying to escape grim medical destinies are left to reckon with, and that has to be addressed on its own terms.

Epistemological breakthroughs do not belong to experts and analysts alone. The unpredictable and cumulative experiences of people navigating health and humanitarian interventions and their aftermaths can also produce breakthroughs that demand recognition. This practical knowledge compels us to think of people not just as problems or victims, but also as agents of health. It can also help us to better understand the larger systems and policies in which lives actually unfold. A life is lived out and endured regardless of whether it is written off, ostracized, or degraded in the technocratic discourses of the status quo.

When People Comes First emerges from the lessons its authors have learned through sustained engagement with the altered human, institutional, and technological landscapes of disease and health in poor settings today. The book's case studies attend to people's struggles for survival and a future, and also to the larger discourses, structures, and economies that shape life chances—that is, to the ways in which politics matter. As we know from our various experiences in the field, unexpected events happen all the time, and different relations of causality are created as people mobilize, seek resources, and confront the vagaries of the market. Thinking through lives and social fields in transit and the categories that are important in human experience can contribute to making global health sciences more realistic and, we hope, more relevant and accountable to those in need.

An Empirical Lantern

This book is the result of a workshop exploring the entanglements of people, disease, health policies, and market dynamics in the present day. The workshop was held at Princeton University in the spring of 2010, and conversations about the chapters have continued online and in face-to-face discussions. The book's contributors work in a variety of academic, activist, and nongovernmental organizations, and the chapters draw from archival, multisited, and long-term field research, and from professional and consultancy work in the fields of development, international health, and human rights.

We all share an intellectual curiosity and sensibility that privileges ethnographic approaches: charting the lives of individuals and institutions over time and chronicling people's points of view and their varied interpretations of their conditions, all the while denaturalizing operational categories and illuminating the concrete ways in which meso- and macro-level actors impinge on local worlds and become part of global orders, if only transiently. Attending to the omnipresence of social relations and humbly aware of our own situatedness as researchers, we strive to produce nuanced portraits of people, experts, institutions, and situations. This approach also entails comparing phenomena across regions and different analytical points of view; historicizing social processes and recognizing that they are embodied and marked by time; and probing established social theory and striving to create alternative figures of thought. While we value multidisciplinary collaboration in the production of knowledge relevant for public debate and policy, we acknowledge unknowns, the limitations of expert knowledge-making, and an inexhaustible richness at the core of the people we learn from.

Several of us teach courses in global health, medical anthropology, research methods, and the social studies of science and technology. We are all committed to addressing, in our teaching, pressing sociomedical realities. Some of us are helping to launch global health programs and to internationalize education in our universities. As we reflect on the gaps between technical know-how and health outcomes, we are also creating pedagogical pathways through which this generation's overwhelming interest and on-the-ground involvement in global health can be harnessed toward a deepened understanding and meaningful action. We share a healthy skepticism of established hierarchies of knowledge-making, recognizing that innovation can come from surprising places.

We advocate "thinking-in-cases" (Geertz 2007:214). Much global health scholarship is invested in developing models—more or less hypothetical—of optimal interventions, and in identifying and evaluating programs that supposedly "work," and that might therefore be replicated or scaled up across a range of often widely divergent social contexts and geographic locations (Biehl 2007; Cueto 2007; Stepan 2011). Against the dominant epistemic and political modes that enable these operations, *When People Come First* offers ethnographic case studies as an alternative heuristic. The form of the case brings granular ethnographic evidence to the forefront of analysis and enables analogical thinking. Close attention to particular realities on the ground and to the metrics in which they are cast highlights the productive and uneasy coexistence between global health systems design and the alternative models people craft for "engaging the real . . . worlding the world" (Geertz 2007:222).

Each contributor has chosen a specific problem in global heath as his or her focus of inquiry. And each case is representative of a broader phenomenon or a slice of reality that can, in being studied and described, provide a ground for social critique. The case becomes a means whereby both the researcher and the reader gain a sharpened understanding of why particular outcomes emerge or what determines the plasticity of a given reality. This in turn allows problems and questions to be reframed in concrete terms, illuminating the entanglements between systems and human experiences. The written case—a condensed ethnography of sorts—is a way of interrogating evidentiary practices with an eye to what is at stake, not just for patients and other kinds of beneficiaries, but for all the actors involved in the enterprise of health and care.

The book's case studies are drawn from field research involving state and nongovernmental agencies, public-private partnerships, and clinics and communities in Brazil, Chile, the Caribbean, South Africa, Botswana, Ghana, Mozambique, Uganda, and India. Cases are indices of key problematics in global health, but they by no means exhaust the field. They tackle issues such as the possibilities and limits of technology-centered approaches to disease control and eradication, the migration of evidence-based medicine into cost-effective global health policy, the moral economy of vulnerability, and the politics of global health knowledge. Cases also examine how massive treatment rollouts, specifically in response to HIV/AIDS, impact care, health systems, and well-being in resource-poor contexts; the work of nongovernmental organizations on neglected tropical diseases; and the lack of systematic attention to noncommunicable and chronic conditions, such as cancer and mental illness. A final set of cases considers market-based solutions to tuberculosis treatment; the emerging science of global chronic disease care; and how the demand for pharmaceuticals as a human right, as in Janira's case, blurs the border between the clinic and the court, forcing us to consider the limits of reigning concepts of health and quality of care.

If this book has a bias, it is against a too uniform and unilateral diagnosis. As we chronicle in our works, disease is multilayered and multiply determined, people are plural beings and not reducible to populations, and local realities still very much frame, constrain, and orient interventions, be they vertical or diagonal. The agency of local actors is not limited to their blind acceptance or refusal of whatever form of knowledge, technology, or care is provided by extralocal interests. Rather, people's agency is bound to preexisting forms of exchange, politics, and desires as they find expressions, both new and old, in the changing landscape created by global health initiatives.

We identify with the humanism and critique of economist Albert O. Hirschman, who wrote: "I have always had a certain dislike for general principles and abstract prescriptions. I think it is necessary to have an 'empirical lantern' or a 'visit with the patient' before being able to understand what is wrong with him. I know well that the social world is most variable, in continuous change, that there are no permanent laws" (1998:88). Our goal is to advance methodological and analytical frameworks that focus on people and the dynamism of social fields. We explore on-the-ground involvements that address the successes and failures of health efforts, the politics of control *and* nonintervention, the effects of heterogeneity, the primacy of the personal and the role of the interpersonal, and, finally, human inventiveness in the face of impossible choices and even untreated pain.

The human populations that constitute the subjects of health and development plans are not just the source of problems or so-called cultural obstacles. Their experiential and practical knowledge, all too readily dismissed by the champions of quick technical fixes and measurable, generalizable results, can transform paradigms and may well provide the keys to effective solutions. At stake is the development of institutional capacities that go beyond the repetition of history and help to defend, in Hirschman's words, "the right to a nonprojected future as one of the truly inalienable rights of every person and nation" (1971:37).

We have organized the essays in the book under three general headings: *Evidence*, *Interventions*, and *Markets*. The first set of essays (by Cueto, Adams, Amon, and Fassin) traces specific global health institutions, epistemes, and programs to their historical, political, economic, and disciplinary roots. The second set (by Reynolds Whyte and colleagues, Pfeiffer, Livingston, and Moran-Thomas) examines how global health interventions (various and piecemeal and often tied to neoliberal principles and strategies) become part and parcel of public health landscapes and life chances in resource-poor settings. Finally, a third set of essays (by Ecks and Harper, Han, Whitmarsh, and Biehl and Petryna) explores the legal, political, social, and medical realities that accompany the expansion of therapeutic markets and their encroachment in public health.

At the opening of each section, we provide an overview, reflecting on the central themes of each contribution and how it fits into the broader scheme of emerging global health regimes. We also highlight the conceptual importance of each case study and the insight that emerges through its interplay with other cases in the section and in the book as a whole. The afterword (by Fischer) brings the book's main findings to bear on new frontiers in the life sciences.

In attending to the implementation of policies and their embodied responses, the book examines the value systems undergirding incentives, expertise, technologies, measurements, and outcomes. In the process, models of causality and claims of success are scrutinized, and new possibilities for research, policy, and care are brought into view. What or who must be valued in order for knowledge to count as global health science, and what or who remains subjacent or unaddressed? What forms of patienthood and political belonging take shape when new medical technologies are deployed via global health interventions? How can donors and governments be held accountable in the long run, especially in financially volatile times? How can human rights and equity concerns be integrated into global health research and policy? These unanticipated problems and questions have to be addressed now, as lifesaving imperatives are being converted into pharmaceutical and geopolitical capital.

People's everyday struggles and interpersonal dynamics have a way of eluding expert projections and short-lived experimental approaches. The task of the social sciences and humanities in the field of global health is to break through these projections (Whitmarsh, this volume) and to produce different kinds of evidence as we approach bold challenges such as historical health disparities and the pharmaceuticalization of health care. We must also engage crucial questions about the role of the state and the market in global health design and delivery, and investigate what happens to citizenship when politics is reduced to survival—all while maintaining a deep and dynamic sense of people in local worlds (Biehl and Petryna, this volume).

A historical and critical assessment of global health knowledge and tools combined with dedicated ethnographic research is a vital antidote to the quick theoretical fix that has taken its place in our culture alongside the quick technical fix. For the contributors to this book, people come first. Upholding the right to microanalysis, our chapters bring into view the fields and ideas that people invent and live by: call it contrapuntal knowledge. This respect for people, their travails and aspirations—combined with attention to how health policies are put together, take institutional hold, and function in the messiness of idiosyncratic human milieus—makes a great deal of difference in the kind of knowledge we produce.

Simply engaging with the complexity of people's lives—their constraints, resources, subjectivities, projects—in unfixed and multilayered social worlds requires us constantly to reset our conceptual compasses and standards of evidence-making. What would it mean for our research methodologies and ways of writing to consistently embrace this unfinishedness, seeking ways to analyze the general, the structural, and the processual while maintaining an acute awareness of the inevitable incompleteness of our own accounts?

In making these peopled fields—always on the verge of disappearing from view—public, the authors of *When People Come First* want to elicit a different sense of what might be possible. As Hirschman writes, "In all these matters I would suggest a little more reverence for life, a little less straitjacketing of the future, a little more allowance for the unexpected—and a little less wishful thinking" (1970:338).

Ethnography in Global Health

Ethnographic evidence consistently *dies* within the dominant conceptual paradigms of global health. The multiplicity of problems ethnography uncovers has nowhere to live in the numerical counting of drugs delivered, in the recording of dire (and often faulty) mortality statistics, and in the biased selectivity of randomized experiments. In an atmosphere that gives its first allegiance to quantifiable, volume-based audits or replicable scientific knowledge, ethnographic evidence is readily seen as anecdotal and exceptional, unreliable on account of its granularity or the wiliness of its subjects.

Yet, to make the case, we need a human story. To draw public attention, to politicize a cause, to enlist donors, to name and shame, to justify sweeping ideas and large-scale interventions, nothing seems to work better than a compelling story of crisis. The call to intervene is strongest when it evokes empathy for a particular human need. As anthropologists have painstakingly noted, this humanitarian storytelling is quite selective. An unattended-to inequality of lives is at the core of a Western moral economy in which an ethics of suffering and compassion freeze-frames people and compromises a politics of rights and social justice (Fassin 2011; Redfield 2005; Bornstein and Redfield 2011; Feldman and Ticktin 2010; James 2010; Nguyen 2010).

With our empirical lanterns, we see people refusing to be stratified out of existence and trying to be singularized out of the molds of abandonment, salvation, or rescue into which they are cast. The fine-grained ethnographic excesses of lives and stories are often smoothed over or averaged out by coarse-grained statistics and plans. Ethnographic granularity impedes generalizable knowledge, so the official story line goes. Our view, to the contrary, is that ethnography often debunks generalized knowledge, if only retrospectively or too late. The ethnographic, we argue, offers a sharper resolution of how things are, what sustains their intractability, and how they might be otherwise. People's practices of survival and inquiry challenge the analytical forms we bring to the field, forcing us to articulate more experience-near and immediately relevant conceptual work. How to operationalize ethnographic knowledge, and whether this move compromises what can and cannot be asked in the field, is a crucial and enduring question.

Consider the widely cited study by economists Edward Miguel and Michael Kremer (2004) on curing worm infections in rural Kenya. Kremer and Miguel found that treating Kenyan schoolchildren with extremely cheap deworming medication increased their school attendance by roughly 10 percent. A *New York Times* op-ed piece heralded the study as "landmark" (Kristof 2007): with just a bit of cheap medication, poor countries could increase school attendance by leaps and bounds. Given the affordability and stunning success of the treatment, many commentators suspected that families who had not benefited from treatment during the study would very happily adopt this new technology.

But Kremer and Miguel observed a puzzling turn of events after the trial ended and when they followed a group of families outside the original cohort (2007). Families who were friendly with families in the deworming treatment group were *less* likely to treat their children than those who were friendly with families in the control group. They were also less likely to deem the medication effective at improving health. If deworming medicine is the panacea for anemia and school truancy, then why were better-informed families not treating their children?

Miguel and Kremer do not pinpoint the reason for the negative effect of this word of mouth. But they conjecture that the power of communication networks and people's own understanding of worms as a social disease (not predicted in the study design) might have been at play. We have once again a case in which interpersonal relations and the needs and concerns of people on the ground, as well as their own sense of the complex ecology of disease, health, and medical technology, elude controlled studies. With their strict methodological imperatives, global health experts often sacrifice the ethnographic evidence or counter-knowledge that is available as experiments and interventions (ever more closely linked) unfold—at the expense of better understanding and, ultimately, more meaningful and long-lasting outcomes.

The *unpredictable social* is not just an obstacle to or a means for perfecting theoretical tools and experimental strategies. How to account for persons in the context of their homes and relationships, and how to involve local communities in the very design and implementation of feasible (rather than technology-enamored) interventions, are continuous political, medical, and ethical challenges. With international and national health policy's success largely framed in terms of providing and tallying the best medicines and newest technology delivered, what space remains for the development of low-tech or non-tech solutions (such as the provision of clean water) and the strengthening of local health systems and prevention efforts that could prove more sustainable than high-tech solutions alone? How can we escape the dystopic futures of present pragmatics?

In this book we think of ethnography as an early warning system. People on the ground recognize what's troubling them. And it is somewhere in the middle of their social lives that ethnographic work always begins. Ethnographers are uniquely positioned to see what more categorically minded experts may overlook: namely, the empirical evidence that emerges when people express their most pressing and ordinary concerns, which then open up to complex human stories in time and space. Life stories do not simply begin and end. They are stories of transformation, linking the present to the past and to a possible future.

The argument that ethnography is not replicable tends to solidify a technocratic monopoly on truth and, really, misses the point of what ethnographers can convey. The simple fact that we are interested in particularities, contexts, awkward scales, and even the virtual, does not make the work of ethnographers any less rigorous. On the contrary, it raises the bar. The complex social realities of "target populations" and the midlevel actors on whom the burden of implementation lies beg for analytic frameworks that weave them together, and for innovative genres that will allow people-centered evidence to add up, to travel, and to *matter* publicly and comparatively.

When People Come First provides a place where ethnographic evidence can live and expand without the demands and constraints of hegemonic modes of truth-making and evaluation. Against the taken-for-granted and obvious, the book's case studies problematize the ways in which global health initiatives work or fall short. They attend to the altered landscapes left behind after programs scale up or down or move on and elicit how people go on with their lives and imagine alternatives. Ethnographic cases untangle people from their shadow realities and representations, capturing, for a moment and over time, institutional designs, diseases-in-motion, and survival, implicated as these are in scarcity, politics, technology, and money. Taken together, these accounts affirm the urgency of a crosscutting framework that integrates health, development, and social justice. By shifting the emphasis from diseases to people and environments, and from trickle-down access to equality, we have the opportunity to set a humane agenda that both realistically confronts the deep challenges the world faces and expands our vision of the future of global communities.

There is no universal formula for relevance, and ethnographic research should not be valued or discarded solely on the basis of its immediate utility. The realities social scientists unearth are often urgent, but they are also historically deep and carry the potential of discernment that is so critical for movement forward. In our work, we must continue to challenge orthodoxies of all kinds and seek original ways to communicate the categories that are significant in human experience, even when the powers that be dismiss this as anecdotal, nongeneralizable, and inherently impractical—and we must seek ways of translating and communicating that experience so as to compel the worlds of science, policy, and human rights to reckon with it. If this kind of engagement leads to the subtraction of quick-fix theories and policies, and to the advent of new ways of theorizing and reconstructing worlds, so much the better.

Notes

1. Orixás are spirits or deities, manifestations of God in the Yoruba religious system, which appear in Afro-Brazilian religions such as Candomblé and Umbanda.

2. See http://nyudri.org/initiatives/deaton-v-banerjee/.

3. See http://www.hbs.edu/rhc/global_health.html.

4. See http://www.pih.org/pages/who-we-are/.

I

EVIDENCE

Overview

Enter history and you find the missing politics, then and now. When we look at international health interventions historically, it becomes clear that the political and economic requirements of the day and the ideological whims of the elites in charge determine how priorities are set and why they are abandoned. As social scientists unearth the recent history that explains how people become target populations in global health, unexpected anthropological terrains come into view: we find ourselves face-to-face with profound disconnections between how campaigns are designed and the complex ways in which they are actually received and critiqued. The counterknowledge of the people who are actually at the center of things is thus integral to the structures and effects of interventions and has the potential to protect us from the repetition of history.

In his chapter, historian Marcos Cueto explores the politics that shape the world of global health, especially with regard to the treatment of malaria in the 1950s and its iteration in the 2000s in the form of Roll Back Malaria (RBM). The World Health Organization (WHO), the institutional catalyst of international health initiatives, is at the center of Cueto's account. He vividly describes how the changing interests of the funders and collaborators involved in particular state-market interactions significantly influence how technology and health interventions are imagined and deployed.

In the 1970s, on the heels of the WHO's failed DDT-centered malaria eradication program, efforts in international health and the magic-bullet model behind them came under heavy critique. During the 1980s and

1990s, however, the United Nations found itself in dire financial straits, unable to collect money from its most powerful member country. As the Reagan and Bush administrations chose to undermine the role of international political arbiters in favor of market forces, the WHO rose as an important institutional channel through which to explore the efficacy of neoliberal approaches to international health and humanitarianism in general. It was in this climate that the WHO was forced to change leadership and to move toward greater integration with the interests and practices of the private sector.

In this history, we see a shift from centrally planned to decentralized interventions and an increasingly heterogeneous field of actors and strategies on the ground vying for funds and access. Within this anarchic environment, burdens of proof and evidence of success are often moving targets. Changes in goals (from eradication to control and back to eradication) lead to similarly circuitous changes in strategies (from spraying to treatment to vaccines; from prevention to treatment and back). As Cueto shows, Roll Back Malaria needed to position itself as a magic bullet in order to retain its position and funding. RBM's failure to reach its self-imposed goals, the attempts to relegitimize the program through a variety of evaluative practices, and the subsequent issuing of new goals all hint at an institutional landscape of global health in which funding and political clout themselves become the objectives of intervention.

Through Cueto's historical X-ray of a particular intervention by one of the institutional backbones of global health, we see the machinations and politics that allow institutions to remain relevant and powerful within an ever more contested field of players. This case study also shows how the current configuration of global health, with its emphasis on Public-Private Partnerships (PPPs), arose not simply from firmly held ideological convictions at the WHO, but as a response to a number of external pressures, chief among them a shrinking budget and an antagonistic political arena. The growth of PPPs owes much of its impetus to this mentality, in which the grand scheming of health system building meets the technical and financial know-how of the private sector. We learn how a particular ethics of global health, always looking outside and up toward funders and politicians, began to take hold. Lost in this calculus, as Cueto and the other contributors to this book demonstrate, are the on-the-ground realities and difficulties with which local partners must contend. A micro-level analysis of macro-level politics thus begins the work of providing critical accounts of these processes and of alternatives being imagined.

* * *

Global health institutions, epistemes, and programs have to be traced back to their political, economic, and disciplinary roots. In her critical ethnography, Vincanne Adams studied a resiliency-training program for school-age children in New Orleans and a safe-motherhood training program for Tibetan health workers. Both programs required health workers to participate in the new and unfamiliar economy of information on which the legitimacy of the programs rested. And in both cases, the demands imposed by the now-predominant evidence-based medicine approach transformed not only the evaluation of the interventions, but also their methodologies, goals, and subjects. The New Orleans program could only be deemed reliable, credible, and, ultimately, fundable, through the acquisition of privately produced and internationally standardized assessment tools. In Tibet, the original project had to be radically altered on statistical grounds: it was not possible to determine whether the intervention was more effective than chance because "not enough women" died. Following the advice of a Maryland research consortium, the program—now upgraded to a "study"—was made "more scientific," more globally comparable, by abandoning training in safe motherhood and focusing instead on infant mortality for which "better numbers" were available.

In this regime of veridiction and falsification, evidence-based medicine has migrated to the realm of health interventions and has quickly positioned itself as the default language of a growing "NGO industrial complex." We now see in policy the same logic of the production of experimental subjects and experimental sites that we see in medicine. The confluence of evidence-based medicine (with its standardized approach to clinical research and practice) and the advent of private funding and neoliberal measures of accountability and efficiency have established a set of demands that the traditional players in global health have been ill equipped to handle. Global health data-making has become a profitable business.

As Adams's study shows, this new landscape of evaluation is displacing the previous goals of interventions, making the purveyance of actual health services secondary to the development of reliable methodologies, the generation of comparable data, and the training of a workforce capable of deploying interventions with similar results at a later date. Abandoned in this move are the experiences of the nominal targets of interventions. The focus is no longer on the sick and their caregivers, nor is much consideration given to the long-standing effects of programs on the lives of people and on public institutions.

Ethnographic accounts of global health projects allow us to demystify claims as to the natural givenness of evidence-based medicine and to determine who constructs them, and how. They provide a window into the workings of new methodological imperatives and their impact on programs, experiments, and practitioners. The voices of people affected by these programs should be recovered, but that is not the end of the matter. Ethnography also brings into view how projects themselves become the object of intervention and gives insight into the ramifying consequences of this shift. This line of inquiry sheds fresh light on the kinds of experts and economies that arise from the modes of governance and values that global health interventions subscribe to.

* * *

Joseph J. Amon's chapter further explores how knowledge functions, both as a rhetorical device and as a principle orienting global health policy. His focus is on the ways in which certain bodies of knowledge become privileged domains in the fight against HIV/AIDS; how these knowledges are intrinsically entangled in the politics, economics, and morality that underpin efforts to combat the disease; and how they are built on a language of human rights that often obscures effective avenues of care. Amon calls for a people-centered approach to policy decisions, countering other models that would label case-based evidence as anecdotal and that opt instead to allow politics, ideologies, or the market to guide health interventions. Combined with legal analysis, such an approach highlights how the protection and enforcement of some rights in a vacuum, and to the exclusion of others, risks jeopardizing not only individual programs, but also the provision of care in general.

Amon argues that the "right to know," whatever its form or object (knowing the serostatus of oneself and others, for example, or knowing about HIV/AIDS and its prevention), offers only temporary control over isolated aspects of the disease. Nor is knowledge about prevention and treatment sufficient on its own, for it does not guarantee care or compliance. An emphasis on piecemeal solutions also obscures other aspects of the epidemic, such as its intersection with structural forms of violence, thereby making meaningful and effective interventions even more difficult to establish. Amon thus advocates for a right to know about the barriers that impact one's care, a right to access to treatment after one's status has been known, and a right to protections under the law for one's personal property and against domestic violence and discrimination, as well as a right to confidentiality. These are what he calls "structural rights."

By bringing the voices of those living and dying with AIDS to bear on the legal and structural analyses of policy, critical studies of global health not only rescue voices left behind by other epistemologies but also offer a way to uncover the inadequacies of current approaches and to orient the development of new ones. Under the right "to be known" that is advocated here, what is so often dismissed as anecdotal becomes instead the nuanced locus of evidence that brings failing systems, simplistic diagnoses, and ineffective treatments into the light of day. Knowledge thus becomes something more than a rarefied technical object produced by programs or states, to be consumed by their populations (HIV positive or otherwise). Rather, it is a relationship between interested actors built on critical thinking that can ground vapid talk of rights, transforming rhetorical gymnastics into sturdy and meaningful understanding and a means to collective well-being.

* * *

The complex ways in which certain discourses become, simultaneously, productive and limiting forces in global health are also at the center of Didier Fassin's study of the politics of childhood in the context of HIV/AIDS in South Africa. Fassin employs the concept of "moral economy" to address the ways in which the tragedy of orphanhood became crystallized as a notion; the constellation of moral sentiments within which it has become entangled; the political debates in which orphanhood has been deployed and transformed; and the interventions that have relied on it as an orienting principle.

The construct of children as worthy recipients of protection from disease by society (as victims whose visibility opens new spaces for action) is accomplished through the portrayal of others as negligent and unworthy. This adversarial moral opposition is the result of the history of HIV/AIDS in South Africa, of old prejudices and misconceptions stretched over new social and biological realities. In this context it would seem that children can become valorized victims only if adult men and women are understood to be predatory, lascivious, or weak; the possibility of intervention on behalf of the purified child subject is realized through the erasure of a complex history that entangles men, women, and children, a history that impinges powerfully on the course of the AIDS epidemic. This construct, Fassin argues, is emblematic of the aspirations and contradictions of modern-day humanitarianism.

Here as elsewhere in global health, the vocabulary of emergency hinges on a temporality that insists upon a break from the past. Such an appeal, while effective in marshaling action, serves to mask other factors that may be contributing to the unfolding of the epidemic and to mask as well other actors desperately in need of help. Discourses and interventions couched in the tragedy of AIDS orphanhood thus often disregard South Africa's violent past and present, and the loss and breakups of families that resulted from apartheid's political violence and the continuing effects of economic insecurity. In the past as in the present, extended family and close communities often have been called upon when a child loses his or her parents, changing the concept of "orphanhood" at its very roots. Although the emergence of orphans as the face of HIV/AIDS is laudable in that it introduces previously disregarded subjects, it is a concept sustained by many of the same misconceptions that have plagued previous approaches to the disease and that are all too often the products of long-standing racist attitudes.

Fassin positions his case study at the intersection of several historical moments and scales of analysis. This perspective allows us to understand the ways in which certain discourses come into being, circulate, and are transformed over time. We become conscious of both the actors who wield them and the actors who are affected by them, and we begin to understand how these discourses may guide action or inaction. The notion of moral economy provides an important framework through which to analyze the problematization of some people at the expense of others, the network of exchange and symbolic equivalences that turns some into innocent victims worthy of care and others into villains to be disregarded or condemned. The ethnography Fassin offers demands that we recognize public fictions as such and become aware of the power that sustains and perpetuates them. It is this depth of inquiry that makes possible intelligent critique and raises hopes for genuine transformation.

—*João Biehl and Adriana Petryna*

1

A Return to the Magic Bullet?

Malaria and Global Health in the Twenty-First Century

MARCOS CUETO

At the turn of the twenty-first century, international efforts to combat malaria, one of the deadliest and most insidious rural scourges in modern history, entered a new phase, marked by the emergence of new medical technologies and the greater involvement of global agencies and local health workers. Initially, these changes raised hopes that a holistic intervention against malaria would replace the "magic bullet" approach that was launched in the mid-1950s and put an end to the apathy that had followed the failure of that initiative to achieve results. However, after a few years of innovation it now appears that most donors, as well as major international health agencies, including the World Health Organization (WHO), have returned to advocating top-down programs that resemble those of the 1950s.

An examination of recent successes and failures in malaria control illuminates contemporary challenges and suggests that traditional assumptions and a reliance on the medical technology advocated by some experts still play a key role in the design of international programs. The relevance of history to policy discussions also becomes evident. My purpose in this chapter is to examine the recent cycle of malaria elimination and control efforts and to raise some questions about the future of global health.

The policy changes I discuss occurred against the background of the slow but steady growth of a killer that is second in its global impact only to tuberculosis. Despite a general decline in malaria morbidity during the 1960s and 1970s, especially in semitropical and temperate climate zones, the number of cases and deaths increased in the following years. Among the social factors that explain malaria's increase in the developing world were floods of refugees fleeing civil wars and famine, the marked precariousness of medical systems during a period of structural adjustment, and the growing number of unemployed rural people moving to previously uncultivated lands where infection rates were higher and medical care was scarce.

In 1988, a malaria epidemic in Madagascar resulted in twenty-five thousand deaths. By the early 1990s, the disease had resurged in almost all of the regions where it previously had been controlled, so that almost half of the world's population was again living in malarial areas. Around 1993, over 50 percent of the population living in savanna and forest zones of Africa was infected. In this area of the world—which had not been fully involved in the previous malaria eradication campaign—malaria was the main cause of death in young children, killing one in twenty before the age of five.[1] At the time, it was estimated that, of the 100 million clinical cases worldwide, 80 percent occurred in Africa. Between 1994 and 1996, malaria epidemics in fourteen countries in sub-Saharan Africa caused a high number of deaths, many in areas previously free of the disease.

At present it is estimated that, globally, more than a million malaria-related deaths occur each year (about four-fifths of these in Africa), and that about 247 million people worldwide became ill with malaria in 2006.[2] In addition, about three billion people, more than half the world's population, are at risk of infection. In the Americas, according to Pan American Health Organization figures, about 38 percent of the population lives in malarial areas. Malaria disproportionately affects the rural poor, who are more exposed to infection, have the least access to services, and suffer more from the disease's consequences.

The Boom and Bust of International Health

Between 1955 and the early 1960s, WHO was the unquestioned leader of a worldwide malaria eradication campaign that embodied the hopes of the recently created field of international health. Although some precedents can be found, it was only after the Second World War that international health emerged as an epistemic community, a subdiscipline in American schools of public health, and a web of multilateral organizations that formed part of the United Nations (UN) system and worked in close association with the foreign policy of the US Department of State. Among these organizations were WHO and the United Nations Children's Fund (UNICEF), created in the late 1940s. After flings with European social medicine, they became champions of an American-inspired illusion that social engineering could solve the problems of underdeveloped countries and thus stave off the communist revolution advertised by the Soviet Union.[3]

To complement the work of these organizations, major industrial countries reorganized and upgraded their bilateral aid organizations and coordinated the roles played by private foundations. An important outcome of these rearrangements was that bilateral and private organizations assumed a low profile, yielding center stage in terms of prestige and leadership to the multilaterals. This web of institutions collaborated in the launch of a major global effort to eliminate malaria, a decision made in the 1955 World Health Assembly that took place in Mexico City, in what was the most ambitious international and coordinated attack on disease ever undertaken.[4] The campaign was based on DDT spraying and the use of new antimalarial drugs, and it aimed to interrupt transmission of the disease in all endemic areas within five to eight years. (The deadline was later postponed.) This goal explicitly excluded tropical Africa. A 1956 report by an expert committee considered efforts to eradicate the disease in Africa "premature," and instead suggested the implementation of a number of pilot pre-eradication projects.[5]

The decision to eliminate malaria was based on a number of assumptions that are important to review here, and that in one form or another reappeared on the eve of the twenty-first century. One of the main assumptions of the campaign, and of international health in general, was that technology could overcome any obstacle posed by social conditions and processes—water use, housing standards, lifestyles, and the like. According to this construction, the malaria parasite and the mosquito that spread it were the real problems, and they could be addressed by quick technological fixes, namely insecticides and antimalarial drugs. Little attention was paid to social and institutional factors, such as the state of the health system in rural areas or the level of education of rural inhabitants. As a consequence, an understanding of local cultural beliefs and intercultural education were de-emphasized.

A second assumption was that disease caused poverty, not the other way around. The conviction was that nature was bigger than society—in other words, that mosquitoes and parasites were the main phenomena that impeded the evolution of the so-called third-world nations. It followed that up-to-date medical technology and expertise would solve the main health and social problems in these societies as soon as well-designed and cost-effective magic bullets could be implemented (an idea that would echo in popular expectations that long-term public health structures could evolve from short-term interventions, such as making specific drugs available).

A third assumption revolved around new medical technology itself. It was portrayed as so detached from lay knowledge that only a group of experts ("malariologists") could design and implement the campaign. It was, in other words, the international givers who knew what was best for the local receivers. A corollary idea was that medical technology could only be managed by an elite group of experts, so that a public health program was necessarily an innovation that came from outside and from well above the level of the local communities that it aimed to benefit. Moreover, it was believed that the new cadre of medical experts were uniquely qualified to convince policy-makers that it was crucial to invest in health. Only experts would know how to craft a compelling and hegemonic alliance between multilateral organizations, bilateral assistance programs, private foundations, national governments, and leaders in the field of international medicine.

Linked to this assumption was the conviction that malaria was mainly a global economic problem since it affected the export capacity and buying power of workers in developing countries, and that elimination of the disease would therefore contribute to the health of the world economy. In addition, the thinking went, disease control or elimination could be achieved without major public health improvements in poor countries (for which there were no resources available). Linking medicine, economics, and politics, international health touted its approach to the disease as an exemplary application of realistic humanitarianism (and, thus, as something that should not be criticized or resisted).

By the mid-1960s, these assumptions could no longer validate the antimalaria operation, which seemed futile to both multilateral and bilateral agencies because of cultural problems such as the resistance of people to the chemical contamination of their environment. The power of technology as an antimalaria tool had, in this case, been overstated. Although reports had warned against an overreliance on technology since the beginning of the campaign, insecticide-resistant mosquitoes and drug-resistant parasites began to emerge everywhere, rendering the operation useless. Concern for the environment increased after 1962, with the publication of the bestseller *Silent Spring*, in which Rachel Carson questioned the wisdom of releasing chemicals into the environment without understanding their effects on ecology or human health. The book suggested that DDT was a cause of cancer and a threat to wildlife, particularly to birds. Among the many consequences of the book was a public outcry that led to a DDT ban in the United States in 1972. In addition, in a climate of controversy over family planning, malaria eradication was portrayed as counterproductive because, if achieved, it would worsen the overpopulation problems of developing countries. As a result, international funding for antimalaria programs fell off rapidly.

The 1969 Boston meeting of the World Health Assembly (WHO's governing body) reversed its malaria eradication policy by approving a resolution calling for containment of the disease. This had the benefit of establishing an uneasy coexistence between those advocating control and those favoring eradication.[6] WHO's decision was accepted by other international health agencies but was questioned by some developing countries, which continued to argue for eradication[7] even as articles in mainstream journals questioned the eradication approach.[8] An editorial in the *Lancet*, for example, carried the self-explanatory title "Epitaph for Global Malaria Eradication?" In 1974, a new Director-General asked the WHO Executive Board: "Was malaria eradication a foolish enterprise? Where, when, and how did the program go wrong?"[9] Regrettably, however, the failure to eradicate malaria did not prompt a thorough assessment of the experience or give rise to comprehensive countermodels for malaria control, and it resulted in even less effort being devoted to building health system capacity from the ground up. For some years, a disorganized and confusing coexistence between control and eradication persisted. In practical terms, it amounted to little more than local health centers offering diagnosis and dispensing medication.

In the 1970s, WHO began to insist on better mechanisms for continuous surveillance of malaria and criticized nationally designed malaria eradication services for their attempts to remain "autonomous," independent of the work of local health services devoted to a series of issues that were in fact not unrelated to malaria. Some international health leaders and health workers around the world became convinced there was no magic bullet for malaria. Technologically driven "vertical" mass campaigns were not sustainable or feasible. They could deliver only temporary success. Instead, the disease needed to be attacked on many fronts with strategies adapted to diverse ecologies and cultural settings, undertaken in the context of permanent rural health services, and tied to significant improvements in the living conditions of the rural poor. The resulting campaign was to prove a learning experience for many experts who questioned vertical, magic bullet programs and who, from the mid-1960s on, began to promote the development of basic health services at the local level. Many criticized the passive surveillance approach (case detection followed by treatment) taken by most malaria workers, but they did not propose an alternative at the time.

Only a few antimalaria programs in poor countries were able to fully participate in the new and more comprehensive international health programs, that is, in the development of the concept of primary health care (PHC). Some individual health workers hoped to use efforts against endemic diseases like malaria as an entry point for testing PHC's effectiveness at meeting its stated goals, such as exposing and ending the inadequacies and inequities of health and social systems that predispose people to illness, but this approach never gained popularity among agencies.[10]

The Transition to Global Health

During the 1980s and early 1990s, it was difficult to overcome a growing sense of futility. Low priority was given to malaria work, despite the complex challenges posed by the disease and its increasing gravity. In the early 1980s, there was little research underway on antimalarial drugs, with the exception of some work by Chinese researchers and by the Special Program for Research and Training on Tropical Diseases (funded by various agencies housed at WHO) on the drug artemisinin. This work would later prove essential since in the 1980s, some Asian countries, especially in the Indochinese peninsula, began to experience serious difficulties with parasite resistance to chloroquine, the drug of choice since the 1950s. Chloroquine would gradually lose effectiveness in many other parts of the world as well. In addition, growing resistance to mefloquine (another first-line drug that was developed in the 1970s at the Walter Reed Army Institute of Research as a synthetic analogue of quinine) was noted a few years after its introduction in the early 1980s. In 1989, the World Health Assembly asserted that malaria control should be a priority and a crucial component in the implementation of primary healthcare.

WHO sponsored a conference of health ministers in Amsterdam in October of 1992 to discuss a coordinated attack on the disease. It subsequently adopted a Global Malaria Control Strategy advocating early diagnosis and treatment of cases, various preventive and protective measures, and the early containment of epidemics, as well as the strengthening of local health services and human capacities in basic and applied research.[11] (It is important to mention that among the participants at the Amsterdam meeting was Pascal Lissouba, the president of the People's Republic of Congo, a significant presence since African malaria had not been given much attention before by international agencies.) Subsequently, the World Health Assembly, the Economic and Social Council of the UN General Assembly, and the General Assembly itself fully endorsed the new strategy. According to the final report of the Amsterdam meeting, one of the main obstacles to reorganizing and revamping malaria programs was the lack of national political determination to confront malaria, "stemming in large measure from doubt and disillusionment created by past setbacks."[12]

The strategy was also the product of regional conferences, organized by WHO's regional offices and attended by the heads of national malaria programs, in Brazzaville and New Delhi in 1991 and in Brasília in 1992. Still, the strategy echoed the broader international concerns of PHC, since the 1993 World Health Assembly approved a declaration calling on the WHO Director-General to ensure its implementation in the context of primary health care. Moreover, clearly implying that the magic bullets of the past partly explained the failure of malariologists, advocates of the strategy made clear that they did not promise a single and immediate solution, that eradication was not a realistic goal, and that many standard practices based on eradication principles were, in fact, inefficient. One of these standard practices involved spraying all malarial areas in a given country, when a program of selective spraying would be more effective and sustainable. The strategy's objectives were to prevent malaria mortality and *reduce* malaria morbidity (not to eliminate it) and to promote intersectoral collaboration (in contrast to the lack of coordination that had characterized previous efforts).

A WHO document gave support to the strategy, stating, "The time has come for a renewed attack on malaria."[13] This was the beginning of a reorganization of national malaria programs in many developing countries. In 1996, the WHO African office, under the leadership of Ebrahim Samba, director of the successful campaign against onchocerciasis, launched—with the help of the World Bank—an African initiative for malaria control.[14] The next year, African medical scientists organized a meeting in Dakar that led to the Multilateral Initiative on Malaria (MIM), which aimed to increase research on the disease. Also in 1997, the US National Institute of Allergy and Infectious Diseases launched a ten-year research program for malaria vaccine development; American scientists were certain that it would not take long to design a vaccine.[15]

The year 1997 saw the advent of important alliances. One was the MIM, initially funded in part by the British Wellcome Trust, which focused on improving African scientific capacity and coordinating research collaboration among national and international agencies. Another important program was the Medicines for Malaria Venture (MMV), launched in 1999 as a nonprofit foundation devoted to discovering, developing, and delivering new and affordable antimalarial drugs. Its members included the Rockefeller Foundation and the Federation of Pharmaceutical Manufacturers Associations.[16] This mix showcased the new and increasingly complex relationship between big pharmaceutical companies and the emerging domain of global health.

Little malaria work occurred inside WHO, partly because the agency was facing serious financial troubles (as were other multilateral UN agencies), and was under criticism from the US Department of State during most of the 1980s and early 1990s. These were the final days of the Cold War, which saw the dissolution of the Soviet Union and the reemergence of neoliberalism, with presidents Ronald Reagan and George H. W. Bush questioning the very need for a United Nations. Many American neoliberal politicians championed unilateralism in US foreign relations, criticized the UN system for becoming a home for radicals and an example of the wastefulness of funding public-sector-like institutions, and proclaimed that humanity was entering a new phase of globalization that rendered multilaterals irrelevant.

An important change in WHO, and for malaria work, occurred in 1998, when Gro Harlem Brundtland began her tenure as the fifth Director-General of WHO[17] and the first woman ever elected to head a UN agency. Brundtland was a physician with a master's degree in public health from Harvard University, and she had been prime minister of Norway.[18] She had acquired a global reputation during the 1990s when she headed the UN's World Commission on the Environment and co-organized its landmark meeting, the 1992 Earth Summit in Rio de Janeiro. It was this meeting that popularized such code words as "sustainable development" and "global warming."[19] Brundtland and her supporters would later give their imprimatur to the notion of "global health," praising the new concept as one that would transcend the concerns of individual nations through cooperative actions and solutions designed by experts, usually from the private sector, where, supposedly, good management practices were the norm.

Many experts saw Brundtland's election to head WHO as an opportunity to reform the beleaguered agency, whose two previous administrations under the Japanese Hiroshi Nakajima had been severely criticized by the US Department of State. Not least, Brundtland also raised hopes that, because of her perceived neoliberal views, she would be able to attract fresh financial resources to support international health work. As Richard Feachem, the former director of Health, Nutrition, and Population at the World Bank and the main author of the 1993 World Bank report *Investing in Health*, declared, "WHO just elected the best possible leader that it could elect . . . her leadership heralds an era when WHO can be a truly powerful and influential agency."[20]

Brundtland immediately made clear that she expected to make significant institutional changes: "WHO . . . must become more effective, more accountable, more transparent and more receptive to a changing world."[21] She set herself two complex tasks: a vigorous internal management reform and direct engagement with the agencies trumpeting "globalization," especially the World Bank. From her perspective, these two goals were complementary. WHO must reform itself internally while also reaching out to become a player in global health. Brundtland also shook up the agency by demanding efficiency, adherence to timetables, and accountability. Her internal management reform was financed by sizable funds made available by a number of European governments, the US government, and some American private donors.[22] In 2000, one of the emblematic World Health Reports published under her command redefined the role of governments in public health: rather than operating programs, their main functions were to be stewardship and supervision (for example, the regulation and licensing of private practitioners) and the promotion of the interface between the public and private sectors in health work. Shortly after Brundtland launched her reforms, an editorial in *Science*, signed by, among others, the economist Jeffrey Sachs and Barry R. Bloom, dean of the Harvard School of Public Health, stated that Brundtland was "reinventing" WHO and called on the US government to pay its $35 million pending contribution to the agency as an investment in health.[23]

Integral to the new Director-General's second task was improving WHO's ability to respond rapidly and effectively to outbreaks of serious diseases such as malaria. In part because of WHO's financial problems, but also because such arrangements had become the new model of social engineering in the neoliberal era, the new Director-General favored the creation of more public-private partnerships (PPPs). PPPs could bring together dissimilar partners and stakeholders—multilateral and bilateral agencies, pharmaceutical companies, NGOs, and different levels within WHO (headquarters, regional offices, and country offices)—to find the most effective combination of agents to address a particular health problem.[24] PPPs were able to collaborate with institutions outside of Geneva and to appeal to private-sector funding agencies and corporations because they enjoyed considerable influence within them, had the means to direct their investments toward very specific goals, and could manage budgets in a transparent way.

Brundtland adopted and expanded the PPP model. Shortly after she was elected Director-General, she threw her support behind the recently created PPP Roll Back Malaria (RBM) program. It began operations as a "cabinet project"—that is, its head reported directly to the Director-General rather than through a cluster unit, as had the old malaria eradication programs of the 1950s. The British provided the initial stimulus for the project. Its first leader was David Nabarro, a charismatic former professor at the Liverpool School of Tropical Medicine and an officer in a British bilateral agency, the Department for International Development, who had joined WHO in 1999. Nabarro had been head of the large British delegation at the 1992 Amsterdam meeting, where the new control strategy was adopted. Much of the funding came from the United Kingdom as well, with the British playing a role similar to that played by US bilateral assistance in the 1950s. The UK bilateral assistance agency provided US$19 million in the first year and over $100 million overall.[25]

Although in later years the program suffered from a certain lack of organization and of focus in its goals, RBM's main priorities were firmly established at three events. The first was a meeting in Birmingham in 1997 at which the representatives of the G8 group of industrialized countries agreed to create RBM. Within a few months the decision took the form of a partnership between WHO, the World Bank, UNICEF, the United Nations Development Program, USAID, and the British bilateral agency.[26] The second meeting took place in Abuja, Nigeria, in 2000, and was instrumental in persuading fifty-two African heads of state to fully endorse RBM. The third, a meeting that shaped the mandate of RBM, was the summit organized by the UN in 2000, which established eight Millennium Development Goals (MDGs).

The main objectives that derived from these meetings were the following: a 50 percent reduction of malaria mortality by 2010 (or halving global malaria infections by 2010); a 60 percent increase in access to prompt treatment of the disease by 2005; a 60 percent increase in access to insecticide-treated mosquito nets (ITNs) and a 60 percent augmentation in appropriate treatment for pregnant women and children by 2005; and a prompt reduction or waiver of taxes and tariffs for ITNs, insecticides, and antimalarial drugs. A sixth objective, to combat "HIV/AIDS, malaria, and other diseases"—which many considered over-ambitious—formally reinforced the target of reversing the incidence of malaria worldwide and halting the disease by 2015. In addition, it suggested the possibility of a two-thirds reduction in the under-five mortality rate from malaria by 2015 and, in cooperation with the pharmaceutical industry, the provision of access to affordable, essential antimalarial drugs in developing countries. One implication of these goals, which was not given sufficient attention at the beginning, was that there would be a significant improvement in malaria reporting, especially in Africa, where such records had been fragmentary and irregular. This was true not only as regards malaria but also in the case of other diseases such as AIDS, where a reduction in the infection rate and the eventual discovery of a vaccine were anticipated.

More broadly, these goals signaled a new philosophy in antimalaria work. RBM would not be merely a revamped eradication program but a completely new health-sector-wide approach to combating the disease. RBM would also avoid becoming a short-term effort divorced from other health systems. Its program was broadly intended to improve malaria control activities across health systems.[27]

As RBM was being unveiled, an important innovation was also underway in the area of malaria treatments. Chloroquine, the drug used since the 1950s that had become ineffective in many parts of the world, began to be replaced by drug combinations that contained the core ingredient of artemisinin, a plant extract long used in Chinese herbal medicine. The new public health focus on malaria created new interest in the disease on the part of medical researchers and pharmaceutical manufacturers. (Between 1975 and 1999, only four of the approximately 1,400 new drugs developed worldwide were aimed at treating malaria.)

Artemisinin-based therapies were fully endorsed by WHO.[28] Unfortunately, the use of the drug alone proved ineffective after a few years. In 2006, WHO announced that, after some effort, it had convinced thirteen major pharmaceutical companies to phase out single-drug artemisinin medicines for the oral treatment of malaria, on the grounds that their use hastened the development of resistant malaria parasites, and to instead focus their malaria-related marketing efforts primarily on artemisinin combination therapies (ACTs). ACTs combined two medicines that worked in different ways, making it unlikely that the malaria parasite would acquire a resistance to the compound. With these new drugs, malaria workers were following a model developed for the treatment of tuberculosis, HIV, and leprosy, in which a combination of two drugs proved highly effective in preventing the evolution of resistance. ACTs were likewise much more efficient at curing uncomplicated malaria and were well tolerated by patients. They became the standard treatment.

This new approach to malaria was validated by the work of prestigious scholars such as Jeffrey Sachs, who entered the field of international health, which many experts at the time advocated calling by the new term "global health." Sachs authored or coauthored a series of influential articles on malaria published around 2000 that aimed to elucidate the link between the disease and poverty and that estimated the cost of the disease to Africa at US$12 billion per year.[29] He believed that malaria was, in fact, responsible for retarding economic growth in developing countries and that if annual donor contributions from industrial nations for malaria prevention programs were to increase in a significant but realistic way, millions of Africans could escape the cycle of disease *and* poverty.

Sachs rose in prominence with two appointments. First, in 2000, he became chair of WHO's Commission on Macroeconomics and Health, which was launched by Director-General Brundtland and entrusted with the goal of identifying those health-related investments that would have the greatest positive impact on economic growth in developing countries. Second, from 2002 to 2006, he was director of the UN Millennium Project and MDG advisor to then secretary-general Kofi Annan. With Sachs's work—as with malaria eradication efforts in 1955—the economic argument in favor of energetic measures to control malaria took a convincing political shape. Again, no one questioned the nature of the connection between malaria and poverty; simply put, malaria caused poverty, not the other way around.

Another important change occurred in the area of insecticides. Since the late 1990s, there had been a campaign to restore the use and prestige of insecticides in public health. This meant a reversal of the trend that began in the 1970s (later partially supported by the Persistent Organic Pollutants Treaty signed in Stockholm in 2001) to eliminate, restrict, or phase out global use of DDT, mainly because of its long, toxic history. Even in the early 1990s, articles published in mainstream journals were still suggesting a relationship between DDT and human cancer.[30] By the early twenty-first century, however, some agencies and scholars had come to believe that evidence for the adverse effects of DDT should not preclude its use in antimalaria activities and that, with supervision, it would be safe for indoor spraying in endemic regions. In 2006, WHO approved and advocated its use according to safety specifications.[31]

RBM thus reversed the prevailing attitude of resignation of health systems in the face of malaria, placed malaria on the international agenda, infused donors with new energy, and contributed to a significant increase in international expenditures for antimalaria efforts. (These almost doubled in the first five years of RBM, from US$67 million worldwide in 1997 to $130 million in 2002.) The trend toward more international funding for malaria continued in the following years, culminating in a dramatic rise with the establishment of the Global Fund to Fight AIDS, Tuberculosis, and Malaria.[32]

The Global Fund was originally proposed in 2001 during a meeting of the G8 industrialized countries, who agreed that existing agencies would not, by themselves, be able to conquer the world's three so-called most important diseases (AIDS, malaria, and TB). The Global Fund, which began to operate a year later, was to be the principal means of attracting more financial resources and of directing those resources to the countries most in need, of reinforcing PPPs, and of disbursing grants in an open, transparent, and accountable manner. The Fund established its headquarters in Geneva and held the legal status of a private foundation. Representatives of corporations, donors, recipient governments, and NGOs formed its board. In 2003, the US Congress approved significant sums to support the Fund, amounting to almost half of all the money it would distribute.[33] As a congresswoman from California argued, this was to be an investment in national security because "disease knows no borders."[34] Her statement also underpinned a growing consensus over the notion of "global health."

The Global Fund employed a novel approach to international health financing that aimed to strengthen local capacity, complement available resources, and promote the transparent use of financial resources.[35] Independent review processes evaluated the technical quality of proposals, management practices, tangible results, and the ability of a country to take over ownership of a project after external funding had ended. Decisions were to be made after weighing merit, capability, and urgency.

One of the requirements of a Global Fund application was that it specify a multisector country-coordinating mechanism (CCM), representing both public and private sectors and preferably including government ministries, NGOs, groups of individuals affected by the disease, faith-based organizations, and academic institutions.[36] This gathering of diverse stakeholders was designed to improve coordination, avoid duplication of work, and develop a consensus on a country's programs. In the first two rounds of funding, nearly two-thirds went to AIDS programs, 17 percent to malaria, and 14 percent to tuberculosis. Most of the countries that were awarded HIV/AIDS funds intended to use a significant portion of their grants for antiretroviral treatment. Grants for malaria control both expanded the distribution of ITNs and provided treatment for the sick. Directly observed therapy, short course (DOTS) was promoted in tuberculosis programs. In the years around 2005, the Fund was the source of about two-thirds of all international funds collected and distributed to fight malaria.

A Bumpy Road for Revamping Malaria Work

Despite these resources (or maybe because of the way in which they were used), RBM began to face criticism. According to its detractors, funding was insufficient to reach the goal of controlling the disease, as the number of cases continued to grow dramatically, especially in Africa.[37] Another criticism was that education efforts and community participation were de-emphasized, while the use of ITNs was overemphasized, especially as bednets were not always effective in poor environments either because people did not receive the information and education on how to use them properly or because they were used inconsistently.[38] Although RBM was well aware of some of the cultural and political challenges that had frustrated former antimalaria efforts and had officially discarded vertical interventions, its ITN initiatives all too often began to take on the role of magic bullets.

More controversial was the issue of cost recovery (user fees) for ITNs. Donors and experts became divided on whether mosquito nets should be distributed by "social marketing." Some proposed that they not be distributed for free but sold for nominal sums. The supporters of this option argued that the poor would only value and use goods they had paid for.

Other public health scholars believed that this option would negatively affect access and equity. According to these critics, "social marketing" would benefit the "richest of the poor," namely city slum dwellers and people in the larger rural towns, but not peasants living in smaller communities, who were the principal victims of mosquito-borne diseases. The debate continues to this day, but most public health workers have an eclectic and flexible attitude toward the issue.

The controversy and criticism faced by RBM led, in 2002, to a thorough external evaluation commissioned by the British government (the largest financer of RBM). Its head was Richard Feachem, then professor at the Institute for Global Health at the University of California. The evaluation clearly spelled out RBM's limitations. It was ineffective because its loose and complicated government structure caused confusion, and its inadequate monitoring and evaluation system made the work of country units inconsistent and inefficient.[39] An additional problem was that the senior manager in charge of the whole operation changed four times during its first years of existence. This meant instability, little clarity about who should make the decisions, and an erosion of credibility. Feachem's evaluation team considered whether RBM should have been established in the first place and whether it should continue; despite the problems enumerated, the answer to both questions was "yes."

RBM followed many of the recommendations outlined in the evaluation and underwent a thorough reorganization. (It interesting to note that the effort was pursued after Gro Harlem Brundtland left WHO in 2003.) It created an independent governance board, placed more emphasis on prevention (including the distribution of ITNs, wider use of rapid diagnostic tests, and the safe use of insecticides, including DDT), prioritized work with children and pregnant women, promoted research into and production of ACTs, supported the search for a vaccine, and sought new partners (beyond its few core founders). The latter activity implied recruiting more multilaterals, bilaterals, NGOs, and private donors. RBM also set a new deadline for its main goal: a significant reduction of malaria cases by 2015.[40] In the following years, that goal was refined to call for a reduction in the burden of malaria of at least 75 percent by 2015. As a result, RBM was able to restore its legitimacy and recover the confidence of donors.[41] Revamping RBM was possible because of the legitimacy that

PPPs still had with international agencies and industrial countries, as well as the growing support of the Global Fund.

However, some questions about RBM and the Fund have not been fully answered to this day. For example, are grants recreating "vertical" disease-specific control programs and dismissing broader "horizontal" approaches? Is the Fund giving sufficient attention to the need for more health workers and for essential health infrastructure? Are CCMs being formed quickly merely for the sake of submitting grant proposals to the Global Fund?[42] Is there really a process of encouraging national and local ownership of disease-control programs? Will these programs have a life after the outside funding is gone? Is the Fund a springboard for investments in health care systems, or does it promote stand-alone interventions?

In the case of malaria, more specific questions can be posed. Health systems need to engage in a genuine effort to decentralize and thus empower local health workers, but how is this to be achieved in countries characterized by political centralization, authoritarianism, and precarious health services? What can health workers and the Fund do to confront conditions that encourage the spread of malaria, such as the civil strife that too often displaces populations and leads to "illegal migration"? What is to be done about the breakdown of basic services, especially in rural areas, produced by neoliberal policies? Is RBM addressing the social conditions that make people vulnerable to communicable diseases? Military expenditures are still gigantic in poor countries, far out-sizing health budgets. What is the role of RBM or the Fund in modifying changes in spending priorities? What are the effects of governmental cuts in social and health expenditures linked to the structural adjustment programs of the World Bank and the International Monetary Fund? These and other questions remain to be answered.

In 2004 and 2005, new criticism was leveled at RBM. It was alleged that any hope that the project would achieve its goal of reducing the incidence of the disease by 2010 was unrealistic. A critical editorial in the *British Medical Journal* with the telling title "Roll Back Malaria: A Failing Global Health Campaign" reported a grim statistic: "The annual number of deaths worldwide from malaria is higher now than in 1998."[43] According to a 2005 article in the *Lancet*, "Five years on from the Abuja Summit, it is clear that not only has RBM failed in its aims, but it may also have caused harm."[44] An editorial in the *New York Times* entitled

"How Not to Roll Back Malaria" stated, "Seven years ago, with much fanfare, international health and development agencies unveiled the Roll Back Malaria campaign, which was supposed to cut malaria deaths in half by 2010. Yet progress has been worse than sluggish: there are actually indications that more people are suffering from malaria now than when the campaign started."[45] Another sharp criticism was that RBM had been slow in providing effective drugs (ACTs) to malaria victims, probably because of the cost of distributing these medicines. This was partially due to local infrastructural problems that had not been taken into account in the planning stage. Public health systems in developing countries usually have an inefficient system of drug delivery, marked by over-prescription in urban and periurban areas and an irrational use of drug-stocks, factors that undermine the credibility of health programs.

For critics, scarce financial resources were the major challenge for the future. Governments of the countries receiving aid provided insufficient funds and RBM risked becoming a top-down intervention promoted from abroad. The assessment of RBM's troubles appeared more clearly in an independent evaluation covering the 2004–2008 period that was conducted by a consultancy firm based in New York and specializing in PPPs. This assessment, the project's second since its inception in 1998,[46] introduced new terms such as "long-lasting insecticidal nets" (LLINs), and confirmed the return of pyrethroids and DDT with a new and subtle acronym (IRS, or indoor residual spraying). Once again, RBM's legitimacy was validated. As an indirect outcome of the criticism of malaria work, the new Director-General of WHO, the Korean Lee Jong-wook, began searching for a strong new leader for its malaria program. In 2005, the Japanese Arata Kochi, who had previously run WHO's STOP TB program, was appointed as the new head of the program. During his tenure at STOP TB, Kochi had turned what had become a lackluster effort run by a two-member staff into one of the agency's resounding successes. He was ousted from that job partly because of his disagreement with private donor foundations. A few months after his appointment to head the malaria program, Kochi confronted the big pharmaceutical companies. He issued an ultimatum to the industry to immediately stop selling single-dose artemisinin because it contributed to parasite resistance. As a corollary, he argued for the urgent need to abandon artemisinin monotherapy and switch to ACTs.[47]

Despite these criticisms, RBM and the advocates of magic bullet approaches would receive support from old and new players in global health. In 2005, President George W. Bush launched the President's Malaria Initiative, a five-year, US$1.2 billion program to combat malaria in the hardest-hit African nations, which emphasized the free-of-charge distribution of LLINs and the use of IRS.[48] In the same year, the World Bank announced its Booster Program for Malaria Control in Africa, which had a ten-year horizon. UNITAID was created in 2006; it was promoted by Brazil, among other nations, and hosted and administered by WHO, though formed by several agencies. With a smaller budget than that of the previously mentioned initiatives, its mandate was to obtain, supply, and negotiate price reductions for drugs, and to diagnose and treat HIV, malaria, and tuberculosis in poor nations.

A Return to Eradication?

Against this background, in October 2007 Bill Gates made an announcement at a malaria forum convened by his charitable foundation that shocked international agencies. He called for the complete global eradication of malaria. (Previously, Gates had launched a Malaria Vaccine Initiative in 1999 with a US$50 million grant.)[49] Gates argued that the effort could build on RBM's Global Malaria Action Plan (elaborated in 2008, celebrated by the second evaluation report, and endorsed by the UN). Many public health scholars supported Gates's call, believing that having an ambitious goal would be instrumental in overcoming the limitations of current efforts in a number of ways. It would make more visible the reductions in morbidity and mortality achieved in some countries, take advantage of a politically favorable climate for specific interventions in less-developed countries, capitalize on the willingness of stakeholders to extend the effective control already applied in key areas so as to achieve global coverage, and encourage the development of new drugs and of a first-ever vaccine. More recently, in 2010, the Gates Foundation announced that it would more than double its donations for medicines and vaccines, including those dedicated to the prevention and treatment of malaria, over the next decade, to at least US$10 billion. The foundation endorsed vaccines as the most cost-effective public health measure and assumed that a malaria vaccine, then in development by GlaxoSmithKline, would be approved by 2014 and would save the lives of some of the one million children, mostly in Africa, who would otherwise die annually of the disease.

Newly elected WHO Director-General Margaret Chan and RBM endorsed Gates's call and subscribed to the new goal of eliminating malaria, despite the reservations of some WHO officers.[50] WHO convened a panel of experts early in 2008 to examine the feasibility of eradicating the disease. They were less enthusiastic than the Director-General, concluding that there was a scientific basis for malaria elimination in some places, but that the effort's goal, scope, and deadlines needed to be more precisely defined. According to the experts, a reorientation from malaria control to elimination was feasible in countries where the malaria caseload had been reduced to a level that would allow individual follow-up with each malaria patient, but global eradication could not be expected, mainly because of the limitations of the existing eradication technologies.[51] A cautious but positive editorial in the *Lancet* celebrated the goal in the following words: "By calling for eradication they have rightly challenged the global health community to ask itself whether it should not be more ambitious."[52] Likewise, an important malaria journal created a new thematic series entitled "Towards Malaria Elimination" as a forum on how to achieve malaria eradication, starting with specific endemic settings.[53]

The Gates plan also had its critics. The two main arguments against it were, first, that the hope of producing the right eradication technologies in sufficient quantity in the next few years was unrealistic, and, second, that malaria control, or eradication, could not be framed as a matter of technology. For example, Arata Kochi, the head of WHO's Global Malaria Program, argued that promoting eradication was counterproductive because it would foster the false hope that a miracle was in the making and lead to the abandonment of control measures.[54] According to Kochi, with enough money and the better use of current tools such as bednets, medicines, and DDT, malaria could be reduced by 90 percent. Eliminating the last 10 percent, however, would in his view be a gigantic and expensive task beyond the power of medical technology or health agencies. Kochi believed, in fact, that the Gates Foundation's growing focus on malaria research ran the risk of concentrating on a few technological interventions, endangered the autonomy of scientists assessing the best programs, and undermined the leading role of WHO in the antimalaria effort. He was also concerned with more mundane issues, such as how to make the usually slow public sector more flexible and responsive to changing demands in malaria control and how to engage local health workers in sustained, long-term efforts. The latter were crucial, as in many developing countries health workers did not always adhere to recommended treatment and referral guidelines for children with fevers, administered therapy on the basis of narrow diagnoses, and tacitly disagreed with referral guidelines.[55]

The concerns of Kochi and of a few other critics (such as Awash Teklehaimanot, director of the malaria program at the Earth Institute of Columbia University, who argued that the resilience of the disease was being overlooked) generated some debate but, in general, are considered minor dissonances within a hegemonic trend. The response to such criticism suggests that, as in the 1950s, discordant opinions are being largely ignored.

Final Remarks

The changes I describe in this chapter can be sorted around three pivotal moments: first, in the 1970s and 80s, there was a tendency to discredit technologically driven malaria interventions, and this led to a period of confusion; second, in the 1990s and in the early years of the twenty-first century, RBM promoted progressive technological interventions designed to eliminate malaria as a public health problem; and third, we have seen a recent revival of at least some of the assumptions that reigned over international health during the 1950s, for instance, the notion that solving the problem of malaria is a matter of applying proper technology and massive funds. The last two moments coincided with the end of the Cold War, the revival of neoliberalism, and the emergence of new social-engineering tools of "global health" such as PPPs. Currently, technological weapons aimed at defeating the threat of the malaria parasite and mosquito appear to be universally endorsed, while associated social, political, and cultural factors are downplayed, just as occurred with the overemphasis on DDT in the 1950s.

During the posteradication era, from the late 1960s to the early 1990s, malaria work stopped being a priority, and the little that was done frequently produced only scattered advances in drug development, vector control, and preventive measures. Along with this lack of commitment went a lack of interest in fully assessing past antimalaria efforts and, thus, the loss of any useful lessons that might have been learned from them. I argue that the current revival and growing hegemony of the notion of "malaria eradication" frequently ignores the limitations of previous attempts, has been advanced without attention to its relationship with a developing notion of "global health," and usually fails to recognize the political and social factors that make living conditions miserable for the poor.

The new eradication effort differs from the 1950s efforts in its leadership. First, it does not place such single-minded reliance on a class of metropolitan experts and medical doctors from developed nations, usually trained in US or western European universities. There is now more sensitivity toward local actors and policy-makers and a greater interest in cooperating with them. Second, the new eradication effort comes with a new set of international alliances that is far more complicated than the "international health" scene of the 1950s. In the past, WHO and UNICEF were the clear leaders. In today's global health environment, private and bilateral donors, as well as major pharmaceutical companies, appear to carry the same weight as multilaterals, and WHO and the public sector have shown a willingness to relinquish some of their leadership in both national and global health efforts. However, problems remain in this era of new alliances. Although many of the leadership positions in international agencies are held by African experts, there is still little real community participation or engagement at the local level. According to a recent study, some of the major difficulties in malaria prevention in Africa are related to a lack of public understanding of the mode of malaria's transmission, the popular belief that malaria cannot be prevented, suspicion of medical malaria treatments, and the frequent misuse of bednets.[56] These observations confirm what the failure of the malaria eradication program launched in 1955 has demonstrated: namely, that any malaria prevention program should be based on the local social and cultural features in which it aims to operate.

Notes

1. World Health Organization (1993a).
2. Ibid.
3. Cueto (2007).
4. Nájera (1989).
5. Dobson et al. (2000).
6. The new policy appears in World Health Organization (1969).
7. *New York Times* (1969).
8. *Lancet* (1975); Reeves (1972).
9. Cited in Bruce-Chwatt (1980).
10. WHO Study Group on Malaria Control as Part of Primary Health Care (1983).
11. World Health Organization (1993b, 1994).
12. World Health Organization (1992).
13. World Health Organization (1993a).
14. *African Health* (1998).
15. Desowitz (2000).
16. Crossette (1998c).
17. Crossette (1998b).
18. Olson (1998).
19. World Commission on Environment and Development (1987).
20. Abbasi (1999).
21. World Health Organization (1998).
22. The Norwegian government awarded WHO US$7.5 million and the Rockefeller Foundation gave US$2.5 million specifically to recruit expert personnel. Lerer and Matzopoulos (2001); Crossette (1998a).
23. Bloom et al. (1999).
24. Buse and Walt (2000); Muraskin (1996). This had been the model used before in programs that did not achieve a high international profile, such as the Special Program for Research and Training in Tropical Diseases (TDR), the Onchocerciasis Control Program in Africa (OCP), the Global Alliance for Vaccines and Immunization (GAVI), and even UNAIDS.
25. Crossette (1998c).
26. Global Partnership to Roll Back Malaria (2001); Nabarro and Mendis (2000). For a discussion, see Bremen et al. (2000).
27. Nabarro and Tayle (1998).
28. In 2001, WHO and Novartis, the manufacturer of the artemisinin-based medicine Coartem, established a special pricing agreement: Novartis provided the drug at cost price (US$0.90 and US$2.40 for the child and adult treatment courses, respectively) for use in the public sector in malaria-endemic countries. Through the special price agreement WHO and UNICEF procured the drug for governments of malaria-endemic countries, United Nation agencies, bilateral agencies, and NGOs.
29. For example Gallup and Sachs (2001); Sachs (2002).
30. Garabrant et al. (1994); Wolff (1993).
31. Rehwagen (2006); WHO Global Malaria Programme (2007).

32. http://www.rollbackmalaria.org/gmap/1-4.html [last accessed July 1, 2010]. Funding for malaria continued to increase significantly, reaching an estimated US$1.5 billion in 2007.

33. US Congress (2003).

34. Ibid.

35. McNeil (2002).

36. Brugha et al. (2004).

37. Narasimhan and Attaran (2003).

38. Molyneux and Nantulya (2004).

39. Malaria Consortium (2002).

40. Coll-Seck et al. (2008).

41. *Lancet* (2000).

42. Lu et al. (2006).

43. Editorial, *British Medical Journal* (2004).

44. *Lancet* (2005).

45. *New York Times* (2005).

46. World Health Organization (2009).

47. Boseley (2006).

48. Loewenberg (2007).

49. Enserink and Roberts (2007).

50. Mendis et al. (2009).

51. Ibid.

52. *Lancet* (2007).

53. Tanner and Hommel (2010); Tanner and de Savignya (2008).

54. Bate (2008).

55. Walter et al. (2009).

56. Maslove et al. (2009).

2

Evidence-Based Global Public Health

Subjects, Profits, Erasures

VINCANNE ADAMS

> It's true that JAMA seldom publishes qualitative studies. A qualitative study can say that an exposure-outcome relationship occurs at least occasionally, and can describe some of the circumstances, but it cannot determine incidence, prevalence, independent risk factors, effective prevention or treatment, etc. At JAMA we are much more interested in studies at the other end of the research pipeline, meaning studies that show how to prevent or treat a known health problem.
>
> —*Editor of the* Journal of the American Medical Association, *in response to a query about submitting a qualitative, ethnographic article on violence and human rights in reproductive health, 2010*

The topic of this chapter is the impact of "evidence-based medicine" (EBM) on global public health.[1] An epistemic transformation in the field of global health is underway, and I will argue that the impact of evidence-based medicine has been twofold: (1) the creation of an experimental metric as a means of providing health care (following Petryna 2009);[2] and (2) a shift in the priorities of caregiving practices in public health such that "people [no longer] come first." The production of experimental research populations in and through EBM helps constitute larger fiscal transformations in how we do global health. Notably, EBM has created a platform for the buying and selling of truth and reliability, abstracting clinical caregiving from the social relationships on which they depend.

The Rise of Evidence-Based Medicine

Most contemporary health scientists would agree that evidence-based medicine, as currently known, emerged in the 1990s (Timmermans and Berg 2003; Timmermans and Mauck 2005; Sackett et al. 2000; Evidence-Based Medicine Working Group 1992), although some have noted that the foundations of EBM may be located in the mid-nineteenth-century (Sackett et al. 1996) rise of scientific epistemology based on inductive empirical reasoning (see Gordon 1988) and the creation and use of an "experimental field" (see Shapin and Schaffer 1986). Modern EBM's technical raison d'être has primarily been to address the persistent problem of nonstandard variation in clinical practice. The assumption in EBM is that a "conscientious, explicit, and judicious use of current *best evidence* in making decisions about the care of individual patients" will eliminate this problem and improve health care delivery and outcomes (Timmermans and Mauck 2005).[3] In sum, the goal has been to create a stronger "scientific" foundation for clinical work by focusing on new kinds and meanings of "evidence." I note at the outset that many have pointed to other compelling forces behind the birth of EBM, such as the rise of mandated cost control and resource limitations under "managed care" systems in industrialized nations. The perceived benefits of evidence-based medicine are significant and worthwhile, despite skepticism among some who doubt that the ideals of EBM will be achieved.[4] Here I will focus on the rise of EBM in terms of its outcomes and implications beyond these debates.

Of importance in the shift to an era of "evidence-based medicine" is that while evidence can take many forms, in EBM, the statistical, experimental, and epidemiological models of evidence are taken as the *gold standard*. In fact, evidence in EBM is codified: "Level 1" evidence in EBM (on a scale of 5) is derived from the properly designed randomized controlled trial (RCT). "Level 5" evidence, the least useful, derives from "opinions of respected authorities, based on clinical experience, descriptive studies, or reports of expert committees."[5] Between these extremes are the kinds of evidence derived from what EBM writers consider quasi-well-designed studies (controlled, cohort, case-control, multiple time series, etc.), but which are missing some critical component of the gold standard. In this approach to health care, the type of evidence that counts the "least," if at all, derives from what gets called "anecdotal" information and is relegated to a level below 5. Like the untouchables of India's caste system, "anecdotal" evidence is seen to lie beyond the pale of quality. "Anecdotal" refers to information based on the observations of nonclinical experts, unsystematic interviews, and eyewitness testimonials (Brownson et al. 2003).[6] This kind of evidence is interesting and empirical, but not useful in the RCT. In EBM, studies that foreground the individual speaking subject as the primary source of truth have virtually no purchase, nor do those additional truths garnered from the families, communities, or relationships that help form that speech. Certain kinds of evidence are essentially irreconcilable with EBM's definition of reliable evidence, except insofar as such words can be made to fit in a quantitative way into the RCT design, or otherwise to corroborate RCT findings with a bit of ethnographic "color."

That the use of EBM is on the rise is clear. The epigraph at the start of this paper was written by the editor of the *Journal of the American Medical Association* in response to a colleague whose ethnographic research on the politics of sex selection and gender discrimination in assisted reproduction in the United States was considered inappropriate (or at best a long shot) for the journal. The editor states explicitly that "a qualitative study can offer evidence that something occasionally occurs," but it cannot establish *reliable* evidence of the sort that really counts when it comes to effective prevention or treatment.[7] Years of achievements of health policy, not to mention feminism, are summarily cast upon the ash heap of irrelevance here. This is not to say that I disagree entirely with the editor, for it is evident that some things indeed cannot be known except through techniques akin to RCT research, and journals like *JAMA* have *always* prioritized quantitative over qualitative studies. What is new today, however, and hinted at in the editor's response, is that for evidence to be *reliable* today, it must be pushed through the engines of scientific scrutiny in new ways. Specifically, for evidence to say anything valid about "how to prevent or treat a known health problem" it must speak the language of statistics and epidemiology, or, to be even more specific, it should use the methods of the randomized controlled trial. In this ordering of priorities, one finds a simultaneous discrediting of other forms of knowledge and evidence and other ways of conveying truth that have historically been invested with value in both deciphering ill health and evaluating the clinical outcomes of health interventions, especially in the global health context.

Viewed from the perspective of EBM advocates like *JAMA*'s editor, only randomized controlled studies can show that an intervention *really* works. RCT study designs are the most reliable way to be certain that what one is seeing is more than either a matter of chance or subjective perception and more than the occasional experience of a small and statistically insignificant group of individuals. RCT research knows its findings are reliable. Why? Because RCTs tie efficacy to statistical truth. That is, results of RCT studies are considered objective (they appear as unbiased, numerical facts) and they are considered valid (they use statistical configurations to present their truths). To contest these truths, one would have to doubt the reliability of both statistics and the objective realities they reveal. Although social science critics have contested this view, noting that the outcomes of such studies are in some sense prefigured through the anticipatory logic of the statistical method (that is, their outcomes are produced by the very structure of the research design as opposed to being discovered by it),[8] EBM advocates take the statistical method as the most unbiased technique for evaluating health interventions.

To date, fundamental challenges that compel the shift to evidence-based methods in health care have been largely articulated around concerns over the validity and generalizability of empirical claims about outcomes. RCT models of research provide a convenient and reliable way of encoding and specifying a language for overcoming these challenges and achieving the goals of Best Medical Practices. As a result, it becomes increasingly the case that medical interventions that do not lend themselves to evaluations using RCT designs must be seen, from the EBM perspective, as being of *poor quality* and, by default, unreliable, and therefore of little use in determining policy, practice guidelines, or fiscal support.

I suggest that EBM approaches have become not just routine but rather tyrannical in the world of clinical health care in the industrialized nations. Not surprisingly, they are aggressively promoted as the new gold standard, not just in clinical medicine, but in territories that spread far beyond the US bedside to a wide variety of disciplinary and interventionary fields, including public and global health. The review panels that vet research grants and make funding decisions in global health (from large governments, bilaterals, and multilaterals, as well as foundations) have trended toward favoring projects that employ RCT in the belief that results from these projects will be more reliable because they can be more easily evaluated. While it is not entirely surprising that this is the case for research, it is surprising that health intervention projects are being subjected to similar demands to use RCT-style designs. In the United States, EBM is used to determine the best clinical practices and the optimal insurance policies. In global health, we are seeing similar trends with equally strong impact at intervention and policy levels. Even traditional humanitarian interventions that involve no research component are increasingly called to task over the question of whether their impact and effectiveness can be assessed using evidence-based standards of evaluation. New regimes of accountability using EBM standards have emerged as a kind of "audit" necessity in organizations far and wide, from the Gates Foundation and Save the Children, to the NIH and the WHO. The results of this shift are worth exploring.

In what follows, I recall the effort begun years ago by the World Bank anthropologist Michael Cernea in his volume on international development, *Putting People First*, as I attempt to answer the question posed by our conference organizers: What kind of medicine and what kind of research are called for if we wish to ensure that people come first? Subsidiary questions emerge from this as well: What kind of subjectivity must be produced in order to do EBM in global health? What kinds of economic engines are fed by this shift and who profits from them? What kinds of evidence must be disregarded in order for RCT-style evidence to matter more in the shift to evidence-based medicine in global public health? In the shift to valorizing one kind of evidence over other kinds of evidence, the unintended outcomes that arrive in the wake of this new regime of truth making in global public health need to be accounted for. This essay is only a first step in that effort.

Evidence-Based Medicine in Global Public Health: Producing Subjects

The contours of the transition to EBM in global public health settings are instructive and suggest an impact that is both epistemological and practical. First, EBM arrives in international health as part of the uptake of EBM by public health (in EBPH [evidence-based public health]) and alongside a shift in the field away from traditional "international health" toward what is called "global public health" or "global health science" or simply "global health" (Adams et al. 2008).

At my own university, a new multicampus Global Health Sciences program has been recently launched. Among its many rationales is the notion that clinicians who have long worked in the fields of health development will benefit from interchanges with bench scientists, pharmaceutical researchers, and industrialized nation public health experts as they grapple collectively with some of the most intractable problems of poor health on a global scale. Biochemists and molecular biologists undertaking research on infectious diseases find it increasingly necessary to work in globally remote sites in order to fully understand the etiologies and pathologies of viral, retroviral, and bacteriological pathogens and treatments that have a large and productive life outside of their laboratories. Infectious diseases travel rapidly around the globe, and researchers are finding that treatment programs designed for one location are useless in others. Such travels bring these bench researchers into contact with international health experts who have spent decades trying to eradicate and prevent transmission of these diseases in places where they have become endemic.

Pharmaceutical researchers are also finding themselves increasingly involved in international health work. Often, through the collaborative infrastructure of public-private partnerships, these researchers struggle to locate drug-naive populations for clinical trials and to explore the dynamics of drug therapies among populations that are often in dire need of these drugs. At the receiving end, public and international health experts in underdeveloped and resource-poor countries find themselves having to negotiate with pharmaceutical research projects run by pharmaceutical contract research organizations (CROs) and with federally funded pharmaceutical research teams from wealthy nations (Petryna 2009; Biehl 2008). Together, they must navigate through, or around, existing government-run public health infrastructures and policies in countries where research subjects are in plentiful supply but where thorny concerns about ethics, inclusion, and risk are still being worked out (Petryna et al. 2006; Petryna 2009).

Bringing models of traditional bench and pharmaceutical sciences research to international health is also in part a result of the perception that more scientific rigor has been needed in the world of international health, just as it was and is needed in clinical, bedside medicine at home. The meeting of bench and pharmaceutical scientists with international health experts has produced many fruitful and productive collaborations, but among the most significant is a "scientization" of international public health. That is, Global Health, as a new field emerging from the foundation of International Health Development, carries with it the notion that EBM-driven programs will satisfy the need for more scientific rigor in their international health development efforts. The use of evidence-based medicine will make global health look and feel more scientific because it will *be* more scientific in its practices. Already, most programs in global health have begun to train a cadre of intervention-oriented researchers who can think through international health by way of RCT-based languages and skills.

At the same time, the marriage of bench science and pharmaceutical researchers with traditional international health programs, and the scaling-up of use of RCT-model research in this effort, has also resulted in a shift away from certain forms of taken-for-granted "caregiving." In place of the intervention programs that aimed at eradicating and treating disease by way of a variety of efforts aimed at maximizing impact for the largest numbers of people, a more ambitious mandate now circulates in global health, calling for "intervention-as-research" that aims to answer not the simple question "What works to improve health for the most people possible?" but rather "How can we be sure that our outcomes are not an artifact of chance or personal bias in perception?" The simple counting of those who are helped or made healthy is today insufficient, because now most, if not all, international health care interventions are asked to be attentive to a larger set of methodologies that allow for greater precision in the assessment of outcomes. Measurements modeled after the RCT enable researchers to determine the *statistical* significance of outcomes in ways that are believed to show evidence of impact that is uncontestable. Along the way to getting this kind of evidence, however, some things might be compromised in the very prioritizing of what interventions can or should be done.

From the perspective of those who like to use RCT models, these methods are valuable because they offer a comparative platform that produces reliability based on statistical constants. The RCT proves efficacy in a number of quite specific ways—through the use of controls, randomization, generalizability, power calculations, and, above all, the use of only quantitative forms of data. RCTs define the variables that matter in terms of what can be counted, disregarding other kinds of information that might be attached to the intervention or outcome as irrelevant to the study. Using models that can be replicated in other geographic areas, other villages, other countries, EBM public health researchers believe that they will be able to demonstrate the efficacy of some interventions over others with a higher level of accuracy than in interventions where efficacy was claimed but results could not be replicated over time or in other locations. The assumption is that although we may think that a program has worked, we cannot know for sure until we have subjected it to a rigorous test, using controls and large sample sizes. Similarly, what worked in Uganda may not work in Russia but we will learn *why* only if we keep in place the components of a well-designed RCT across these vast cultural and geographic territories.

In EBM-driven Global Health, the ability to evaluate and generalize results across vast differences and contexts of culture, geography, politics, economy (and one could go on) is thus not a problem but an advantage. Seemingly insurmountable differences in contexts and circumstances are the reason to rely on things like RCTs. However, determining whether or not an intervention has a measurable impact is never a simple task. Beyond obvious concerns over which outcomes should be measured and for whom these outcomes matter, social scientists have offered numerous critiques of so-called successful health interventions, noting that although successful by some measures, they often produce unintended consequences that render their overall success ambiguous (Justice 1989; Ferguson 1994; Nichter 2008; Biehl 2008). In fact, much of the corpus of social science research in international public health has been specifically devoted to this topic, and, in the end, much of this work has been used in international health planning in order to revise and reformulate intervention approaches (from the work of George Foster all the way to Paul Farmer).

Generalizability is also a tricky epistemological undertaking. Outcomes can be measured in a variety of more or less contested ways, but in EBM an outcome is generally considered valid only if it meets very specific criteria: if it has an established comparative case (using a control or comparative group); if it has statistical power (a large enough *n*); and if it can be shown to be reproducible in other settings using the same standard methodology. In other words, the logic of the RCT uses a set of criteria that are peculiar to itself in order to establish validity. Outcomes are tautologically measured by one criterion above all others: namely, by the degree to which the intervention is designed as a randomized controlled trial; or, failing that, by the degree to which it has *some* design components of the gold standard. Thus generalizability, which is established by following standard methodological protocols, becomes one of the most important determinants of the value of any particular health intervention. Not surprisingly, the validity of context-specific interventions that demand methodological specificity is apt to be questioned. That is, regardless of how well any particular intervention seems to work in a specific location (e.g., giving out free condoms in rural Nepal to prevent STDs), the notion that a local success is a positive outcome is supplanted by the notion that unless it used the controls, randomization, and statistics that guarantee generalizability, it is of minimal usefulness. Thus, a study that compares the distribution of free condoms with the use of social marketing strategies to sell condoms to prevent STDs in neighboring villages is seen as much more useful than a study that simply documents lowered STDs in a village where free condoms have been distributed. But a study that compares two methods of distribution and then randomizes these distribution methods across multiple villages and generates enough individual outcomes on STDs to compare villages would be the ideal method for establishing what really works to reduce STDs in relation to condom distribution.

What is lost in this leap to the use of rigorous statistical methods is the recognition that sometimes context itself determines what methods can and cannot be effective. The conditions of life and living in the places where interventions are offered often make studies that have all (or sometimes any) RCT components extremely difficult, if not impossible. Using RCT as the standard and then trying to deploy RCT-type interventions in places where they are not appropriate sometimes means ignoring the unforgiving realities that inhibit ideal RCT design. Other times, it means giving up on such designs altogether and accepting that the outcomes of one's intervention may never be taken seriously in global health publication circles. Thus, for instance, in the hypothetical case above (of condom distribution), problems of "contamination" between distribution villages either have to be addressed (making the RCT impossible) or ignored (making the RCT flawed). If one did distribute condoms in a village and noted declines in STDs, it would be difficult to make the case that this observation had scientific value. It would merely be a subjective observation until one added in measures of comparison, control, randomization, and large "n"s that can be powered.

The challenges that face attempts to implement RCTs in global health go beyond this set of concerns. All kinds of empirical realities may impinge on the ways that RCT data is produced, and they may condition the outcomes that one sees. Questions about the social and infrastructural dynamics that get involved in managing the distribution, consumption, and use of condoms (to continue with the hypothetical case), and the meaning of cash versus gift transactions in relation to notions of sexuality in villages (based on religion, family pressure, sentiments of love, and the like)—and these are just examples—might, if pursued, lead one to the conclusion that reducing STDs has nothing to do with how condoms are distributed, but rather with things like the religion of the person distributing them, the color of the packaging, the commitment to healthy families over and above the cost of condoms, or the social and behavioral obligations that come along with receiving gifts from a health center. All of these considerations may be vital to explaining rates of STD reduction, or the lack thereof, but unless the RCT study is designed to include them all, there will be no way to know this, and assuming that the RCT has captured the essential variables that matter may lead to misleading claims.

While RCT-research advocates argue that any and all of these potentially confounding conditions could be adapted to, or incorporated within (or somehow managed away by), well-designed RCT planning, what instead happens is that such confounding variables are often treated as "static" in the system and ignored. What really matters is getting sufficient numbers. In an RCT numbers seem to carry intrinsic validity. If there are sufficient numbers, this by itself lends the study a perceived reliability that transcends questions about how those numbers were produced and what they actually stand for. Any notion that context-specific, tailor-made, and nonreproducible interventions and findings might just be the most efficient way to conduct international public health interventions falls by the wayside as generalizable results formulated around the RCT standard take precedence.

Approximating the Ideal: EBM in Public Health

There is a history of controversy over the marriage of EBM with public health. Even within countries like the United States this merger has not been easy, and many of the ongoing debates are pertinent to efforts to understand the globalization of these methods. Public health scholars and researchers have raised concerns over the quality of EBM as implemented in hospital clinical care and over the validity of its evaluations. In fact, over time, the notion of the "rigor" of EBM in public health has undergone some changes. Whereas the best evidence-based *clinical medicine* was seen as relying on randomized controlled trials of medical treatments, "evidence-based public health" (EBPH) was initially thought to be capable of achieving only an approximate version of EBM, and not necessarily rigorous RCT work. Notably, it was thought that the link between intervention and outcome might become visible only after a longer period of time had elapsed than would be allowed for in a controlled study. It was noted as well that in most public health worlds, multiple disciplines were involved in an actual intervention, thus complicating randomization—among other things (Brownson et al. 2003; Briss et al. 2004). Initially, what proponents of EBM in public health called for was a "quasi-experimental" design. They acknowledged that interventions often lacked "true" comparison groups (Brownson et al. 1999). Journal articles sought to promote standardized ways of assessing public health interventions and of assessing the literature produced about them, so as to make the best of what was implicitly seen as a messy situation (Briss et al. 2004). Granted, real-life public health scenarios did not look or feel like the laboratories or the clinics where EBM techniques were born, but, with effort, it was felt that they could be made to approximate these research spaces, conceptually and epistemologically.

It is important to remember that one branch of public health that is equally important in international health already relies heavily on the use of statistical methods: epidemiology. Long-standing debates between social scientists who study or use epidemiological methods had aroused some awareness of the pitfalls and limitations of using statistical methods to account for complex social phenomena (Janes, Stall, and Gifford 1986; Susser and Susser 1996; Treichler 1999; Trostle 2005; Shim 2005). Researchers noted that the use of statistics at the population level could serve both a political function (in advocacy) and a depoliticizing function (by rendering social problems "objective" facts). They also argued for methods that mixed a variety of strategies to create more complete pictures of outcomes, including ethnography, rapid assessment, and case studies. Some have documented how the use of epidemiological models negatively impacts clinical caregiving (see Gifford 1986 for an excellent example). However, these critics did not anticipate that the uptake of RCT-style research in EBPH might colonize all other research, under the mandate that all international public health interventions should look like experiments. The use of statistical models in public health work is complicated by the adoption of RCT as the gold standard, as researchers of all kinds are asked to embrace the idea that in order to be scientific their interventions must be designed like clinical trials. This goes far beyond using statistics to make strong analytical claims; it requires doing research to get statistics in a whole new way. At its worst, the advent of such experimentalist platforms for research has made the job of producing statistics as important as, if not more important than, the actual medical goal of the interventions they hope to implement.

Over the past decade, it has become increasingly imperative for public health efforts to front-load their efforts with more rigorous and scientifically competent design strategies. Although this is not yet universally true, the messy world of public health has begun to look, here and there, like a bench science laboratory. Today, it is common to see public health interventions that use randomization with comparison or controls as part of their delivery strategy. Public health epidemiologists have, at times with celebratory zeal, taken the basic four-phase RCT model designed for pharmaceutical research and adapted it for behavioral and public health interventions. Increasingly, the earlier "quasi-experimental designs" that preceded EBPH have lost legitimacy, and the literature based on such designs has been judged of limited use (Briss et al. 2004). Simultaneously, public health has witnessed a ratcheting-up of efforts to make all intervention studies conform to the rigors of phase I-, II-, or III-style research interventions.[9] The shift to using an experimental platform for public health interventions is now considered not only possible, but preferred.

Many contemporary journals of public health (the *International Journal of Public Health*, the *WHO Bulletin*, the *International Journal of Health Services*) and the standard clinical journals (*BMJ, JAMA, NEJM*) are filled with public health research publications based on RCT designs. Titles often include the phrase "A Randomized Controlled Study of [fill in the blank]." In these journals and bulletins, "research" articles are designated as such on the grounds that they use this study design, while other articles (based on observations, social behavioral analysis, etc.) are identified as "news reports" or "editorials." The latter are not "research," and are thus treated as if they are of questionable reliability when it comes to evaluating health care achievements. Described as "qualitative studies," these "soft science" pieces are treated as fun stories that are empty of real scientific value. This is true despite the fact that such findings are often based on rigorous empirical methods, just not the methods of the RCT. Whereas a mere ten years ago, one would be hard-pressed to find a single published article that used an RCT study design for a public health intervention, such studies are now commonplace. The RCT imprimatur seems the most certain route to publication in most of the reputable journals that deal with either international or public health.[10]

What is important to recall in all this is how dramatic the transformation has been. In the past, international public health publications typically offered straightforward impact reports. How many children were immunized? How many people were using contraception? How many clean water systems were built? How many hygiene programs were delivered through outreach? Obstacles to interventions, or interactions between one health problem and another, were presented in articles that described the complex local context of global programs and the reasons projects worked or failed.[11] These simple but obvious, and often context-specific, ways of addressing efficacy were sufficient for many years and for many people. This was particularly true in the small NGO world, where reports were generated for donor organizations in ways that highlighted the specific outcomes and inefficiencies of a target program or community.

Nowadays, similar efforts are seen as woefully deficient. Labeled "reports from the field" or published under the heading "News," these simple counting exercises are seen more as an attempt at public relations than as an approach to producing compelling scientific results on which to make claims about outcomes or about the benefits of one type of intervention over another. Meanwhile, a different kind of study is called for when facts about the impact and effectiveness of programs are at issue. Global public health interventions must show that they do more than simply count the number of immunized babies, safely delivered mothers, diarrheal deaths prevented, or hygiene and nutrition lessons taught. An intervention must demonstrate that it achieved results because it was designed as an experimental study to begin with. These results can be useful only if they show that they were better than chance (randomized), and better than nothing (controlled), and, above all, generalizable.

Randomizing the Whole Country: What Counts in Counting Health Outcomes

Thus global health emerges today as an experimental research endeavor. Glancing through journals, we find that everything from "rates of diarrhea" to the "use of antiretrovirals" to "the benefits of combining HIV treatment with contraceptive planning" is now being investigated in randomized controlled research trials.[12] Researchers must give some interventions to some people and either something else or no intervention at all to others, and then they must make sure that these groups of people don't cross-contaminate, and then that their subject numbers are large enough to show significance or, as I was told by a program officer with regard to my own research (to which I will return below), enough to do "a good power calculation." If it is possible to run statistical analyses and power calculations on the results . . . then *voilà*: good science and (therefore) good global health.

An exemplary case of this was shared with me by a colleague. It involves a public health policy project being conducted in an island nation. This study, which I will call the Island Insurance Study (IIS), focuses on the impact of health insurance schemes on child health. The intervention is grounded in politics that are, to my mind, laudable: it is designed to show, with measurable outcomes clearly hypothesized from the start, that the government (and its various lender nations) should view providing health insurance coverage for basic care as an "investment" rather than a "cost," and therefore as worth the expense. Specifically, the IIS aims to show, using RCT designs, that paying for health insurance is not only cost-effective but beneficial for the health of children. IIS has been implemented in all public health and clinical-care centers across the nation and scientifically designed with three arms: (1) an intervention arm in which expanded insurance coverage is provided, (2) an intervention arm in which providers are compensated at higher rates for better care, and (3) a control arm in which clinics and patients receive neither benefit. The intervention is designed as a research project in which, as the primary researcher on the project proudly announced to me, "the entire country has now been randomized." It is a spectacular achievement.

In the IIS project, outcome measures are based on physiologic and cognitive assessments, derived from data collected at all of the clinics. Although clinical services are provided throughout the country, these services are being reconceptualized specifically in order to enable the creation of an experimental platform for research, with each kind of care delivery serving as either control or contrasting arm. That is, no health care will be provided unless it serves as a tool for data collection. The project is referred to by its author as an "experimental evaluation" of the policy impacts of these different forms of health care provision. It is simultaneously a study that will demonstrate the value of evidence-based public health research in creating evidence-based public health policy. Finally it will provide valuable insights about which insurance strategies produce the best measurable health outcomes for the public. The deployment of EBPH thus has interesting implications in that it enables interventions to serve two masters simultaneously: both to evaluate health outcomes and to build and sustain a research infrastructure.

Intervention-cum-research projects in global public health often use the notion of a "natural laboratory," suggesting that the social world can generate laboratory-like data. Often, outcome "measurables" are seen as the end product of the intervention as much as the health outcomes themselves. Good data, it would seem, is as valuable as (in some studies perhaps more valuable than) a positive health result. The data that is particularly sought after is the kind that can be used to generate statistically robust calculations and comparisons that, once analyzed, can tell the truth about which interventions are most effective at a population level. Often, this means creating a research platform that eliminates the need for data collection about complex social realities, and using select variables as proxies that will tell us indirectly about these larger and complex social realities. For example, in the IIS project, the intention is to use an RCT design to make claims about entire populations, but the evaluation indicator most readily available is children. Because children are seen as an easy target for data collection, they are being used here as proxies for everyone else in the system. Similarly, the study selects "tracer" conditions for measuring physiologic outcomes—proxies for general states of health and diseases. In this case, the tracer conditions are pneumonia and diarrhea (with a wide spectrum of biomarkers). To measure cognitive outcomes, a battery of intelligence and psychological tests are used that assess well-being and the "normal" development of children. Being able to show that some children have better physiologic and cognitive outcomes than others will be, in other words, a positive result for the intervention, and the intervention is therefore designed around an imperative for measurables—data sets that can be obtained in sufficiently large numbers to ensure some degree of reliability. In order to get good numbers, all sorts of proxies must be used. Reality is best captured in the RCT in small measurable bites rather than in its vast and unmeasurable complexity.

What is interesting to me about the IIS intervention is that right from the start it displaces old straightforward questions about what justifies projects like this. While it is clear that the project hopes to improve the health of children, and that it is noble in this effort, it is not clear to me that the IIS design is the best way to do this. Why not roll out insurance schemes across the country and then compare health statistics ten years down the road? It is a large and potentially messy way to generate data, and it won't be based on use of controls, but it might show dramatic health outcomes anyway. Doing an RCT instead is justified on two grounds: first, to establish an experiment that will show, definitively (in the terms of EBM), what kind of insurance helps most, and, second, to establish that this form of research is possible in large-scale public health projects. My point would be to note that interventions designed in this way actually change the kinds of questions that can be asked. If ten years ago an intervention would have been designed simply to see whether children would benefit from having health insurance by counting reported diseases and collecting morbidity and mortality numbers, today's intervention must do much more than this. It must be designed to show difference in outcomes in different populations based on the variables of the experimental design of the intervention. Not only are children allowed to be proxies for entire populations, but some kids will have to show that they do more poorly than others. We will have to accept numerous premises concerning proxies and control groups that may raise questions about the research design, but at present this model for research is seen as, again, the gold standard. It is useful thus to explore what else gets produced in generating truth about health and health care in this particular way. Each and every intervention goal is recalibrated to meet the needs of the statistical model, while other possible ways to get the sought-after truth of whether or not insurance helps keep kids healthy are potentially pushed off the table.

In addition to evaluating the benefits of one kind of intervention versus another or versus no intervention, the IIS, like other RCT interventions in global health, will also attach itself to the partner-in-crime of EBM: cost-effectiveness. That is, in the new EBM of Global Public Health, economic calculi are affixed to interventions in ways that make cost something that must be accounted for in the same ways that things like "rates of diarrhea" are counted (and studied statistically). This makes sense, because one wants to show that spending money on health care (however much or however little) "pays off" in health dividends in the end. But this tethering of health to cost variables constitutes another way that EBM is changing global health and how we go about trying to help people achieve health.

Not surprisingly, cost-effectiveness is not the only fiscal concern of the IIS project. The IIS, like other global health interventions today that strive for EBM standards, has to spend a lot of money on data collection, processing, and analysis. The data processing for the IIS study, involving the massive use of biomarker and cognitive assessment instruments, large-scale data-entry teams, and epidemiological biostatistical analysis, is being undertaken by a locally based subcontractor. The intervention itself will help stimulate the local economy, which is surely not a confounding variable, but it is a fact that points to important new demands that are being placed upon anyone hoping to do Global Public Health in ways that will be recognized as scientific, useful, and valid.

My point, as an observation more than critique, is that the experimentalization of the entire clinical health-service system in the country where the IIS intervention is being done is an accomplishment that is not simply the product of a desire for reliable and effective health care delivery. It is also the product of a convergence of specific neoliberal political and economic trends. By neoliberal, I refer to the normalized privatization of public institutions, in which creating pathways by which public-sector activities can be transformed into private-sector, profit-garnering infrastructures is the norm. In this transition, the problem of accountability to a market becomes a nonnegotiable priority. The effort to roll out and scale up use of EBM in Global Public Health comes as a package in which the management of cost (of intervention as well as of doing the research) is inextricably sutured to the ways the research/intervention is designed.

This suturing of fiscal to scientific kinds of health data in and through the research enterprise shows up in the new medical industries that come into being in countries where "scaling up" research and biopharmaceutical infrastructures is a priority (Sunder Rajan 2006). It results in the capitalization of health-sector research and in a consequent tethering of health to biological models that can deliver high-cost research opportunities. It also shows up in more subtle ways in the global health world: as when interventions themselves must incorporate *labor-* and *cost*-intensive research measures. Finally, the impact of neoliberal trends toward privatization of the health sector shows up in the presumption that the best public health must be ever-attentive to the question of cost-effectiveness—that is, to insisting that economics and sustainability are a health priority (as opposed to recognizing that some things just cost a lot and can't pay for themselves, or that they will require a long-term commitment before they achieve self-sustainability).[13] Thus, even though the IIS intends to show that a *government* health care insurance program will improve health, it is deeply committed to working within a US model of entrepreneurial research that is rapidly privatizing and creating for-profit infrastructures for health research in and through commitments to Global Health.

The shift I am pointing to is one in which fiscal concerns have become a foundational, and perhaps tyrannical, presence not only in what we study, but also in how we study it. For the sake of efficiency, projects like the IIS are now required to work with large corporations because they are capable of processing voluminous quantities of data, for a price.

Simultaneously, research-based interventions are asked to consider cost-effectiveness as a variable that penetrates and pervades all that is done. These are, I believe, outcomes of the adoption of neoliberal ways of doing things in Global Health, and they are tied to the methods of EBM and RCTs.

A prime example of what happens when all health concerns are tied to a market or economic model is the use of DALYs (Disability-Adjusted Life Years).[14] Designed to measure the impact of illness and disability on a community and to help prioritize investments of health intervention aid, DALYs are a tool for gauging a sociological phenomenon (quality of life) on a quantitative scale (according to the value in productivity of that life). That is, DALYs equate quality of life with a fiscal criterion for the value of life. Critiques of the shortcomings of DALYs are plentiful. Nichter (2008) summarizes them well. Still, few note the seamless way in which the insertion of such metrics into the messy world of international or, now, global health lends credibility to the idea that everything (from the impact of disease to the impact of an intervention) can be measured quantitatively. This notion has emerged from within a nexus of neoliberal priorities that privilege fiscal bottom lines above any and all other possible bottom lines. To see how the institutions of evidence-based research further contribute to this particular form of neoliberalism, consider another project.

Evidence-Based Medicine in Global Public Health: Producing and Privatizing Profits

In 2008, I witnessed an effort to bring a resiliency-training program to low socioeconomic status (SES) school-age children in a large US city. The public school systems in this city are among the least successful in the nation, judging by performance measures, and this is attributed to such factors as entrenched poverty, high levels of violence, limited to no social or health services within the schools, and high rates of ongoing trauma. I first heard about the desire for this project from a city resident who had worked in the schools and had seen the children's needs first hand. In response, I joined a collaborative partnership that included a non-profit resiliency-training organization that had done extensive work with children, and a research team that had experience working with NIH funding in large-scale intervention research programs. The team that came together to design the project was headed by a clinician-epidemiologist who was joined by the nonprofit director, a well-known psychology researcher, and a well-established anthropologist (myself). The team's epidemiologist leader set the tone of the research and intervention strategy. The first step would be figuring out the best way to achieve an effective randomization strategy. A control group was needed, but the team did not want to enlist schools or children to participate if they received no intervention. The design eventually used a staggered intervention strategy so that one group could be used as a control initially, even though they would eventually get the intervention. This was a reasonable solution to an ethical conundrum: how to make the research design robust but at the same time avoid denying participants the potential benefit of participation. It is a conundrum that is as serious for community-centered global health intervention studies as it is for hospital-based clinical trials. Of course our study included enough students (a large enough n in each group) to generate reliability and "statistical power."

The second step was to identify *measurable* outcomes, using questionnaires to collect data on a wide range of variables: included were the subjects' development of internal and external psychological assets, their mental-health status, behavioral changes over time, and school achievement. Some of these outcome indicators would be available from the schools (via test scores, attendance records, graduation rates, and rates of expulsion, suspension, and disruptive incidents in the classroom). Other indicators, however, would have to be derived through data collection methods that would involve the use of questionnaires and pre- and postintervention surveys. Our hypothesis was simple: the schools in which we provided resiliency training would have better outcomes on all of these measures than those that did not.

As the anthropologist on the project, I assumed at first that part of our research would involve designing questionnaires for assessing such things as psychological or mental health that were culturally appropriate and specific for this target population. Much to my surprise, I learned that many of the assessment instruments we would use were instead standardized and already in use internationally. Not only would there be no need to tailor questionnaires to local cultural conditions, but the very idea of doing so was anathema to the rationale for using questionnaires as instruments, which was to elicit objective information about psychological states. Tampering with the questionnaires would undermine their utility. I also learned that these instruments had to be purchased for a license fee and a cost-per-questionnaire fee from several companies, one called "ASEBA" (Achenbach System of Empirically Based Assessment) and one called "PsychCorp." We hoped they would offer us the "research-use" rate, which was about half the commercial rate, and would amount to roughly US$1 per questionnaire per child. We also had to consider whether we would need to purchase the scoring programs and data-entry services that the companies offered in order to process the data once we had collected it.

Instruments of research that rely on massive data-collection techniques are themselves a by-product of the notion that reliable evidence comes only from research projects that use statistical methods to document all of their results. EBM, which relies on these techniques of truth seeking, is committed to making the world a better place by collecting more reliable information about what can be known in the real world of personal experience (like the information we hoped to collect using these formal assessment instruments). Along the way, EBM also promotes economies of scale and regimes of truth that introduce a new kind of fiscal profitability to the world of science. If our results were to be reliable and we were going to be "objective," we would have to buy the assessment tools that PsychCorp and ASEBA were selling. (To put it bluntly, these companies own and are in the business of buying and selling reliability and objectivity.) If we used their instruments, our methods, and therefore our results as well, would be standardized, comparable across not only the schools in our study but, in the ideal imaginaries of RCT advocates, comparable across the entire globe.[15]

The logic of "market-driven research methodology" rides on the coattails of an already commodified health care intervention industry. The notion that intervention instruments constitute private property, protected by intellectual property laws and patents, has long been accepted and is key to the market achievements of modern medicine in the developed world. What we are witnessing now is the further migration of this privatization and commodification into the world of social science and health development research. It is no longer only the treatments (drugs and technologies), but also the research and intervention instruments that are seen as patentable private property that needs to be retained by its owner until it is paid for. All of this is augmented by rhetoric that insists on RCT as the unequivocal "gold standard" for truth. Federally supported research projects of this kind do not follow a straight path to serving the public. Rather, they first serve to feed and fuel a growing number of private-sector companies whose main business is to generate instruments and results for evidence-based research interventions.

I note that many researchers and public health advocates stand in an awkward relationship to this economy, frustrated that they have to take part in it, while at the same time feeling some sense of urgency to participate as entrepreneurs in the interest of their own work (which is itself threatened by fiscal cuts in public support for higher education). However ambivalent the feelings of some of the participants in this research economy may be, it nevertheless comes as no surprise to learn that the principal investigators on many projects are also the heads of private-sector research companies that handle subcontracts for data processing and consultation for other interventions in other locales. Universities are providing seminars and training in how to make our research more entrepreneurial and how to develop spin-off companies from our work that might attract investment capital. These new public-private partnerships, as they are often called, fuel a sense of win-win for research enterprises and for researchers alike, but how well this model will attend to the needs of the global poor is not yet well understood.

In global public health, conflict of interest is not yet regulated the way it is in the biotech academic world, which monitors and attempts to regulate the degree to which researchers can profit from the interventions they are studying. Although such conflicts are supposed to be disclosed for projects in the United States, the simple fact that an investigator is earning money is rarely sufficient for a "conflict of interest" judgment. The use of assessments deemed "standardized" instruments in an investigator's area of expertise and simultaneous involvement with the companies set up to make those instruments available is sometimes unavoidable.

In our own project, we figured that we would need at least five assessment instruments, most of which would have to be purchased from private-sector corporations.[16] Only a few of our measures could be obtained via public institutions, such as the CDC or the school district, which held records of nationally standardized assessment tests. In sum, our research would be made "credible" and "fundable" only if we agreed to push it through these required passage points of commerce—in and through the private and for-profit infrastructures of EBM—to the corporations that had begun to emerge as profit-driven subsidiaries of the Global Health World.

The NGO-Industrial Complex and Audit Culture: EBM's Profits

There are many kinds of evidence, and any and all of them could potentially serve different public- or private-sector interests. Nonetheless it is clear that in the push to privatize and to create public-private partnerships, some kinds of evidence are seeing more frequent use than others. An anthology edited by Marilyn Strathern (2000) explains the historical transition toward more evidence-based forms of accountability as an outcome of new infrastructures of "audit culture" tied to late twentieth-century neoliberal reforms. The reduction of complex political, social, and health problems in developing nations to numerical data about things like GDP, poverty rates, and infection rates has long been a stated goal of international aid organizations (Harper 2000, on IMF; Ferguson 1994). Such practices are highly ritualized and culturally normative. And, in complement to what Herzfeld (1992) identified as a rising *bureaucratic indifference* that results from the imperative of the audit, and to Ferguson's point that such practices inherently "depoliticize," it is important to focus also on the ways in which emerging forms of audit are highly productive in their own right. That is, instruments of audit are productive in more than the sense that they produce "effects," and sometimes unintended "effects." They are productive in a fiscal sense as well. While some things are effaced and erased by the audit (like politics and unmeasurable successes and failures), other things are made more visible, and most of these can be made fiscally profitable.

The rising demands of "audit culture" bestow a perhaps undue importance on EBM in the world of scientific medicine. En route, these demands have fostered whole new evaluation and assessment industries, which, in turn, have engendered more and more private-sector companies devoted to generating the kinds of evidence and results demanded by publicly accountable evidence-based medicine and public health. Accountability and evaluation NGOs, for example, are now plentiful, a vigorous growth industry in the world of international health development, and they are altering the contours of global public health (Adams et al. 2008). In the US city where we had hoped to work, I was told that Save the Children paid a private assessment firm something on the order of a quarter of a million dollars to create a report on the impact of their own resiliency trainings. Publicly funded research teams are increasingly compelled, by the litmus of the RCT, to use these research instruments and assessments in order to establish and affirm the effectiveness and impact of their interventions. They have become widely recognized measures of reliability and generalizability and so also serve the purpose of demonstrating *accountability* to donors. These are the pillars upon which audit culture is built. Although some audit instruments are publicly available, many are privately owned, and this is consistent with neoliberal assumptions that private companies are *more accountable* than government-run organizations. Private-sector, for-profit, and nonprofit businesses are, in short, the new arbiters of truth and also the new technologies of profit in evidence-based global public health.

An uptick in the proliferation of NGOs in the world of international health can be dated to the 1970s, along with initial neoliberal and structural adjustment policies that tried to put health development into the hands of local NGO facilitators. What we are witnessing now is the birth of something I have heard called an "NGO-industrial complex" in global public health. At least one arm of this industrial complex is fueled by the rising demand for assessment and evaluation services that define the benefit, or lack thereof, of interventions that now have to come packaged as research projects. Like contract research organizations (CROs) in the pharmaceutical world, some NGOs in the world of public health garner high-ticket contracts for private and public research and intervention, and thus operationalize the business of public health as a private-sector enterprise. NGOs come in all sizes and shapes. Some are for-profit, some nonprofit. Some perform their own interventions; others contract to assess the interventions of other NGOs. Not all NGOs are involved in audit, but audit NGOs and companies that offer services for hard and fast data crunching are proliferating at a very fast rate, and they are being paid in many cases by NGOs that have historically been committed to humanitarian interventions that made only minimal investment in experimental designs.

Two interrelated trends emerge at the present juncture. First is an increasing reliance on experimentally designed interventions as the new gold standard for intervention programs, specifically the RCT model for intervention research. Second is the increased privatization of public health interventions in and through private-sector research groups, NGOs, and companies that offer audit, statistical support, and research design support—a trend that uses multilateral, bilateral, and government funding but responds to private-sector accountabilities. Evidence-based medical standards, and the need for experimentalizing the field of public health, are two components of the shift that enable this privatization and the proliferation of new fiscally driven intervention models.

In Global Health, the transition to more "evidence-based" research is mapped onto a shift away from liberal concerns with preserving public institutions devoted to promoting health over profits and toward neoliberal concerns with promoting private-sector infrastructures that tie health to market accountability. This shift is negotiated in and through the experimentalist rubric of EBM that uses the RCT lexicon of "assessment," "evaluation," and "generalizability" as an essential component of intervention. This is true whether the intervention team operates under the umbrella of public health institutions, academic institutions, or either nonprofit or for-profit NGOs. Despite a long history within the liberal health sciences of quantitative approaches to scientific evidence designed to *protect* health care as a public good (Townsend and Davidson 1982), many of the instruments of today's quantitative science have increasingly aligned with the rise of private-sector investment, leading to a disenfranchisement of both the public sphere (institutions of government) and populist public-sector interests (in health over profits, for example).

Today, evidence-based methods, and particularly the use of these in experimental research interventions that include some measures of cost-effectiveness, by a research team that uses high-cost, high-tech methods of data collection and analysis, are deemed more reliable than other methods that have long held sway in global health. What is not often noted is that this shift brings with it a different kind of accountability. Today, accountability to a market is fused into the heart of the research methodology itself. Not only must researchers show that they are responsible in data collection by spending money on these cost-effective instruments of data collection, but NGOs who often deliver health care are asked to give proof of their market sustainability as private entities. Everyone who wants to get involved in health implementation these days must, it seems, get into the business of assessing interventions, if not health itself, primarily on the basis of these techniques. The turning-over of intervention work to measures driven by the market tends to reduce the work of "experimental research" to questions of fiscal accountability, and RCT models of research help this process along.

Invalidation and Commodification: EBM's Erasures

What sorts of things become invisible as intervention in international public health shifts its ground to occupy and advance an experimentalist platform? In 2005, I documented the ways in which evidence-based medicine derailed a project in which I was involved that aimed to train health workers in techniques of safe motherhood in rural Tibet. Our project, funded by a US government agency and approved by the Tibetan Autonomous Region (TAR) Health Bureau, was nearly ready for launch when we were informed by our funders that our methodology was insufficiently rigorous. Our "numbers," it seemed, would be too low to enable good research. Despite the fact that more women died in childbirth in rural Tibet than in just about any other country (Adams 2005), and despite the fact that our training would be conducted in a large rural prefecture (with roughly eight villages) and was endorsed by the TAR Health Bureau, we were told that in our catchment area "not enough women die to get a robust power calculation."[17] We would not be able to tell whether our intervention resulted in a reduction in maternal mortality or whether any such reduction was simply due to *chance*.

In order to keep our funding, we were advised to work with a research consortium NGO based in Maryland, which could help us restructure our project so as to render it "more scientific." Our funding administrator referred to our need to generate results that could be generalizable beyond the Tibetan context. Our Maryland NGO research consultants advised us to abandon the training for safe motherhood project and to focus instead on infant mortality (because the numbers would be better and because geography prevented our extending our study to a significantly larger area to get more women in our sample). Since we did not have in hand a training program focused on infant diseases, however, and since we had a commitment to the TAR Health Bureau to work on safe motherhood, we had to be more creative. In the end, we agreed to undertake a randomized, controlled clinical trial comparing the efficacy of traditional Tibetan medicine with that of a Western drug that prevents hemorrhage in delivering women. The study would be conducted in several hospitals in Lhasa, and it would involve a large team of data collectors, randomization, and controls. Meanwhile, the people on the team who had committed to helping the Health Bureau train rural workers in safe motherhood splintered off from our project and set up a separate NGO to do this work with private funding.

Although the investigation we pursued in Tibet had little relevance for the Health Bureau, and in fact delayed the safe motherhood intervention until a different funding source could be found, the *research* project was successful. It was a negative study, in that we were *not* able to show that Tibetan medicine worked better, but the project was considered successful to our funders in the sense that we were able to do an RCT. We trained a small cadre of Tibetan and Chinese health employees in methods of reliable statistically based, IRB-approved RCT research. The most compelling criterion of success was thus the research, and not the cure per se, or even the health outcomes. We were showcased by the US funding agency for having set up a Tibetan IRB at the Lhasa Health Bureau. Our impact on Tibetan health concerns was, however, decidedly mixed.

Evidence-based medicine has become a screening mechanism, a sieve through which truths about health, and judgments about the effectiveness of health interventions, must pass. EBM has also become an end in itself. This sieve/end point enables funders to shut down projects or keep them alive based on how strictly they conform to the model of best-practice EBM and EBPH research. EBM in all its forms becomes conveniently linked, as an apparatus of audit, to the growing NGO-industrial complex—the subsidiary growth industry in public health infrastructures that is being turned over more and more to the private sector.

Petryna notes that "clinical research is now a worldwide data-making enterprise" (2009:187) that spills far beyond the contours of the pharmaceutical sector. It generates growth coincident with the growing need for more scientifically rigorous models of health intervention. But it also "weeds out" other kinds of activities and resources. Contract epidemiology firms and assessment firms that get bids to go in and "evaluate" school resiliency-training programs, or to measure the impact of public health interventions, or to do the data processing for large public health RCTs, are often in the position of hoping for outcomes that may differ from those most often prioritized by public institutions (and I would add some humanitarian aid institutions as well). Research firms are often more interested in getting results that show the study was done well, as opposed to caring primarily about whether the outcome of the study actually improves health. As a result, other evaluation and intervention methods that have long been used may be marginalized or discarded outright. Interventions of the kind that cannot be subjected to experimental evaluation become not obsolete but seen as somehow of poor quality, as experimentally designed interventions become promoted as the gold standard.

If doing EBM in Global Public Health changes the kinds of questions we ask in our research as well as the way we think about interventions and health-delivery efforts, then it also changes how we think about outcomes. Other kinds of outcomes and intervention strategies that do not meet these standards tend to fall by the wayside as if they can't tell us much about anything. Some possible interventions are made to seem useless and cavalier from the perspective of using an evidence-base; you can do them, but you can't really know for sure that they help. This includes things like paying for the training of rural health workers so that they can learn safe delivery techniques even though we cannot prove that their interventions work better than chance; paying for government health care insurance even though it cannot be shown to reduce morbidity using the limited set of measures in the RCT-designed intervention.

What happens to populations whose health needs are not ideal targets for experimentalist research and intervention projects? How does one even show that such interventions are vital to health and survival when they can't be measured using RCTs? What and who will attend to the needs of those for whom one cannot find "generalizable" or comparable health solutions? Questions about who evaluates the evaluators, and who audits the auditors, are seldom asked. Concerns that don't fit into RCT-style research tend to drop off the radar, become relegated to an insignificant backwater of public health because they cannot be made to fit into the mainstream of evidence-based public health. Despite the optimism among EBM supporters who argue that any and all of these things could be studied using experimental research methods, the reality is that the bar of RCT is simply too high for many lived realities and determinants of health in most of the world. And then, there are all the things that simply can't be counted, or that, even if they could be counted, in being counted would be turned into misrepresentations of their true relationship to health. What I am arguing here is that there are unintended outcomes involved in reprioritizing health goals so that they meet the EBM standard for research interventions. I would ask: Does this growth industry actually assist or impede the work of caregiving?

Within the world of international health development, many of the people involved in implementing and evaluating programs are aware of the contested nature of evaluations. Patton (2004) noted growing concern over the standardization of monitoring and evaluation procedures in HIV/AIDS research and warned that using experimentalist linear methods of evaluation poses numerous problems. He observed that the needs of local operating clinicians and health providers often differ from the needs of a research program: "the data most useful to local programs fail to provide what international donors want" in the form of global comparative data sets on outcomes. He concluded, "Donor reporting and accountability demands burden the system and engulf local data collection efforts to such an extent that evaluation is little used for program improvement." Most evaluation strategies obscure the stories of real people and real-life circumstances in favor of numerical facts. Patton's greatest concern was over the use of linear, quasi-experimental models of evaluation:

> The dominant concept of evaluation . . . is a traditional inquiry into an autonomous intervention delivered in a linear-outcomes model to isolate and attribute its impacts, including conducting quasi-experimental designs. I am openly skeptical about the utility of such designs in these circumstances. Indeed, the controls needed to even attempt such designs risk having the evaluation design interfere with the effective creation and implementation of complex and dynamic systems interventions that are too messy and emergent to be appropriately evaluated by static designs and linear, mechanistic attribution models. (Patton 2004:169)

The still-emergent sense that Patton expresses, that program monitoring and evaluation must be seen as a complicated task involving the exploration of entire systems, complex specificity, and impacts beyond the catchment of the experimental design, has met with a huge amount of skepticism from many researchers in global health sciences. Advocates of experimentalist-driven research often respond to such concerns with skepticism of their own, noting that much of what gets published and reported in international public health circles tells us little if anything that is reliable. Unless research is designed effectively to provide significant and reliable data, the information it generates cannot be used in turn to generate responsible policy or intervention plans. A good example of this is an article titled "Weighing the Gold in the Gold Standard: Challenges in HIV Prevention Research," an editorial review in the journal *AIDS* (Padian et al. 2010). The authors looked at thirty-seven published HIV prevention studies and, rigorously evaluating the quality of the research designs in relation to the results, reported that 90 percent of the studies had "flat" results, meaning that regardless of published claims, a study could not show positive results either because it began with a flawed concept (an intervention that was not proven to be useful), or because "aspects of the study design, implementation, or context limited detection of a true effect." The focus of the article's critique is the last shortcoming: the fact that most studies to date were designed poorly, meaning they were not up to the RCT standard—a failing that, the authors argue, "squanders resources and costs lives." Like the tyranny of Damocles's sword, the RCT hangs over our heads as the standard we must all live up to or, failing, be brought down by.

The Disappearance of Subjects, Relationships, and Caregivers

In scientific discourse, credibility often hinges on the scientist's ability to control bias and reduce the complexity introduced by multiple perspectives. [Thomas] Kuhn discussed scientific knowledge production in terms of the nature and logic of what is deemed scientific, as well as the "techniques of persuasive argument" offered by scientists. However, Kuhn was ultimately unwilling to question scientific rationality, a skepticism that

underpins constructionist claims. . . . Ian Hacking argues that
people and their behavior are interactive kinds, capable
of looping effects that change them, individually and as a
group, as a result of classification. They can potentially
destabilize knowledge categories that are meant to be
stable. . . . Because of looping effects, the targets
of the social sciences are on the move.

—*Kelly Knight (2010)*[18]

One of the problems EBM faces in the world of global public health is
that it needs, in the words of Kuhn, Hacking, and Kelly Knight, above,
stable objects, but in that world, most of the objects of health care are
neither stable nor firm. They are tied inextricably to things social, political, and cultural; and they are, as Hacking notes, always "on the move."
Things like RCTs use an experimental method to create a sense of certainty and stability around their objects of study, whether in terms of
measurables, outcomes, or effectiveness. The RCT method provides an
illusory sense that there is firmness and stability in the intrinsically messy
social world of people, health, and disease. In a rapidly privatizing economy and in a world where competition over resources is intense, EBM
is also seen as the solution to several problems in public health: (1) the
need for accountability and assessment (the auditing of interventions,
which has historically been absent); and (2) the need for an objective platform for globally comparable research, such as generates objects of intervention and measures of effectiveness that seem to have stability regardless of culture, politics, social hierarchies, national institutional variability,
and inequality. But in the effort to create such stable objects and methods, some ancillary institutions and interests are created and fed (NGOs
and private-sector research investments and profits), and some things are
erased. I turn now to collecting the threads of the things that are potentially erased.

I have argued that there are phenomena in the world of global public
health that cannot be measured by the use of EBM's RCT methods. I
suspect that because of Tibet's infrastructure, population demographics,
and level of development, it will never be possible to randomize enough
of rural Tibet to undertake a RCT of safe motherhood interventions.

There may never be a way to know if the disadvantages suffered by those "randomized" to control status in the IIS intervention are suffering in ways that cannot be accounted for in the RCT design, or if an inability to demonstrate cost-effectiveness necessarily means that providing insurance is not a good idea. Some of the ways in which underprivileged school children in one US city experience a lack of resiliency around trauma may never become visible if we are required to use an assessment instrument calibrated to the national average. Nor will we be able to tell what impact our "controlling" of some schools will have on the children in those schools; for we are not measuring *that* impact. The problem with evidence-based public health research is that much of what we can learn from those who are the "targets" of medical interventions simply does not fit and cannot be made to fit into the epistemological architecture mapped by the RCT. Variability in the nature of health problems from place to place, from person to person, or indeed in the perception of what exactly is causing people to suffer, are all made to seem insignificant in research designs of EBPH. In some rather important ways, these erasures point to the disappearance of a subject—and to the disappearance of his or her social worlds.

As recipients of public health intervention turn into research subjects (a problem noted by Petryna for those enrolled in pharmaceutical research), their ability to contribute truth to the interventionary playing field is reduced. They are able to speak now only through the fine-grained amplifier of the EBM research model. If the things they say don't fit the study's template for responses standardized for generalizability, they are winnowed out in the data-cleaning process. Relationships that play important roles in people's health, including such contexts as families and communities, are not easily standardized, and therefore they are often ignored or made irrelevant to study designs.

But subjects do matter, and subjects who speak in their own peculiar ways and who are embedded in highly mobile social relations particularly matter. In fact, it is possible that their testimonies should be ranked more valid than what RCTs tell us. Robert Castel (1991) noted this in his analysis of risk discourse in clinical medicine. Early on, he warned about the historical displacement of the notion of a medical "subject" by the notion of "risk factors," such as are needed for the surveillance of populations. In Castel's view:

The new [preventive strategies of social administration] dissolve the notion of a *subject* or a concrete individual, and put in its place a combinatory of factors, the *factors* of risk. Such a transformation [...] carries important practical implications. The essential component of intervention no longer takes the form of the direct face-to-face relationship between the carer and the cared, the helper and the helped, the professional and the client. It comes instead to reside in the establishing of *flows of population* based on the collation of a range of abstract factors deemed liable to produce risk in general." (Castel 1991:281)

Castel's concern over the erasure of a critical relationship of caregiving under new regimes that prioritize population risk assessments over specific and immediate instances of harm (to self or others, what he calls "danger") is similar in form to that of the subject and his or her social worlds under the hegemony of EBM and the RCT. Relationships of caregiving foreground the specificity of particular cases and of the kinds of individual needs that are visible only in the face-to-face encounter between healer and patient. Such relationships are variable, and, above all, they evidence a kind of particularity, as medical anthropologists have been demonstrating for many decades now. Context matters, and individuals matter, as do the kinds of variations that emerge within specific social encounters that vary from person to person, group to group, context to context. People and their engagements with health do not inherently or easily form "data points" that can be used as measurables. But many researchers nonetheless find ways to identify the easy data points and hope that whatever factors appear *subjective* and *socially complex* will somehow fall away quietly as the RCT model takes shape in research planning. Even if it were desirable to include all of these subjective and socially complex factors, it would be impossible to take all these variables into account in the streamlined world of EBM RCT work, but it would be equally problematic to assume that because these realities don't fit the statistical straitjacket we want them to wear, they are therefore empirically invalid as evidence of what works, or fails to work, in global health.

It is difficult to imagine the epistemological displacement that would have to occur in order to generate a research or intervention paradigm that could carry as much credence as EBM or even a part of EBM. I suspect that a new kind of "community-based medicine" approach might provide a clue in its ability to prioritize the contours of the setting in which research takes place as a means of interrogating and designing research strategy (Malone in Offen et al. 2008; Minkler 2004). Some community-based research builds political issues and variable conditions into its method as an inherent empirical foundation upon which to determine, in an objective way, what may or may not work (Epstein 1996, 2009). Results from one site may or may not be generalizable to other sites. Each problem may demand its own solution. Assessment has to be local and specific, even subjective, and sometimes contrary to the rules of statistical reasoning. Partners In Health's human-rights approach to health care and the work of many nonprofit NGOs that operate small-scale intervention and aid projects in single locations, single countries, or single communities clearly have impacts that go largely unrecorded in the annals of academic and multilateral work. Research projects like these are, like the subjects they aim to study, always on the move, in Hacking's sense. They are capable of changing to accommodate more realistic approximations of reality and truth than can be produced through the experiment of the RCT. It is worth thinking about what sort of counterregime might be possible when concerns like this are kept in mind.

It is also worth remembering that even when EBM marginalizes the case study, the anecdote, and the particularity of different voices, this sort of data still matters. And it matters for more than its public relations value. It matters because it tells us how things really work, no matter how nongeneralizable such insights may be. Adriana Petryna's insight that what we need to do in some sectors of global health is to undertake a "rescue of perception" is apt. We perhaps need to recognize that these spaces, relations, and lives that fall off the maps of RCT research, perhaps constitute a different kind of "evidence" in a different kind of "evidence-based medicine."

Notes

1. I am indebted to several institutions for funding for the research upon which these insights are based, although none of the funding was directed specifically at exploring this topic, including the NSF, NIH (NICHD, NIA), Wenner-Gren Foundation for Anthropological Research, and the Institute on Global

Conflict and Cooperation (UC). I am also indebted to input from a variety of colleagues whose insights have helped shaped this paper, particularly through their contributions to a previous panel at the American Anthropological Association on Experimentalism (organized by João Biehl and Alex Choby), as well as to colleagues Kelly Knight, Ian Whitmarsh, and Deborah Gordon, and the participants in the workshop "When People Come First: Anthropology and Social Innovation in the Field of Global Health," Princeton University, March 11–13, 2010.

2. Petryna (2009) has explored this thoroughly in the case of globalized pharmaceutical research, which is directly tied to the phenomena I discuss here.

3. Brownson et al. (1999:87) define it as "the delivery of optimal individual patient care through the integration of current best evidence on pathophysiological knowledge, cost effectiveness, and patient preferences." They note that it involves primarily the ability to track down, critically appraise, and rapidly incorporate scientific evidence into practice.

4. There are critiques from within medicine about the difficulty of implementing strict EBM practices. Sackett et al. (1996) offer a critical exploration of the compounded nature of this problem in resource-poor settings.

5. Taken from the US Preventive Services Task Force, Agency for Health Care Research and Quality (http://acc.org/qualityandscience/quality/evidence.htm).

6. I note that there is an ample literature on evaluating social science and behavioral research (Giacomini et al. 2000).

7. The editor directed the author to a reference for producing high-standard qualitative research, noted above (Giacomini et al. 2000).

8. This point is made by Foucault, and follows the work of science studies scholars, beginning with Ludwig Fleck and later Thomas Kuhn, who noted that the concept of a "discovery" of solutions or answers is a misnomer in well-designed scientific research, since outcomes of interventions or trials are already in some sense built into, embedded in the design of the research that prioritizes only this intervention.

9. RCT research for clinical trials is defined by the National Institutes of Health as being appropriate for clinical drug trials as well as epidemiological and/or behavioral interventions. However, most RCT-designed studies in epidemiological behavioral health programs (seen in public health) use some form of one of these, and often use the final (nondefined phase III model). These are:

> *Phase I* clinical trials test a new biomedical intervention in a small group of people (e.g., 20–80) for the first time to evaluate safety (e.g., to determine a safe dosage range and to identify side effects).
> *Phase II* clinical trials study the biomedical or behavioral intervention in a larger group of people (several hundred) to determine efficacy and to further evaluate safety.
> *Phase III* studies investigate the efficacy of the biomedical or behavioral intervention in large groups of human subjects (from several hundred to several thousand) by comparing the intervention to other standard or experimental interventions, monitor adverse effects, and collect information that will allow the intervention to be used safely.

Phase IV studies are conducted after the intervention has been marketed. These studies are designed to monitor effectiveness of the approved intervention in the general population and to collect information about any adverse effects associated with widespread use.

NIH-Defined Phase III Clinical Trial. An NIH-defined Phase III clinical trial is a broadly based prospective Phase III clinical investigation, usually involving several hundred or more human subjects, for the purpose of evaluating an experimental intervention in comparison with a standard or controlled intervention or comparing two or more existing treatments. Often the aim of such investigation is to provide evidence leading to a scientific basis for consideration of a change in health policy or standard of care. The definition includes pharmacologic, nonpharmacologic, and behavioral interventions given for disease prevention, prophylaxis, diagnosis, or therapy. Community trials and other population-based intervention trials are also included (from NIH Public Health Service Grant http://grants.nih.gov/grants/funding/phs398/phs398.doc).

I also note, from talking with researchers in behavioral health research, that the notion of what constitutes phase I, II, or III research design is somewhat variable. For some, phase I entails doing the intervention to see whether there is a measurable (statistically significant) impact, not necessarily with a control group; phase II entails doing one intervention and comparing it to something else that involves a larger or different kind of intervention (likened to evaluating different "doses" of a drug); and phase III entails comparing interventions and using a control (or placebo or "no") intervention.

10. Although it is new, I believe the *Global Public Health* journal (Columbia University) may prove an exception to the norm.

11. I refer here to the *International Journal of Public Health*, the *Journal of Health Services*, the *WHO Bulletin*, even *Social Science and Medicine*, and other international health bulletins.

12. Many of my examples come from the research proposals I have reviewed for various UCSF and NIH funding agencies and for projects within UCSF's Global Health Sciences.

13. It is, in part, as a result of the social scientific critique of failed health development programs (Mark Nichter, Judith Justice, Arturo Escobar offer popular examples) that international health programs have adopted more rigorous standards for evaluations of interventions. These usually include not only health outcomes but cost-effectiveness outcomes.

14. James Pfeiffer explained to me (personal communication) that this model was developed by Chris Murray, who is now part of Health Alliance International, a public-private partnership in Seattle, where the focus has been to develop what they are calling "Implementation Sciences."

15. This standardization is also produced by the critique that psychological sciences are too "soft" (as Allan Young noted in his study of PTSD).

16. The instruments include ASEBA (the Achenbach System of Empirically Based Assessment), YRBS (the Youth Risk Behavior Survey), CCSC (the Children's Coping Strategies Checklist), SSIS (adapted from Social Skills Rating System), and HSSSC (the Harter Social Support Scale for Children).

17. Cited in Adams 2005.

18. She is referring to Thomas Kuhn's *The Structure of Scientific Revolutions* (University of Chicago Press, 1996 [1962]), and Ian Hacking's *The Social Construction of What?* (Harvard University Press, 2000). This quotation is taken from Kelly Knight's doctoral dissertation, "Tricky: Evidence, Facts and Reproduction among Homeless Women Addicts in California" (University of California San Francisco, Program in Medical Anthropology 2010).

3

The "Right to Know" or "Know Your Rights"?

Human Rights and a People-Centered Approach to Health Policy

JOSEPH J. AMON

Human rights abuses fuel vulnerability to HIV infection and act as barriers to universal access to prevention, treatment, and care. This has been recognized in numerous international declarations, and attention to human rights has been incorporated into the mission statements and work plans of grassroots groups and global organizations alike. Yet *how* recognition of this relationship is translated into action varies, as do the ways in which the *language* of human rights has been employed by HIV programs and campaigns.

"Treatment" activists, human rights advocates, and HIV programs of varying types (from evangelical and other faith-based organizations to youth groups to multinational development organizations) sometimes unite to promote rights (such as the right to treatment) and sometimes diverge in their interpretation of rights (e.g., the right to condoms or methadone as an effective HIV prevention strategy, or the rights of LGBT people). United Nations agencies and governments, including those governments traditionally less sympathetic to human rights, have increasingly been forced to define and defend their HIV efforts using the language, if not the principles, of human rights.

For some organizations, rights are a rallying cry. For others, they are a legal framework or an operational approach. At times the invocation of rights seems to be perfunctory or disingenuous. Certain rights are emphasized while others are ignored or even denied. In this complex arena of competing human rights claims, how does one evaluate the relevance, force, and effect of these claims? What evidence is marshaled to support claims to rights, and how does this evidence differ from that used by other actors in efforts to shape global HIV policy? The objective of this chapter is to explore different contexts in which the claim of one particular right, the "right to know," has emerged, and how this claim relates to the experience of people living with HIV. The "right to know," defined variously and used to advance competing and controversial agendas, is then contrasted with efforts encouraging individuals to "know their rights."

Introduction

At the start of the HIV epidemic, ignorance and fear of a new and deadly disease meant that when rights were invoked, it was often for the protection of those who were *uninfected*. What was at issue was their access to information about the status of those who were *infected*. Within this environment there emerged the notion of a "right to know," specifically, a right to know the HIV status of *others*. This claim led to calls for mandatory HIV testing and disclosure in a wide variety of settings, including among health care providers and patients, employees and employers, school children and officials, and among intimate partners.

In 2001, the World Health Organization (WHO) introduced a "right to know" with a dramatically different meaning. It launched a campaign based on the idea that every person has a right to know his or her *own* HIV serostatus. However, the focus of this campaign, coming from an organization that rarely invoked human rights, was constructed, in part, to counter HIV and human rights activists who advanced the rights of individuals to informed consent, privacy, and voluntary counseling and testing—advocacy that officials at WHO felt was slowing the acceptance of routine HIV testing services.

Not long after WHO's campaign was launched, UNICEF introduced a "your right to know" campaign. In contrast to WHO's campaign, UNICEF's effort focused on the right of adolescents to comprehensive information about HIV prevention. This version of a "right to know" was also contested, this time by governments that sought to limit or deny information about HIV treatment or prevention—either broadly or to specific populations.

Amid these battles to define and lay claim to a "right to know," individuals living with HIV campaigned for expanded HIV prevention programs and greater access to affordable antiretroviral drugs. These campaigns sometimes included a rallying cry calling for people living with HIV to "know their rights," emphasizing not only a right to HIV prevention and treatment, but also rights to be free from violence and discrimination.

The ways in which these claims emerged and were defined reveal not only how human rights were understood and considered "useful" at specific stages of the global HIV pandemic, but also how different types of evidence and sometimes competing principles contributed to global HIV policy setting. In the response to HIV, science and ideology have often clashed, especially when HIV programs have sought to address illegal or "immoral" behavior. Less visibly, conflicts between public health and human rights actors have also occurred. While both may champion pragmatic and evidence-based responses, public health officials often focus on proximal causes, while human rights advocates emphasize distal ones. At times public health officials see attention to accountability and human rights as an obstacle to fast action or, to the contrary, to diplomatic or "scientific" dialogue. Human rights advocates, in turn, may struggle to produce the type of evidence public health officials demand to support their claims of effectiveness. An examination of these debates illuminates how and why "people-centered" data matter, and why "knowing your rights" is a more valuable response to HIV than a "right to know."

The Right to Know Others' HIV Status

> Most people would expect it was their right to know
> if a prospective sex partner was HIV-positive.
>
> — "HIV and the Right to Know" (New Zealand
> Herald, October 7, 2005)

In June 1981, the Centers for Disease Control published a report about five men, "all active homosexuals," who were critically ill from a rare pneumonia. An editorial note suggested a link between the illness and "some aspect of a homosexual lifestyle" or a sexually transmitted disease. The report was the first account of AIDS in the United States.

Within two years, the so-called gay plague was known to affect a wider group, pejoratively known as the 4-H Club: homosexuals, injection (heroin) drug users, consumers of tainted blood products (hemophiliacs), and individuals of Haitian origin. Some identified a fifth "H": sex workers ("hookers"). The first public accounts of AIDS were largely written by physicians and health officials. If the public heard directly from those affected, it was most often from the so-called innocent victims, those infected through blood transfusions or through contact with members of "high risk groups."

Public anxiety, misconceptions, and fear fueled the enactment of restrictive HIV laws and policies in what could be labeled the first wave of AIDS "exceptionalism." Although there was no evidence of airborne or casual infection, the police demanded protection from contact with HIV-positive individuals; HIV-positive children were barred from attending public school; and HIV-positive individuals were evicted from their homes.

The right to be free from mandatory medical testing and the right to medical confidentiality are grounded in broad rights to security of person, to health, and to privacy. In exceptional circumstances governments can compel medical procedures without explicit and informed consent and can reveal medical information, but the standard set for such exceptions is high. To justify such rights violations requires, at a minimum, the demonstration of a pressing public need, evidence that the steps being taken are proportional to that need, and proof that mandatory testing and forced disclosure are the least restrictive of the possible means of achieving the intended goal (in this case, reduced HIV transmission).[1]

The call for a "right to know" others' HIV status was first heard in specific contexts: for example, among patients seeking to know the status of their health care provider, and among health care providers seeking to know the status of their patients. Policymakers and the public also called for mandatory testing of pregnant women and infants, employees, immigrants, sex offenders, and intimate partners. Related to this demand for forced testing and disclosure were efforts to criminalize HIV transmission and to limit the movement of HIV-infected individuals.

Although offering little practical aid—either for individuals or for communities—laws criminalizing HIV transmission have been a persistent element of many governments' response to the HIV epidemic. In the past five years there has been a new wave of such legislation in Africa.[2] A proposed HIV/AIDS law in Uganda is typical. It criminalizes the *intentional* and *attempted* transmission of HIV, despite the fact that such provisions duplicate already existing provisions in the Ugandan penal code, are contrary to international guidelines on HIV and human rights, are difficult to enforce, and can have negative consequences for broader efforts to expand HIV testing and reduce stigma and discrimination.[3]

Moreover, laws criminalizing HIV transmission often disproportionately target women, who as a result of pregnancy-related medical care form the majority of those who know their HIV status. In some countries, women who are pregnant are especially at risk of prosecution, because even maternal-to-child transmission has been criminalized,[4] and this even in circumstances where comprehensive prevention services and safe breastfeeding alternatives are not available. Women are further vulnerable to prosecution because they are frequently unable to negotiate with sex partners for safe sex. Ironically, the faith of public health officials and parliamentarians in the power of a legal remedy is often unjustified, because dysfunctional and corrupt judicial systems routinely fail to enforce existing laws addressing domestic violence and women's property rights, which, if enforced, would lower the risk of HIV infection for many women. Under criminalization laws, the right to know becomes at best an expectation, and at worst a mandate to be tested, doing little to empower individuals or encourage accountability.

In the debate over the criminalization of HIV transmission, legal and public health evidence has rarely been persuasive to government policymakers. Instead, fear-based anecdotes about HIV-infected individuals intentionally spreading HIV are often invoked. In May 2010, I spoke with numerous members of Uganda's parliament and with Ugandan government health officials. Many raised the specter of vindictive individuals deliberately spreading HIV. Few had heard the much more common stories I have heard of individuals living with HIV who struggled to get access to testing, who, having disclosed their status, had been victimized because of it, or who had, out of fear, delayed getting tested and worried about potentially exposing others to infection.

Underlying these debates are questions about how best to "balance" rights—between individuals, for example, and between the interests of the individual and those of the community. Mandatory HIV testing of infants pits the right of a woman to privacy (since an infant who tests positive discloses its mother's HIV status) against the right of the child to early treatment. And this apparent conflict becomes more complicated where treatment to prevent vertical transmission is available, but treatment for women is not, raising concerns about potential risks (such as the development of HIV drug resistance) for the mother against potential benefits to the child. Similarly, disclosure of HIV status among intimate partners raises questions about the interests of individuals in relationships, their relative power, the obligations they have to one another, and the meaningfulness of trust when individuals may or may not know that they are HIV-infected.

In other cases, those advocating a "right to know" seem less interested in resolving competing rights claims than in promoting bigotry or bias. As early as 1987 WHO concluded that screening international travelers was not an effective strategy for preventing the spread of HIV, and both the Office of the United Nations High Commissioner for Human Rights and the Joint United Nations Programme on HIV/AIDS (UNAIDS) have unequivocally stated that "any restrictions on these rights [to liberty of movement and choice of residence] based on suspected or real HIV status alone . . . cannot be justified by public health concerns." Nonetheless, approximately 66 of the 186 countries for which data are available place some sort of HIV-related restriction on entry, stay, or residence, and eleven countries bar all entry for HIV-positive individuals.[5] The United States did not remove its blanket ban until January of 2010. Organizations such as Human Rights Watch, the European AIDS Treatment Group, Deutsche AIDS-Hilfe, and the International AIDS Society, among many others, have sought to remove these barriers and to overturn non-evidence-based HIV policy making, largely by collecting the voices of those affected: students, tourists, businessmen, refugees, and scientists, who have been prevented from fleeing persecution, conducting business, reuniting their families, or attending scientific conferences.[6]

Frustration as much as fear has motivated recent efforts to mandate testing and disclosure. Thirty years into the epidemic, against a background of insufficient funding for HIV prevention and inadequate progress in ending transmission, laws that criminalize HIV transmission appeal to many with their promise of an easy solution that requires nothing but behavioral change on the part of those infected. In some countries, women's groups, convinced that their numbers are disproportionately burdened by HIV and disempowered by male-centric prevention approaches, have, despite potential backlash, led the call for tougher laws mandating disclosure and the criminalizing of HIV transmission.

Understanding these issues and establishing the facts behind competing rights claims often requires an approach more subtle than the routine quantitative survey that is the stock in trade of epidemiologists and health officials. For example, Human Rights Watch, where I work, explored the issue of domestic violence and women's and children's vulnerability to HIV in Uganda in 2002. One woman, Alice, spoke of her efforts to convince her husband to go with her to test for HIV: "He said, 'If I know you're positive I'm going to kill you.' We used to quarrel. He beat me. I never talked about it . . . I can't even test the children because he'll be angry and ask why." Mandating testing and criminalizing HIV transmission may seem like an effective public health approach, but it fails to address the barriers and real risks that people like Alice face when trying to get tested, and when they later try to use the information provided about their HIV serostatus. Although today HIV transmission is much better understood, fear and stigma persist, and they resurface in the popular conviction that the "right to know" another person's HIV status protects public health.

The Right to Know—Your Own HIV Serostatus

> "People have a right to know their HIV status, and testing and counseling should be widely accessible through innovative, ethical and practical models of delivery."
>
> — "The Right to Know: New Approaches to HIV Testing and Counseling" (WHO, 2003)

In contrast to debates around the right to know others' HIV status, there has been a World Health Organization campaign, since 2001, to promote the "right to know" one's *own* HIV serostatus. This effort has been an important part of WHO's push to promote expanded HIV testing; however,

WHO has put forward this "rights-based" claim narrowly, advocating a right to access HIV testing—"to allow people to learn whether they are infected, to consider the implications of their status, and to make choices about the future based on it"—but with no corresponding acknowledgment of a right to access HIV prevention or treatment.[7]

The WHO's emphasis on the "right to know" one's serostatus was grounded in the view that individuals vulnerable to HIV infection, or already living with HIV, are able to realize behavior change unrestricted by structural barriers or factors such as inequality, power, or gender-based violence. In 2004, despite limited and contradictory scientific evidence, then-director of the WHO HIV/AIDS department Jim Yong Kim declared, "Knowing your HIV status is one of the most powerful forces for behavior change."[8]

In fact, the ability that individuals have to act upon their HIV status varies considerably. Most evidence from so-called "general" populations—defined as non-youth, non-migrants, non-minorities, non–sex workers, non-MSM, non-IDU,[9] non-prisoners, and non-disabled (in other words, those relatively less vulnerable to infection)—indicates that while individuals testing HIV-positive may achieve some positive behavior change, particularly when they are in stable and supportive relationships, individuals testing HIV-negative often change their at-risk behaviors little following testing.

The WHO's emphasis on testing and on the right to know one's own status was spurred by calls for change from outside of the agency, including a call from Kevin De Cock, who in the late 1990s began to push for a reassessment of HIV testing norms, highlighting the need for routine testing. In 1998, De Cock and coauthor Anne Johnson decried a new kind of "exceptionalism" that distinguished HIV/AIDS from other infectious diseases. For De Cock the substance of this "exceptionalism" was no longer the stigma surrounding the disease but rather its requirements for informed consent and confidentiality,[10] requirements well grounded in medical ethics and human rights principles.

De Cock and Johnson, while urging a return to "traditional" public health methods of case identification and treatment, were using a language of rights to mask a call for a return to paternalistic models of medical care. Pitting a "rights-based" approach against a "public health" approach, De Cock, together with Dorothy Mbori-Ngacha and Elizabeth

Marum, claimed in 2002 that the emphasis on human rights in HIV prevention obscured the "essential" nature of public health and social justice. They argued that the emphasis by human rights activists on "Western" approaches, such as anonymous testing with informed consent and pre- and post-test counseling, was discouraging the acceptance of HIV testing.[11]

This argument echoed long-standing criticisms of human rights: that rather than being universal, they are reflective of "Western" values; in other words, too expansive. The first recognition of HIV in many countries invoked similar xenophobic, and rights-limiting, responses. Rather than recognizing the indigenous factors facilitating the rapid spread of HIV, blame was first cast on foreigners and "foreign" values—even when the attacks were made by foreigners. In Swaziland, one of the countries hardest hit by the HIV epidemic, UNICEF's former representative argued that the "Western preoccupation" with the need for informed consent prior to HIV testing and with preserving the confidentiality of test results caused "the ignorance and stigma that grew up around AIDS in the West to make its leap to Africa."[12] This argument, blaming consent and confidentiality around HIV testing for the slow response to the epidemic, ignored the kingdom's massive under-investment in health and its severely restricted rights for women. Until recent constitutional reforms, a woman in Swaziland assumed the legal status of a child upon marriage, and there are still no specific laws criminalizing domestic violence. Rape laws exclude marital rape, and one in three women reports having suffered sexual abuse as a child. More fundamentally, this argument ignores the fact that HIV testing was not widely available until after HIV prevalence increased from 4 percent in 1992 to 26 percent four years later.

In our research in China, Human Rights Watch found that, for drug users, it was impossible to isolate the "right to know" one's own HIV status from rights to due process and to be free from arbitrary detention and forced labor. Drug users told us that being tested for HIV often meant being detained by the police and put into a center for drug detoxification or re-education through labor (RTL) for as long as five years. Liu, a drug user in Guangxi province, told us in July 2007: "I had been using drugs and decided to go get tested for HIV. I had just come from having my blood drawn on the CDC [Chinese government Centers for Disease Control] compound, and the police saw that my arm had an open mark and some blood. They stopped me and put me in detox." Another drug user interviewed during the same month told us: "Sometimes I'm afraid I might be sick with AIDS, but I'd rather be sick and free than go to get tested, get arrested, and be sick in detox or re-education through labor [RTL]."[13]

In Zimbabwe I interviewed a woman who told me that after her husband died of AIDS she had been thrown out of her house and had her property taken by her husband's relatives. She said that after a while she found a new partner. "I've been living with a man for six months now. He hasn't been tested. His second wife died, so maybe he is infected. I have been too afraid to talk to him about HIV. He might leave me. He might hurt me. He loves me so much, but I can't tell him that I'm positive. I want someone to share my life with. We use condoms sometimes. Sometimes he refuses and I can't convince him."[14]

Which rights are being protected and which are being violated in this relationship? Without a broader framework of rights, the right to know one's serostatus can, instead of empowering the individual, become a burden that attracts stigma and even criminal prosecution, and does little to open doors to treatment. Where in this discussion over the "right to know" is any attention paid to a woman's right to property, or to live free from violence? Where is there acknowledgment that disclosure of HIV status need not always be direct, but can be indicated in subtle ways: by leaving ART (antiretroviral therapy) medicine out on a table, by a request to use condoms, or by some other coded reference.[15] In light of the evidence that ART can sharply reduce HIV transmission, where funding for further ART program expansion stalls, will individuals or the government be held liable under laws criminalizing "attempted" transmission? The enactment of HIV laws throughout Africa that punish HIV transmission have on the one hand been a validation of the power of women's rights organizations to codify rights into law, but they have on the other hand led many to reassess whether specific HIV laws are always beneficial, and to ask why existing laws protecting rights are not better enforced.

The HIV testing debate has also revealed tensions around policy making in the absence of evidence. When is there an imperative to set policy before data has been collected? How can changing circumstances and differing cultural contexts be considered in the process of setting global policy? As HIV treatment is made more available and the stigma that surrounds HIV diminishes, the experience of being tested changes. Research results from studies conducted in areas with lower levels of stigma and a higher level of community-based support cannot always be extrapolated to countries where the level of stigma is high, and support is lacking. The result is that quantitative studies can suffer from the same lack of external validity that often causes agencies such as WHO to dismiss qualitative (and human rights) research as "anecdotal."

The "Right to Know" versus "Know Your Rights"

> UNICEF is working with adolescents in various countries and settings on a communication initiative called "What every adolescent has a right to know." Founded on the principle that adolescents have a right to access vital information, this initiative actively engages adolescents in the development of innovative communication strategies to reach the most vulner- · able youth with information and skills for HIV/AIDS prevention.
>
> — "Right to Know" (UNICEF, 2004)

Another UN agency, UNICEF, has also promoted the "right to know"— understood now in the sense of a right to know accurate information about HIV. The right to access information is widely acknowledged to be an integral component of the right to health, one that requires states to refrain from "censoring, withholding or intentionally misrepresenting health-related information, including sexual education and information."[16]

Throughout the history of the HIV epidemic, some governments have limited their populations' access to information on the transmission, prevention, and treatment of HIV. Human Rights Watch has documented, for example, abstinence-only education campaigns that have limited the information available to adolescents in both the United States[17] and in Uganda.[18]

In 2005, Human Rights Watch reported on Uganda's redirection of HIV prevention programs for adolescents from comprehensive information on HIV, including information on sexual abstinence and condoms, to an exclusive focus on abstinence before marriage. Uganda had previously been praised for its high-level commitment to and frank acknowledgment of AIDS, for its grassroots support for people living with HIV, and for making available comprehensive information about the disease.[19] In our report, we documented how the government, with US funding, had replaced comprehensive information with information limited to abstinence, and how inaccurate information on the effectiveness of condoms was included in school education materials.

The change in policy, accompanied by hundreds of millions of dollars in funding, was not based upon evidence of the effectiveness of abstinence-only approaches—no such evidence existed—but upon an ideological and paternalistic view that ignored the rights, and needs, of children. UNICEF's initiative, in contrast, was designed to realize the right of children to information. However, like WHO's campaign to promote a "right to know" one's HIV serostatus, this campaign emphasized a right to information without reflecting upon the structural and human rights barriers that would affect attempts to act on the information gained. Many adolescents have appropriate knowledge of HIV prevention but are constrained in their ability to apply it. The result can be a dynamic of self-blame and self-conceptions of failure.

An alternative to "your right to know" campaigns are broad-based human rights campaigns that tell people to "know your rights." These campaigns are implemented in combination with a spectrum of related interventions, such as treatment literacy (educating people on HIV treatment options), social mobilization (highlighting accountability of government policies), legal services (for people living with HIV and marginalized populations vulnerable to abuse), legal reform, training (of health providers, law enforcement agents, judges, and others on HIV and human rights), and community antistigma and antidiscrimination initiatives. "Know your rights" campaigns clearly identify empowerment as their weapon of choice in fighting HIV vulnerability rather than the acquisition of knowledge or access to testing services. "Know your rights" campaigns also emphasize the need for changes in the structural environments that cause vulnerability to infection. Although occasionally endorsed by UN agencies and governments,[20] these campaigns have most often emerged from grassroots and human rights organizations, and are only rarely funded by donors.[21] An example of this approach is the work of the Treatment Action Campaign (TAC), based in South Africa. TAC is widely acclaimed for its pioneering work on social mobilization, particularly in response to the Mbeki government's denial surrounding HIV and antiretroviral treatment.[22] By highlighting the specific legal obligations of the government of

South Africa in terms of HIV prevention and treatment, TAC was able, through social mobilization and through the courts (in partnership with the AIDS Law Project [now called Section 27]), to compel the government to engage in a dialogue on its HIV response and, ultimately, to provide lifesaving HIV treatment that it had been refusing to provide.

TAC framed a broad-based "know your rights" campaign, which included advocacy of the right to health (including rights to information, access to testing and treatment, and other related socioeconomic rights), but emphasized civil and political rights, such as the right to nondiscrimination, the right to be protected from violence, and rights to speech and assembly. Through this dual focus, TAC expressed a conviction that people living with HIV do not only need their right to *health* recognized but that *all* of their rights must be protected. The broader construction of "know your rights" campaigns also allowed advocacy to evolve in response to changing circumstances and needs.

Related to "know your rights" campaigns have been "rights-based" HIV programs, and calls for the development of "structural-rights" interventions.[23] While structural interventions most often aim to remove sociocultural and economic barriers, rights-based HIV programs that include structural-rights interventions draw attention to the important roles of discrimination, inequality, power, and accountability in shaping HIV vulnerability and effective HIV programming, and they emphasize the *political* determinants of health.

A "People-Centered" Approach

In a decade of work on HIV and human rights, Human Rights Watch has documented the experiences of people living with HIV and AIDS as they confront discrimination in health care settings, in employment, and in housing, and confront violence in their own homes and communities. We have described rape, domestic violence, property grabbing, and wife inheritance; arbitrary arrest, beatings, torture, and the over-incarceration of injecting drug users, gay and bisexual men, sex workers, and other vulnerable groups; arbitrary detention of AIDS activists and outreach workers; and censorship of evidence-based HIV information. And we have documented the ways in which these injustices facilitate HIV transmission.

Our goal has been not only to record the experience of individuals living with or at risk of HIV infection, but also to elevate the reach of their voices, so that they come to inform HIV policy. In essence, we want to generate people-centered knowledge that can shape HIV policies, practices, and initiatives to be more effective, and to advance human rights.

One such voice is that of my friend and colleague Beatrice Were, from Uganda, one of the most courageous and inspiring people I know. Beatrice has been outspoken in her criticism of Uganda's so-called ABC approach (which encourages people to be abstinent, to be faithful, and to use condoms, often in that order of moral hierarchy). She told me, "I was abstinent until I married. I was faithful in my marriage. It did not prevent me from being infected with HIV. When my husband died, his parents took my property, they took my children. They tried to marry me off to his younger brother. But I went to the court and fought back."

Another voice is that of an HIV-positive Thai drug user, Chai, who was told—in contradiction to official Thai policy and medical best practice and ethics—that his drug use rendered him ineligible for lifesaving HIV treatment: "The doctor said if I use drugs, I can't have ART."[24]

A seventy-five-year-old woman in Zimbabwe told me about her struggle to care for her children and grandchildren amid the upheaval of the Zimbabwean government's mass evictions and collapsing economy: "I owned two cottages [shacks] that I rented out. I used the money for food, water, school fees for my grandchildren, and to keep my own house up. During the tsunami [mass evictions], they made us tear down the cottages and then they charged us fees to remove the rubble. Now I rent out three rooms in my house, and I live in the one other room without a roof with my daughters and grandchildren. I had seven children. Five have died from AIDS. Some of my grandchildren have died of AIDS, too. I was taking care of one and his mother came and took him away and said, 'I'm not going to let him stay with you and die like all of your children.' "[25]

Anastasia, a sex worker in New York City, explained how police harassment limited the effectiveness of the city's condom distribution program and affected her ability to protect herself from HIV: "If I took a lot of condoms, the police would arrest me. If I took a few or only one, I would run out and not be able to protect myself. How many times have I had unprotected sex because I was afraid of carrying condoms? Many times."[26]

The still-widespread lack of access to affordable antiretroviral medicine and quality health care for people living with HIV throughout the world is a significant problem that relates to the right to health and life. But rarely do medical and public health officials cite the factors that so many people have described to me as the major barriers they face to HIV prevention, treatment, care, and support: discrimination, violence, fear, and persecution. Human rights campaigns focusing on these issues are often seen by public health authorities as too complex and far removed from individual behavior change to have significant impact on the HIV epidemic over the short or even medium term. Certainly, challenging often entrenched structural barriers is no easy undertaking and requires work at community, national, and international levels. Changing laws and policies—and then enforcing them—calls for mobilizing political will, resources, and technical expertise. But changing individual behaviors is also difficult and costly, and research has often found only minimal impact from interventions seeking sustained individual behavior change. Providing vulnerable populations with access to legal representation does not, on its face, look like a public health intervention. When it comes to HIV, however, criminal justice reform and legal services may be direct and effective ways of reducing vulnerability to infection and enabling access to care.[27]

Human rights campaigns such as TAC's in South Africa show that human rights–based approaches can have enormous—in fact, game-changing—impact. The converse is also apparent: the absence of vibrant civil-society organizations and human rights activists addressing HIV has in many countries led to ineffective or moribund responses, corruption, and mismanagement. While it is difficult to attribute impact to specific human rights efforts, examples abound of human rights advocacy resulting in the protection of vulnerable populations and the reinforcement of evidence-based HIV programs. For example, after widespread outcry over abstinence-only programs in Uganda, the US Congress in 2008 eliminated abstinence-only funding earmarks. Ongoing advocacy on behalf of drug users in East and Southeast Asia ended a "war on drugs" campaign in Thailand that caused thousands of extrajudicial police killings and accelerated HIV transmission. It has prevented the sentencing of Chinese drug users to "rehabilitation through labor," brought about the closure of an abusive youth drug detention center in Cambodia, and prompted increased investment in evidence-based community drug dependency treatment that can reduce HIV infection risk. Advocacy by human rights organizations led also to the defeat of a bill introduced in 2009 in Uganda that mandated the death penalty for sexually active HIV-positive homosexuals. Strategic litigation has also advanced human rights, and respect, for people living with HIV. For example, in July 2012 the Namibian High Court ordered the government to protect women living with HIV from forced sterilization. In each of these cases, policy change came about through a combination of two factors: people-centered evidence—that is, the first-person voices of those affected—and pressure put on politicians and policymakers to justify policies that violate human rights and hamper effective HIV efforts.

The language of human rights can be easily co-opted when the rhetoric of rights is separated from the voices of individuals. In the abstract, rights rhetoric can be hollow, or even disingenuous, as if designed to restrict rights rather than to empower and protect. Broad campaigns to "know your rights" can advance rights and promote effective responses to HIV, while narrow campaigns that emphasize a "right to know" without connecting it to the promotion of all rights will fail to realize the ultimate goals they seek.

The limitations of the "right to know" campaigns conducted by WHO and UNICEF stem from a failure to recognize that what is needed to effectively reduce HIV vulnerability is a commitment to rights that goes beyond the "right to know" and requires action in arenas beyond the health sector. To protect individuals from mandatory disclosure and its negative consequences may require legal reform and, often, legal representation. To promote knowledge of HIV prevention information may require challenging political interests and battling those who privilege ideology over evidence. Linking individuals who know their HIV status to treatment may involve protecting them from discrimination and police abuse. It may require property rights reform for women.

It is not surprising that as different actors adopt the language of human rights to define and justify their response to HIV, they emphasize and adopt different aspects of what is, admittedly, a large, messy, and evolving discourse. While this diversity risks complicating and confusing our understanding of the relationship between HIV and human rights, it is encouraging to see all actors validating the importance of engagement with human rights. Central to translating the rhetoric of human rights into effective action, however, will be attention to the diverse voices of those affected by HIV—that is, to collecting "people-centered" data and building policy around it.

"Know your rights" campaigns that emerge directly from those who are vulnerable to and living with HIV can lead to more effective policies and to empowered individuals. They reinforce the most fundamental principle of rights: that all individuals should be treated equally and with dignity. Dignity is not a commonly cited goal of HIV programs, or indeed of public health programs generally. This fact goes a long way toward explaining why attention to human rights, and people-centered approaches, are needed in a new vision of global health.

Notes

1. For a discussion of this balance in relation to tuberculosis, see Amon et al. (2009).

2. IPPF, GNP Plus, and ICW, "Verdict on a Virus," n.d.

3. There is no evidence that using the criminal law to respond to HIV is effective in protecting public health, and some evidence that it may in fact cause harm. See, e.g., Burris et al. (2007).

4. Paragraph 21 of "The Prevention and Control of HIV and AIDS Act," Sierra Leone, West Africa, signed into law on June 15, 2007 (http://www.sierra-leone. org/Laws/2007-8p.pdf [accessed April 5, 2012]) explicitly criminalizes transmission, while other laws often implicitly criminalize it because of overly broad provisions (for example, the "Law on Prevention, Care and Control of HIV/AIDS" [No. 2005–25] in Guinea).

5. Amon and Todrys (2008).

6. Human Rights Watch, Deutsche AIDS-Hilfe, the European AIDS Treatment Group, and the African HIV Policy Network (2009). Also, in an innovative approach to evidence-gathering, the International AIDS Society requested that individuals submit their experiences of travel restrictions online: http://www.iasociety .org/Default.aspx?pageId=157.

7. World Health Organization (2002a). WHO did aggressively seek to expand access to treatment, but did not frame this in human rights terms.

8. Kim (2004). Kim also noted that aggressive testing must be concurrent with aggressive protection of human rights: "[T]he more routine offer of HIV testing cannot come at the expense of human rights. It can only work with counseling, consent, confidentiality, community involvement and an aggressive effort to fight stigma and discrimination."

9. MSM = men who have sex with men; IDU = injection drug user.

10. De Cock and Johnson (1998).

11. De Cock et al. (2002).

12. Brody (2006).

13. Human Rights Watch (2008b).
14. Human Rights Watch (2006).
15. Klitzman and Bayer (2003).
16. UN Committee on Economic, Social and Cultural Rights (2000).
17. Human Rights Watch (2002).
18. Human Rights Watch (2005).
19. Amon (2006).
20. "Know your rights" campaigns have been identified as important for addressing stigma and discrimination (UNAIDS, 2010); protecting the rights of marginalized populations (UNAIDS, 2010); alleviating barriers to universal access to services" (World Health Organization and UNAIDS, 2010). In 2006, the "Brazzaville Commitment on Scaling Up Towards Universal Access to HIV and AIDS Prevention, Treatment, Care and Support in Africa by 2010" included both a recommendation related to the "right to know" one's own HIV status, and the need for a "universal access 'Know Your Rights and Duties' campaign" (p. 8; http://www.afro.who.int/en/divisions-a-programmes/atm/acquired-immune-deficiency-syndrome/aids-publications/doc_download/3780-brazzaville-commitment-on-universal-access-to-hiv-and-aids-prevention-treatment-care-and-support.html).
21. Examples of organizations that have launched "know your rights" campaigns include the American Civil Liberties Union (ACLU, http://www.aclu.org), the Center for HIV Law and Policy (http://www.hivlawandpolicy.org/), the Community HIV/AIDS Mobilization Project (CHAMP, http://www.champnetwork.org), and the International Planned Parenthood Foundation (http://www.ippf.org).
22. Amon (2008).
23. Amon and Kasambala (2009).
24. Human Rights Watch and Thai AIDS Treatment Action Group (2007).
25. Human Rights Watch (2008a).
26. Human Rights Watch (2012).
27. Todrys and Amon (2012).

4

Children as Victims

The Moral Economy of Childhood in the Times of AIDS

DIDIER FASSIN

The "invention of childhood" in the West (Cunningham 1995), which has generated a considerable amount of debate among historians since the publication of Philippe Ariès's influential book (1965), appears likely to be not only an ethnocentric view (Pollock 1983), but also a deceptively homogeneous concept (Bellingham 1988). The constructivist approach to childhood in fact comprises at least three main theoretical orientations. First, it posits a historical transformation of sentiments, asserting that until the sixteenth century childhood did not exist as a stage of life clearly distinguished from adulthood, and mothers had neither feelings of empathy toward nor attitudes conducive to caring for their children (Shorter 1976). Second, it highlights the role of policing and argues that, from the end of the eighteenth century on, a set of social institutions, ranging from philanthropy and mass education to medicine and social work, normalized families, establishing different models of childhood for the working class and the bourgeoisie (Donzelot 1979). Third, it underscores the transformation of values over time, which by the turn of the century had rendered the child worthless from an economic point of view but priceless from an emotional perspective, again with profound differences based on social inequalities and deep contradictions between private valuations and the welfare state (Zelizer 1985). Thus the history of sentiments, the social history of policing, and the cultural history of economics yield three distinct pictures of the social construction of childhood. They differ in their chronologies and, above all, in the problematics they pose. Is it possible to reconcile them? Do feelings, institutions, and values tell the same story when it comes to the history of childhood? To use another lexicon more familiar to anthropologists—or at least more relevant to my own research—can we formulate a single, integrated concept of childhood that encompasses subjectivity, governmentality, and morality? This is the theoretical question I would like to address.[1]

Contrary to what Lawrence Hirschfeld's humorously provocative title "Why Don't Anthropologists Like Children?" (2002) suggests, the interest of anthropologists in childhood is almost as old as the discipline, going back to the work of Margaret Mead and Bronislaw Malinowski in the late 1920s, but it focused mostly on the various cultural forms of child rearing and socialization (LeVine 2007). In contrast to what occurred among historians and even sociologists, the question of the social construction of childhood as such was rarely discussed until recently, and even pioneering studies of child maltreatment and killing, while not ignoring ongoing debates in neighboring disciplines, seemed more concerned with the depiction and denunciation of abuses than with the way these issues are shaped by policies and inscribed in values both local and global (Scheper-Hughes 1987). The need for a conceptualization of the "politics of culture" integrating the international trends and tensions surrounding the social construction of childhood was perhaps best expressed by Sharon Stephens (1995:8) when she noted that "current crises—in notions of childhood, the experiences of children, and the sociology of childhood—are related to profound changes in a now globalized modernity in which the child was previously located." What historians and sociologists earlier described as a distinctive feature of Western societies has now disseminated worldwide via the transnational circulation of norms and laws, ideologies and sensibilities. The "rights of the child" formulated in the 1989 convention ratified by the United Nations put forward a new vision of childhood, define new obligations for the states, and provide new instruments for nongovernmental organizations. The denunciation of child abuse and child labor belongs now to a global rhetoric that is broadly viewed as common sense, even if violence against children and the exploitation of children remain part of ordinary life in many countries.

It is therefore impossible to study children in contemporary societies without reference to how childhood is "problematized." Retrospectively describing what had been the intellectual project of his life, Michel Foucault (2001:1489) proposed the concept of "problematization," which he saw as a tool to analyze madness, knowledge, medicine, prison, and sexuality alike, cautioning that "problematization does not mean the representation of a preexistent object, nor the creation through discourse of an object that does not exist. It is the set of discursive or nondiscursive practices that makes something enter into the play of the true and false; it is what constitutes it as an object for thought (whether in the form of moral reflection, scientific knowledge, political analysis, or some other category of thought)." The problematization of childhood in contemporary societies is not just about representations more or less loosely related to a cultural context: it has to do also with the sort of moral truth through which we construct children—not only in our familiar environment but also in far-off lands, by means of organizations such as the United Nations Children's Fund (UNICEF) and mobilizations such as the International Program on the Elimination of Child Labor—via compassionate concern toward street children, the dissemination of stories about the sexual abuse of children, and the condemnation of physical punishment by parents as maltreatment. What truth does our practical conception of childhood, as manifested through discourses and actions, imaginaries and emotions, policies and mobilizations, enounce about our world—and in the process, what truth remains untold or even unspeakable? To answer this question, I will explore the moral economy of childhood as it is revealed through the public response to the AIDS epidemic in South Africa (Fassin 2007). It should be noted that much of this analysis could be extrapolated to other African countries, and to a large extent to the rest of the Third World as well.

"Moral economy" is a concept introduced by E. P. Thompson (1971), developed by James Scott (1976), and widely used in the anthropological literature over the past decades. It came into being as a response by neo-Marxist social theorists to the purely materialistic view of class relations and has as its central tenet that peasants and proletarians, both in modern

Europe and the contemporary Third World, do not act on the basis of their immediate physical needs alone, in particular when they revolt. Their acts of protest or rebellion express, rather, a moral concern about the violations of the system of norms and obligations characteristic of traditional economies. This reading necessitates three major restrictions: it excludes values as such; it deals with the economic sphere only; and it is the exclusive privilege of the dominated and the oppressed (Thompson 1991). Extending this restrictive definition to accord with Lorraine Daston's use of the expression (1995), I propose to consider moral economies as "the production, distribution, circulation, and utilization of moral sentiments, emotions and values, norms and obligations in the social space" (Fassin 2009a:1255). Understood in this way, moral economy is constructed around social issues, such as immigration, violence, poverty—and childhood—in particular historical contexts. Tensions, contradictions, and conflicts arise, crystallizing issues and provoking debates. The concept is therefore dynamic and dialectic. I employ it here to explore the interface between the global circulation and utilization of moral sentiments with regard to children and their local production and distribution, as part of a larger project of a moral history of the present focused on "humanitarian reason" (Fassin 2011). The politics of childhood is particularly relevant to our understanding of humanitarianism—its aspirations and its contradictions.

Children were to a surprising degree absent from the AIDS scene during the first two decades of the epidemic in South Africa, as on most of the African continent. This absence may be interpreted in part as a result of the chronological development of the infection, which at first overwhelmingly affected adults; but it was also a consequence of the moral construction of the epidemic, which centered on a stigmatization of sexual behavior that was not compatible with perceptions about children, who were viewed as sinless and powerless. They became major players in the epidemic only in the early 2000s, via the conjunction of three "discoveries" (Fassin 2008): the preventable risk of mother-to-child transmission, and the reluctance of the government to implement programs to provide a new drug called nevirapine; the proliferation of cases of child abuse, which came to light when sordid rapes of infants made the headlines; and, finally, the worrisome increase in the numbers of orphans resulting from the deaths of young afflicted parents. Although quite distinct, the three poignant figures of the infected baby, the maltreated child, and the heart-breaking orphan elicited a common compassionate response in the public sphere. They were viewed as victims—of the indifference of the government, the brutality of adults, and the cruelty of the disease, respectively.

This dawning awareness of issues related specifically to childhood occurred in a context of epidemiological crisis and social drama (Fassin 2004). On the one hand, South Africa, which had surprisingly been spared by AIDS until the early 1990s, was by the end of the decade the country with the highest number of HIV-positive individuals in the world: more than four million people were estimated to be infected, leading experts to anticipate a decrease of twenty years in life expectancy over the following two decades. On the other hand, South Africa became the epicenter of a global controversy regarding the etiology of the disease and the benefits of antiretroviral drugs: by challenging the majority opinion of scientists and physicians, the government provoked an indignant protest from local as well as international actors. Until then largely ignored, in the space of a few months children found themselves at the heart of the AIDS question, when activists and nongovernmental organizations, both inside and outside of South Africa, realized that their innocence and vulnerability could work to generate widespread sympathy for their cause. My objective in this paper is not to challenge this consensus, but to apprehend the nature of the moral unanimity it reflects and to point out what it overlooks. Certainly, in contemporary public health, children come first (as goes the title of a UNICEF song). But at the expense of what and whom?

From Hero to Victim

The opening ceremony of the 13th International AIDS Conference held in Durban in July 2000 was the scene of a classical contest of villain versus hero. The South African president, Thabo Mbeki, played the former, and an eleven-year-old boy, Nkosi Johnson, the latter.

Six months earlier, Mbeki had secretly contacted North American AIDS dissidents, and he now publicly expressed his doubts concerning widely accepted theories about the disease. In a letter to world leaders, he cited features of the epidemic that were unique to the African continent and insisted on his right to explore all possible solutions to control its spread. A few days before the conference, he even convened a panel of experts, including heterodox as well as orthodox specialists, a move that was regarded as a provocation by the scientific and activist communities. In his keynote speech, Mbeki reiterated his doubts, arguing more openly this time that a virus could not be the sole explanation for such a terrible plague and that poverty was certainly a decisive factor in the tragic turn it had taken in developing countries. Infuriated, many in the audience walked out. By contrast, when Nkosi Johnson later took the floor, he received a standing ovation. For most South Africans, he embodied AIDS both as a tragedy and as a cause. He was born to an unknown father in a township near Johannesburg and abandoned by his mother, who suffered from an HIV infection. A white woman, Gail Johnson, who specialized in public relations and was the manager of a health clinic, adopted him. At the age of eight, the child became famous when his adoptive mother denounced the decision of the local school to refuse him admission because of his infection. The protests that followed reversed the decision, and the young boy became a symbol of the struggle against HIV-related discrimination. Several months later, his mother opened the first of a series of homes for HIV-positive mothers and children, which she named Nkosi's Havens, and her son attended the inauguration. Within a few years he had thus become a public figure, arousing compassion and respect. When he spoke at the conference, all listeners were eager to hear his testimony, but Nkosi was uncomfortable in his dark suit and clearly intimidated by the crowd. He spoke inaudibly, stumbling over the words of a speech written by his mother, concluding with a moving message: "Care for us and accept us—we are all human beings. Don't be afraid of us—we are all the same." But the audience did not know what he said until the speech was published in the press the next day.

However, from hero of the cause of AIDS sufferers, Nkosi Johnson soon turned into a victim of the government's policy. The following year, he developed full-blown AIDS himself. From his home, where he was now secluded, he appealed to Thabo Mbeki, using his personal case to plead for universal access to antiretroviral drugs and for the prevention of mother-to-child transmission. The president and his health minister were demonstrably hostile toward the pharmaceutical industry, accusing it initially of overpricing and later of distributing medicines that were at best ineffective, at worst dangerous. For weeks an obscene media watch held

South Africans spellbound with updates on the deterioration of Nkosi Johnson's health, and the press published the messages he had allegedly written to Thabo Mbeki, imploring him to save the lives of the thousands of patients who shared his tragic fate. Journalists systematically contrasted the humaneness and generosity of the boy with the indifference and mercilessness of the president. They underlined the fact that Thabo Mbeki had not even condescended to pay Nkosi Johnson a visit as he lay dying. In the days that followed the boy's death, a controversy broke out when it was discovered that he had been in a coma for weeks and therefore could not be the author of the letters to the president. His adoptive mother had used his image and name in her crusade for AIDS sufferers.

But Gail Johnson was not the only one to exploit the figure of the deceased boy. The Treatment Action Campaign, a federation of nongovernmental organizations waging an aggressive campaign to make antiretroviral drugs available to all patients, made Nkosi Johnson the champion of their cause. For the twenty-fifth anniversary of the Soweto uprising, which marked the beginning of the revolt against the apartheid regime, the campaigners printed a poster juxtaposing the photographs and names of Hector Petersen and Nkosi Johnson. Petersen had been killed by the police during a protest by high school students against the imposition of Afrikaans as the official language of instruction; his death provoked an escalation of violence, and the picture of his corpse carried by a devastated friend became a worldwide symbol in the mobilization against apartheid. The association of the two young heroes and victims on the poster, displayed on walls all over the country, was not surprising. South Africans were by that time familiar with the assimilation of yesterday's struggle against apartheid to today's fight against AIDS. That the significations of the two causes, one against a racist oppressor, the other against a public health policy, were quite distinct is a fact that was overlooked: the perceived emergency seemed to overshadow any attempt to discuss the difference between confronting political violence and facing a deadly disease.

After his death, Nkosi Johnson entered the hall of fame of humanity. Not only did he come in fifth in a poll conducted by a television station to determine the "100 Greatest South Africans"—he was outranked only by Nelson Mandela, cardiac surgeon Christiaan Barnard, the last apartheid president, Frederik de Klerk, and Mahatma Gandhi—but he was also designated an "Angel Hero" by the international program *My Hero*, alongside Mother Teresa, Lady Diana, and Bono. In reality, Nkosi was a hero because he was a victim, and he was a victim because he was made one by his adoptive mother and later by AIDS activists. He became an iconic figure in spite of himself, but even so, he did give children a face at a time when the extent of their plight was not fully reckoned in the toll taken by the epidemic. He represented the innocence of a child infected at birth and the vulnerability of an orphan abandoned by his parents, and yet, through his adoption by a white woman, he also offered post-apartheid South Africa symbolic redemption for its grim recent past. No one ever commented on the structural violence that underlay his biological parents' affliction, and no reference was ever made to the political economy of the epidemic to which he became a martyr. It was certainly much easier to think of AIDS in terms of medicines and care than to face its social meaning—that is, the ways in which inequalities and violence in everyday life heightened the risk of being infected by HIV (Fassin 2003). Nothing was known—and nothing seemed to be worth knowing—about Nkosi Johnson's biological parents. The combination of admiration and compassion that he aroused was more conducive to the production of a moral consensus around his cause, the paradox being that he became a symbol of the struggle to prevent mother-to-child transmission, for which his case was far from being exemplary, since he was born at a time when no preventive regimen was available anywhere in the world, and no child was benefiting from preventive antiretroviral drugs.

Exposed Babies

Indeed, even in the early 2000s, mother-to-child transmission of the virus still posed difficult problems for the medical community (Gibb and Tess 1999). Without intervention, between 15 and 45 percent of newborns would be infected, depending upon whether breastfeeding was practiced and for how long (De Cock et al. 2000). In the mid-1990s, clinical trials conducted in rich countries revealed the efficacy of zidovudine (AZT) in preventing transmission during the last months of pregnancy and around the time of birth, but the extrapolation of these results to developing countries was, for several reasons, not on the agenda (Connor et al. 1994). First, the side effects of the antiretroviral drugs prescribed during pregnancy were unknown, both in the short (congenital malformations) and long term (drug resistance), and would be particularly difficult to control in disadvantaged settings. Second, the efficacy of medical prevention implied substituting bottle-milk for breastfeeding, with increased risks of infection and malnutrition (significant causes of death among infants). Such a recommendation would contradict decades of health education programs that promoted maternal milk. Third, obtaining positive results from antiretroviral regimens (initially zidovudine and later multitherapy) supposed relatively sophisticated technologies and well-trained personnel that were not available in most poor countries. However, these obstacles appeared to suddenly dissipate with the announcement of the results of a clinical trial conducted in Uganda involving a new drug, nevirapine, which offered the triple advantage of being simple, cheap, and safe, according to its promoters (Guay et al. 1999). The enthusiasm aroused was worldwide, but it was especially palpable in South Africa, where several medical teams involved in international trials declared that the "amazing drug" was going to revolutionize the prevention of mother-to-child transmission (*Daily News,* July 11, 2000), in spite of the cautious approach taken by the executive director of UNAIDS at the time (*Sapa,* July 7, 2000). While the government insisted that the benefits and risks of the new regimen had to be confirmed by further scientific investigation and then validated via the normal evaluative process, the Treatment Action Campaign accused the Ministry of Health of voluntarily delaying prevention programs and of perpetrating a "holocaust against the poor" (Fassin, forthcoming). The story of nevirapine soon turned into a national polemic.

This was not the first controversy to swirl around AIDS. A series of scandals had erupted in the second half of the 1990s over an educational program, a presumed wonder drug, and doubts expressed by the government about zidovudine (Schneider 2002). But this time the situation was much more tense and gave birth to a general condemnation of the South African policy, later backed up by decisions in the courts. That children should be a concern was undoubtedly crucial to the mobilization of the public and the success of the cause. For months, newspapers featured front-page headlines such as: "Babies Too Poor to Live" (*Saturday Star,* January 30, 1999), "Babies' Lives in Balance" (*Cape Times,* February 22, 1999), "SA's AIDS Babies Tragedy Grows," (*Citizen,* January 10, 2001), "Baby-saving Program Faces Axe" (*Star,* January 22, 2002), "How Many

More Babies Must Die?" (*Sowetan*, April 5, 2002). Pictures of infants accompanied these titles, sometimes even displayed in the form of a series of small photographs supposed to represent the number of children who would die during a given period as a result of the Ministry of Health's policy. But as a symbol of this cause, it was an actual child, "Baby Tinashe," who formally initiated the first court case brought by the AIDS Law Project, a nongovernmental organization, against the provincial government of Mpumalanga in October of 2001. The six-month-old plaintiff had been infected at birth, and she "accused" public authorities of not having informed her mother of the existence of effective means of AIDS prevention; her ingenuous face filled the full front page of newspapers, under pathetic headlines (*Mail & Guardian*, October 19, 2001). Certainly, featuring infants in such a dramatic way benefitted the cause of AIDS. Who could object to "saving babies," especially when the potentially negative side effects of the nevirapine regimen were not evoked. It appeared that what was at issue was a simple moral choice between good (developing nevirapine programs) and evil (depriving mothers of an effective drug at the moment of giving birth). This simplification and moralization was the more powerful because it was children and even babies who were at stake.

Saving children was not a new theme in public health. It had been in play in the West for more than a century, in the United States (Meckel 1990) as well as in Canada (Comacchio 1998), in Britain (Dwork 1987) as often as in France (Rollet 1990), but also in other parts of the world where the children's causes were taken up as a consequence of local mobilization rather than Western influence (Birn 2005a). In the first half of the twentieth century, international agencies such as the League of Nations Health Organization, voluntary movements such as the Save the Children Fund, and national institutions in many countries developed programs founded on two fundamental assertions concerning children: first, that they were innocent creatures who could not be held responsible for what happened to them, and second, that they were vulnerable beings and needed protection against the hazards of life. These two precepts had for counterparts two related notions: that adults, in particular mothers, were often responsible for the tragedies that befell their children; and that society, either through philanthropy or the state, was obliged to stand in for faulty parents. The moral economy of childhood in the time of AIDS is profoundly embedded in this traditional outlook, especially in Africa.

On the one hand, children are depicted as innocent of the fate that is apt to cruelly fall upon them: they become passively infected at birth; they are born doomed to die early. By contrast, the larger epidemic has been constructed as the result of condemnable behavior, subsumed under the pejorative "sexual promiscuity," which had already served to qualify the sexuality of the working classes and of so-called primitive societies in the nineteenth century. Africans were labeled "promiscuous" in the colonies when syphilis was the principal sexually transmitted disease, and it is this same qualification that serves to explain AIDS, the new plague of the postcolonial period (Packard and Epstein 1991). In the moral Inferno of public health, men occupy the lowest circle of hell, being accused of irresponsibility, disloyalty, violence, and rape, whereas women belong in a somewhat higher circle. The latter are viewed with ambivalence, being on the one hand victims of masculine sexual predation, but on the other potential seductresses and even prostitutes. These representations of both sexes are inherited from a Western imaginary about African sexuality that has been actualized by the epidemic (Butchart 1998). A remarkable consequence of this mindset is that on the African continent, children become victims not just of disease but also of their parents, whose behavior is stigmatized. In South Africa, where the imprint of Christian religion, sometimes in native re-inventions, is especially potent (Comaroff and Comaroff 1991), viewing infants as sinless is an effective means of ascribing sin to adults.

On the other hand, children are pictured as vulnerable, thus justifying the intervention of private aid or public authority: their parents appear incapable of assisting them, being either too ill or simply indifferent or irresponsible, just as they acted irresponsibly when they conceived their offspring without regard to the high risk of transmitting the virus. Defenseless infants must be protected from such ignorance, incompetence, and carelessness. The notion of vulnerability has been widely used in recent decades to elicit compassion for victims in the arenas of social development as well as of environmental hazards, and in association with the symmetric notion of resilience, it has served to encapsulate the ordeal of children in poor settings, mostly from a psychological point of view (Engle, Castle, and Menon 1996). Whereas the idea that babies are vulnerable and should benefit from the protection of adults is indisputable, and whereas it has served as a basis for public health and social assistance programs by states and international agencies, it has tended to eclipse the need for men and women to receive the same consideration. In South African obstetric departments, for example, infants are treated with empathy, while women are routinely insulted and abused (Jewkes, Abrahams, and Mvo 1998). When it comes to the prevention of mother-to-child transmission of HIV, the neglect of women has taken an especially problematic turn. The high priority given to the welfare of children has led to neglect of their mothers' health. First, the initial clinical trials conducted worldwide did not include treatments for mothers. They were designed solely to reduce the risk of transmission to the child, with women receiving antiretroviral drugs only in the last weeks of pregnancy or at the moment of birth. Second, even when the clinical trials involved further therapy for women, the minimal single-dose regimens chosen (and praised for their simplicity and low cost) later caused resistance to the drugs most commonly used to treat AIDS and therefore worsened the mother's prognosis (Lallemant and Jourdain 2010). Both in South Africa and beyond, impassioned newspaper editorials and public debates urging the prevention of mother-to-child transmission never evoked the endangered lives of mothers. The only legitimate vulnerability, it would seem, was the vulnerability of children.

Abused Children

The maltreatment of children is a relatively recent concern in the Third World, but in fact it is also recent in the West (Nelson 1984). Until the end of the nineteenth century, beating children was generally considered to be a normal component of their education and, significantly, the word used to designate physical chastisement was "correction," meaning literally the "putting right" of the child's behavior. Moreover, as far as fathers were concerned, this form of castigation fell not only in the private sphere but directly under the *patria potestas*, two good reasons to keep the state out of it. The mobilization of philanthropic societies against cruelty to children, supported by the emerging profession of social work, led to legislation in Europe and North America that made the excessive punishment of children a criminal act. However, it was not until the mid-twentieth century that the notion of "child abuse" as such became established in public awareness. This followed the discovery by radiologists and pediatricians of a new clinical entity, initially termed the "battered-child syndrome," a development that brought physicians to the frontlines of the child-protection cause (Hacking 1991). The most significant evolution since then has been the sexualization of child abuse—that is, the recognition of a form of violence against children that is specifically sexual, including rape and incest. This development, in large part a result of activism by feminist groups, culminated at the turn of the twenty-first century. Accusations of pedophilia multiplied, the Catholic Church being the most notable target of embarrassing revelations, and the number of legal actions increased, two of the most dramatic being the "Dutroux affair" in Belgium, which concerned a serial killer and child abuser, and the "Outreau trial" in France, which led to the most famous judicial error of recent decades. It is in this context of global sensitization to child abuse and, more specifically, to sexual violence, that the issue of infant rape came to the fore in South Africa in the early 2000s.

Sexual abuse was exposed as a major social problem during those years, giving rise to conflicting interpretations. Was it the result of an increase in effective violence and rape, as some asserted (in which case its coincidence with the beginning of the democratic era had vexing implications)? Or was it an artifact of greater openness about the problem and the increased reporting of the cases (in which case the present regime deserved praise for bringing such a grim reality into the light of day)? The answer to these questions is not easy to determine. Under apartheid, sexual violence was not only repressed by religion and the state, it was also marginalized and denied in all South African communities, including the African townships and homelands (Posel 2005). It is therefore difficult to draw serious conclusions regarding the evolution of the epidemiology of rape and abuse. What is certain, however, is the magnitude of the problem in South Africa today (Jewkes and Abrahams 2002). The number of rapes reported to the police is 210 per 100,000 women, compared to 80 in the United States, and 40 percent of the victims are under the age of eighteen. A national health survey indicates that 4.4 percent of women have been physically forced to have sex, a figure that rises to 7 percent when the definition is broadened to include persuasion against the will of the victim. The proportion of victims, surprisingly, is twice as high for white women as compared to African women. A study on sexual violence yields a figure of 4.5 to 7.2 percent for the lifetime prevalence of rape, and 6.3 to 11.9 percent when attempted rape is included. Two observations should be added here. First, marital abuse is generally not considered in the statistics, in spite of the fact that it seems to be the most common form of nonconsensual sex. Second, the proportion of women having experienced sexual coercion under age 15 is 1.6 percent, of whom more than 80 percent were older than ten, which means that the sexual abuse of younger children is relatively rare.

This is not, however, the picture that emerges from press reports published on the topic: "Child Rape Crisis a Reality, Say Officials" (*Daily News*, December 8, 2003); "Child Rape Is a National Crisis—Police" (*Pretoria News*, December 1, 2004); "Thousands of Children Raped in SA Every Day" (*Saturday Star*, September 3, 2005); "Study Reveals Horrific Facts on Youth—Sex" (*Star*, October 16, 2006); "Baby Rape: The Family Connection" (*Mail & Guardian*, April 13, 2007). This moral panic over child abuse, specifically over infant rape, began in November of 2001 with the story of a nine-month-old girl who was sexually assaulted and seriously injured in a Colored township of the Northern Cape. Six men were involved, including the child's grandfather, and all were drunk when the incident occurred. The child's parents were absent, visiting friends. Under a front-page headline borrowed from the title of a novel by Chinua Achebe, "Things Fall Apart," South Africa's most respected weekly, the *Mail & Guardian*, published a picture of the child's distraught grandmother hiding her face (November 9, 2001). The story revealed all the lurid details of the rape, including the appalling medical certificate. This was only one of several such shocking tragedies involving infants, and each time the press presented to the public the most sordid facts with a mixture of anatomical precision and affected precautions: for instance, "Picture of Child Rape Too Horrific To Publish," followed by suggestive descriptions (*Star*, September 9, 2002). This delectation in the chronicling of horror—which must surely reach its absolute climax in stories of baby rape—is a remarkable aspect of the news coverage in South Africa and, as mentioned earlier, the phenomenon is not limited to local tabloids. There is an unmistakable complacency in the press's depiction of society's degradation. But this form of pornography assumes an especially peculiar and disquieting tone when it is associated with compassion over a case of child abuse, producing a definitely troubling combination.

A singularity of the South African representation of sexual violence involving children is its culturalist turn. It takes two forms. The first is general, consisting in the assumption that African men have an inherent tendency to be violent in their relationships with women. Having been raped by a young man, who was later arrested and convicted, the journalist Charlene Smith recounted her story under the headline "A Society of Rapists" (*Mail & Guardian,* April 7, 2000), which infuriated Thabo Mbeki, who accused her of racism, as the explicit reference was to African men. The association of sexual violence with black males, a common topos both on the African continent and in North America, has been called the "myth of the black rapist" (Davis 1981:172). The second form is more specific, having to do with a certainly more exotic fantasy, namely, the "virgin-cleansing myth" (Leclerc-Madlala 2002). Although no one has ever been able to trace its origin, the dissemination of the myth is widespread, having found its way into local newspapers (South Africa's *Daily News* [December 3, 2001]), with a later emigration to Kenya (*The Mercury,* February 9, 2004), as well as coverage in the international media (including *Le Monde* and CNN). In each instance it is presented as empirically evidenced fact, instead of mere belief. Even the most authoritative medical journals have given it credit, quoting press articles (Pitcher and Bowley 2002) or not bothering to cite any references at all (Murray and Burnham 2009). Whereas experts on sexual violence in South Africa are adamant that the myth is in fact no more than a myth (Jewkes, Martin, and Penn-Kekana 2002), the idea that African men rape girls and even infants to purify their blood and body from HIV continues to circulate worldwide as an established truth. This uncritical explanation of what caused the rapid expansion of the epidemic in South Africa and Africa, which again portrays children as innocents needing protection, not only reflects a deeply prejudiced and deprecating view of African men, their thinking and their sexuality (considered, respectively, as backward and brutal); it also obscures the reality of violence, including sexual violence and its causes (Fassin, Le Marcis, and Lethata 2008). It has been particularly difficult to give a voice to this other, mundane reality.

There is certainly every reason why child abuse should be a preoccupation in South Africa. The sensationalist manner in which it has been constructed, however, stressing the most scandalous acts and spreading the most exotic rumors, undermines public health efforts to deal with the problem. By fixating on horrific but marginal acts and practices, the ordinariness of sexual violence and the social tolerance regarding it are lost from view, just as it becomes easy to forget that in its most common form it is directed against adult women and often involves their male partners. Racializing nonconsensual sex once again stigmatizes Africans, pegging them as morally "different" from the other groups, thus avoiding a necessary reflection on the reality of child abuse across the color line, which is clearly established by statistics. Culturalizing sexual violence erases the historical background of political and structural violence in which everyday violence is inscribed. Although it is meant to be disturbing, the hyperbolic and exotic treatment of child abuse tends paradoxically to reduce anxiety, eluding difficult questions. This complacency has recently been shaken, as the prevailing image of the young as victims of adults has become confused by the troubling discovery of sexual violence between children. "Why Children Are Raping Other Children" (*Pretoria News,* October 23, 2006) and "Now Even Children Are Committing Acts of Rape" (*The Cape Times,* April 2, 2007) read the headlines of newspapers, which increasingly recount stories of abuses perpetrated by adolescents and even younger children, girls as well as boys. No longer exclusively a sexual innocent, the child begins to look like a potential offender.

Uncertain Orphans

Orphans have long been an object of concern in the Western world, and the existence of facilities to take care of them had been established in ancient Greece as well as in Jewish laws, but the development of the orphanhood question as such is related to the emergence of child welfare in Europe and North America during the nineteenth century (Lynch 2000). Philanthropic policies and institutions dedicated to orphans then stressed the unfortunate conditions of parentless children, portraying them as victims of either misfortune or immorality, depending on whether their parents had died or abandoned them, but always eliciting compassion (Panter-Brick 2000). However, historical studies have revealed that most children living in foundling houses had at least one living parent, usually a single mother who was presumed to be incapable of raising her children. Sometimes both parents were still alive, but they were thought to have too many children to care for. This "philanthropic abduction" thus created "imagined orphans," whose real situation as the children of poor families was generally hidden from the public and especially from donors so as to sustain their sympathy and generosity (Murdoch 2006). The blurring of the line between orphans and the poor, the fallacious presentation of children as parentless, their depiction as victims and charity appeals on their behalf—all of these phenomena observed more than a hundred years ago in Britain, for instance—are relevant to our comprehension of the orphanhood question in South Africa and indeed in Africa more generally at the beginning of the twenty-first century.

In the context of the AIDS epidemic the problem has taken a particularly alarming turn. According to international agency projections made at the time of my investigation, the number of orphans worldwide was expected to reach twenty-five million by 2010, 82 percent of whom would live on the African continent (UNICEF 2004). Certain experts even considered this worrisome figure an underestimate and asserted that it should be multiplied by three to take into account children living with parents too ill to take care of them and those who have also lost their grandparents (Whiteside and Sunter 2000). South African calculations indicate that in 2010, 2.0 million children had lost their mother, 3.3 million their father, and 0.8 million both of them. These three variants of orphanhood thus affected, respectively, 19 percent, 32 percent, and 9 percent of eighteen-year-old adolescents (Actuarial Society of South Africa 2006). As early as 2000, the statistics had become so disquieting that a newspaper headlined a proposed "Survival Guide for AIDS Orphans" (*Mail & Guardian,* October 20, 2000). As the justified anxiety about orphanhood was largely built on demographic data, it is certainly useful to take a closer look at the figures and analyze what they mean.

The dramatization of the plight of orphans in South Africa, as on the rest of the continent, gives the impression that the situation of parentless children is radically new, being the consequence of AIDS. This is at least how international institutions and nongovernmental organizations have depicted it, underlining the uniqueness of the tragedy and its consequences for children. But, if we compare two statistical surveys conducted nine years apart on large population samples—the Project for Statistics on Living Standards and Development, carried out in 1993, when the impact of the epidemic was not perceptible, and the Cape Town Panel Study of

2002, when AIDS was the leading cause of mortality for young adults of both sexes—the novelty of orphanhood begins to seem less obvious (Bray 2003). In 1993, 10.2 percent of children below the age of eighteen had lost one or two of their parents; the corresponding figure was 13.2 percent in 2002. In 1993, 58.6 percent had their father or mother or both absent from the home; in 2002, 59 percent were facing this situation. In other words, the proportion of children raised with both parents alive and present was only 31.9 percent in 1993 and 27.8 percent in 2000. The variation is minimal. It indicates that "biological" and "social" orphanhood—terms that differentiate the death and absence of parents—was a significant problem before the emergence of HIV infection. HIV aggravated it only marginally, at least if we consider the period of the early 2000s when anxiety over orphans began to crystallize in the public awareness. But when we pursue the statistics further another interesting fact emerges. Whereas policy papers and even academic writings concentrate on the deaths of young women and the resulting issue of maternal orphans, the two surveys yield figures that surprisingly contradict the commonsense position of most authors. Children who have lost their mother represent 2 percent of the total population in 1993 and 3.2 percent in 2002; those whose fathers are deceased number, respectively, 7.6 percent and 8.9 percent. This means that there were almost four times as many fatherless children as motherless children before the epidemic, and still three times more when it had begun to take its toll. If we look at the figures for absent parents, the situation is the same: both surveys register three times more absent fathers than mothers.

These findings highlight two facts that underlie the controversies over AIDS in South Africa during this period. First, focusing on so-called AIDS orphans implies that orphanhood is almost exclusively a consequence of the epidemic. This assumption contradicts the demographic evidence and constitutes a denial of history. As a result of the oppression and exploitation of Africans under apartheid and even before, most black families were destructured (Reynolds 2000). Fathers often worked in the mines or in industrial complexes distant from their homes; mothers were employed as domestic workers in the cities; sometimes parents died of disease or violent causes; less than one-third of children were living with both parents, while a majority of the rest were being raised by grandparents. Consequently, to attribute orphanhood, both biological and social, to AIDS as most policy papers and media accounts do, is to use the epidemic to obscure South Africa's recent past. Compassion for AIDS orphans thus leads to a kind of depoliticization of the complex issues that families have to face, and that the public health system should confront as well. Second, to concentrate on maternal orphans is to imply that they are a more critical problem from a social perspective than paternal orphans. This perspective is in part understandable considering the role mothers play in rearing children and even in their survival, especially at young ages. However, to neglect fatherless children is to underestimate the statistical signification of male mortality, a mistake that has given rise to polemics in South Africa (Fassin 2009b). When in 2000 the Medical Research Council presented mortality statistics as a consequence solely of the AIDS toll, the government virulently responded, via Statistics South Africa, that violence was still the main cause of death for men. Although both readings were definitely alarming, negating figures relating to homicides and suicides disguised the omnipresent reality of violence, which was so closely linked to history. Emphasizing disease at the expense of unnatural causes of mortality was again to deny the political meaning of death. "Why should AIDS orphans be given special treatment when other parentless children go hungry?" asked Thabo Mbeki in one of his speeches (*Daily News*, April 4, 2007). A critique of the denial of history and of the depoliticization of society was behind his question.

But the problematization of orphanhood in the language of pathos, foregrounding emotional distress and social abandonment, paints an erroneous picture of the usual experience of orphans and has even had unexpected negative consequences (Meintjes and Giese 2006). On the one hand, by highlighting the needs of children and their supposed dependence, they exaggerate an "orphan burden" for the state and more generally for society (Abebe 2010). In fact, quite often, not only do children easily find a home, living with grandparents or sometimes uncles and aunts, as they have done in the past under similar circumstances, but with the social assistance policies implemented by the government, it is on the contrary the extended families that become dependent on orphans, whose foster care grants are a precious resource for those who take care of them (Beegle et al. 2010). Moreover, even child-headed households, which have generated particular concern and even anxiety, are a rare phenomenon—around 0.5 percent, of which nine out of ten have a living parent (Meintjes et al. 2010). On the other hand, by highlighting the desocialization of orphans when the empirical evidence shows that they are most often reabsorbed by their communities, experts' reports and press articles can turn endangered children into dangerous children, apt to be "engaged in prostitution and theft" and "susceptible to suicide and drug use" (Patterson 2003:23). According to a criminologist often cited in policy-oriented documents as well as in academic research, orphans, deprived of parental love and norms, will become involved in "juvenile delinquency and crime" (Schönteich 1999). The grim perspective of orphans growing up as street children and invading the cities or becoming child soldiers as a consequence of the epidemic is also frequently evoked. Thus, orphanhood is transformed into a source of moral panic, with those who were initially regarded as innocent victims suddenly transformed into potential enemies of society. Compassion turns into suspicion and even animosity, as was observed some years ago when the residents of a wealthy Durban neighborhood campaigned for the closure of a recently built orphanage (*Daily News,* August 23, 2001). For these protestors, orphans might be worthy of empathy in the abstract, but they had no wish to see real orphans in their backyard.

Conclusion

That children come first—to paraphrase the title of this volume—is considered obvious in public health from at least two perspectives. On the one hand, in the natural process of maturation, they represent the stage of a person's primary formation and socialization. They come first because childhood precedes adulthood and therefore encapsulates the future of the population—and, even in post-apartheid South Africa, the future of the nation, for children are regarded as a source of regeneration after the infamy of the white supremacist regime. On the other hand, from a moral perspective, they embody both innocence and vulnerability in a context where both are threatened by disease, violence, and poverty. They come first because childhood is sinless and defenseless, calling for protection from society, particularly in a country where religion brings notions of culpability and redemption into the discourse on AIDS. Children thus appear as a consensual object of concern for public health and more generally of compassion for society. And indeed, saving babies, preventing child abuse, and bringing assistance to orphans is an essential mission for policymakers and a collective responsibility for all members of society. But the fact that this is beyond dispute does not imply that we should not challenge the way the mission is conducted, the implicit logics it reveals, the specific interests it may serve, and the contradictions and misconceptions that it may provoke.

The humanitarian problematization of childhood, if one may thus qualify the mobilization of compassion toward children, poses a series of dilemmas that are illuminated by the three issues studied—prevention of mother-to-child transmission, sexual abuse, and AIDS orphans. First, the moralization of the cause introduces hierarchies of moralities: children are viewed as pure victims, which implies viewing adults as guilty; the responsibilities and presumed moral stances of men and women are differentiated, as are those of blacks and whites, poor and rich. In the end, blame devolves onto the dominated. Second, moral emotions are unstable and often reversible. Underprivileged children are pitied as long as one can picture them as virtuous and innocuous; when they come to be viewed as potentially violent and even dangerous, pity turns to fear and hostility. Third, moral economies generally eclipse political economies: commiseration for children, especially when they belong to disadvantaged groups, frequently avoids the necessary analysis of the structural determinants of their exposure to health risks and social hazards. Finally, the moral presentation of children renders them voiceless and deprives them of agency: humanitarianism speaks in their stead and they are confined to their condition of victimhood. To recognize these problems does not imply that one renounces generous commitment to children through benevolent policies and humane care. It is a call instead for combating the illusions through which moral sentiments often tend to obscure social injustice.

Notes

1. The analyses presented in this chapter are based on research funded by a grant from the French National Agency for Research on AIDS (ANRS). I am grateful to Linda Garat for her careful copyediting.

II

INTERVENTIONS

Overview

A critical ethnography of global health must attend to the granular ways in which interventions (multiple and fragmentary and tied to neoliberal principles and strategies) become part and parcel of public health landscapes and social relations in resource-poor settings. The chapter by Susan Reynolds Whyte, Michael Whyte, Lotte Meinert, and Jenipher Twebaze focuses on the micropolitics of HIV/AIDS care in Uganda—the ways in which social networks are produced, expanded, and cultivated in efforts to access health programs and the associated benefits they confer—and how the roles of the state and ideas of political belonging are being transformed by global health initiatives.

The Ugandan health system, at least as it relates to HIV/AIDS, is almost exclusively dependent on international aid projects. It is a "projectified" landscape of care. After the civil war, Uganda's government seized on health interventions to bolster its legitimacy abroad and at home. This welcoming attitude wins the Ugandan government a place in the world of international politics, as it demonstrates at once a willingness to lift itself from its ruinous recent history, and, perhaps more importantly, to comply with neoliberal models of state intervention. At home, the introduction of international actors provides much-needed relief to people living with HIV/AIDS and their families, and enables the government to present itself as at least partially responsible for providing health care to its populace.

Reynolds Whyte and colleagues describe those who benefit from these health initiatives as "clients," a felicitous term that can be understood in two contrasting and interestingly supplemental senses. One, which harks back to Uganda's political past, points to the ways in which these persons, who enjoy little power or resources other than those afforded through social networking, must seek out patrons better positioned within the world of health care in order to gain access for themselves. The other meaning of "client" echoes the voices of neoliberalism, which guide much of global health investment, and refers to persons as clients or consumers of a product (in this case heath care), thereby establishing a contractual obligation between them and the providers of the product. Here health is not a "right" available to all, but a service open to those in the know, and health care interventions increasingly become a survival mechanism that extends beyond the medical and includes labor, food, and education.

Moreover, good clients are expected to be faithful to a program and the services it provides and to recruit others into it, contributing to its growth. An economy of loyalties and of financial, institutional, and medical support is thus created. In this "therapeutic clientship" (standing in for citizenship and governance), the HIV-positive Ugandans can, as much as the funding-dependent NGOs that offer them drugs and care, negotiate and establish their positions by cultivating and extending social relations.

If Vincanne Adams's analysis describes a movement toward an epistemology of health that rejects social positionality and institutional and historical context as sources of knowledge, the chapter by Reynolds Whyte and colleagues demonstrates the ways in which national and international political contexts are experienced locally—and how it is precisely from this base of locality that these politics can be realized, by providing an irreducible logic that is more complex, meaningful, and significant extralocally than what is allowed in other epistemic regimes. Their analysis offers a way to approach persons not exclusively as patients, or as outcomes or failures of interventions, but rather as embedded actors, moving within complexly intertwined social networks. It provides a point of entry to assess the micropolitics in which health and health care are brokered, accessed, and transformed—and it also provides hope that a way will be found to include those who have been left out.

* * *

Despite the deluge of monies and organizations flowing into resource-poor settings worldwide, local health systems continue to be woefully inadequate. Many times, donors' myopic insistence on funding vertical programs and bringing change from the outside comes at the expense of the public sector. In his chapter, James Pfeiffer explores the system of health care that has emerged in postsocialist, democratizing Mozambique after the arrival of the US President's Emergency Plan for AIDS Relief (PEPFAR) aid and looks into the gaps that the Plan's dogged rejection of public-sector expenditures creates for those seeking antiretroviral treatment. We can locate such rejection of public-sector expenditures within the context of structural adjustment policies and the politics that guide—and gird—the flow of resources from rich to poor countries.

The result of this divestment in the public sector is the creation of a fractured and uneven health system in which state-of-the-art facilities for HIV/AIDS testing and treatment coexist with all-but-dilapidated state hospitals, where wealthy donors create showcase clinics in one region while the clinics in a neighboring region atrophy and their long-term sustainability is always in question. In this makeshift system, the focus is squarely at the level of the clinic, where interventions can be followed and their results measured. Attempts to make assessments at a national level are left by the wayside and the myriad social factors that can contribute to positive health outcomes are by and large ignored (or, if acknowledged, not acted on). Health workers are also in short supply outside the spheres dominated by NGOs, because limits are set on wages at public institutions, and because NGOs can afford to pay them more to provide more specialized services.

The workings of international political economy once again become palpable at the local level, as do the fraught and complicated interactions between international donors and host countries. Global health interventions leave people behind, not only by limiting access to the services provided, but also by producing a parallel system of care and governance that undermines other avenues for care that might take into account broader systemic factors. For example, Pfeiffer shows how a poor national infrastructure and terrible economic hardships intersect with everyday patterns of sociality to hinder HIV/AIDS treatment adherence, especially among pregnant women. Pregnant women are at higher risk of being "lost to follow up" (LTFU) because they must confront a number of unique restrictions and risk-laden choices that make treatment access perilous and adherence highly problematic. Faced with hunger, difficulties in accessing treatment, the severe side effects of medication, and the stigma associated with AIDS, too many pregnant women drop out of programs.

Pfeiffer's work draws attention to two important facets of a critical ethnography of global health. First, ethnographic accounts allow for a telling juxtaposition of scales (ranging geographically, from a perspective at the level of the patient and the community to a much broader view that reveals the systemic flaws of the international financial impositions in Mozambique; and in time, from the country's socialist past to its market-fundamentalist present). Ethnography lays bare how interventions are woven into larger spheres of political economy and points to the impact of structural and economic factors on treatment and disease.

Second, certain statistical and quantitative data can be productively reconciled with qualitative ethnographic approaches. If "lost to follow up," for example, is viewed not just as a metric for judging the success or failure of a given intervention but is instead used as a starting point for looking beyond the limits such an evaluation imposes and into the confluence of other factors (national economic systems and infrastructure, for instance) on the lives of the HIV-positive, then new ways of looking at care and accountability might result. Ethnographic evidence can thus be put to use in developing different plans of action.

* * *

In her ethnographic work, Julie Livingston documents the emerging epidemic of cancer in Botswana, and the social capillaries and ad hoc forces of improvisation through which oncological medicine is forged and pain is managed in a context of scarcity. This phenomenon today unfolds against the backdrop of the country's much publicized universal HIV/AIDS treatment program funded by the government in partnership with the pharmaceutical giant Merck and the Gates Foundation. Patients are now surviving their HIV disease only to find themselves grappling with viral-associated cancers facilitated by their history of immunosuppression. Challenging the global health imaginations of medical need that channel care resources disproportionately toward infectious disease, Livingston asks, "How and why does biomedicine proceed in Africa with so little palliation and so much compliance?"

Cancer is something that happens between people and amid institutional efforts to treat it or ignore it. In Botswana's lone oncology ward, where most people come in driven by the intensity of their pain, and where efforts are directed primarily toward its relief and not toward its treatment, this means recognizing that the social existence of the disease and the experience of pain are bound to the material, cultural, and biomedical milieu in which they arise. Pain is thus intimately social and socializable: it mediates relationships, scarcities, health policies, and medical protocols, creating spaces for care and palliation as well as disregard.

Despite the fact that pain is central to life on the cancer ward, opiates are rarely given to those who need them. Lack of access to morphine is the central reason for this. Stocks are difficult to maintain and, due to fears of the creation of a black market in highly addictive drugs, their circulation is tightly regulated to the point of making their prescription, even within the hospital, an onerous task. Moreover, African medical culture in general does not put a very high premium on the relief of pain. As an outgrowth of British colonial medicine, and in its current form as a node for vertical international interventions, health care in Botswana has traditionally operated under the assumption that it is a "zero-sum enterprise."

In such a system, patient comfort is not a priority. Efforts are largely directed elsewhere (as Adams, Reynolds Whyte and colleagues, Pfeiffer, and Moran-Thomas also show in their chapters), oriented toward the demonstration of successful delivery of lifesaving drugs and implementations of large-scale programs. Pain management is often outside the metrics of success of such interventions and thus becomes invisible in a system with very specific evidentiary demands. Moreover, doctors and nurses lack the tools to measure and treat pain medically. These are the systemic silences that muffle the social experience of pain in Botswana and through which palliation can appear only as a frill, inaccessible and unworthy of attention from national and international decision-makers.

Seen ethnographically, biomedicine is inherently a midlevel trial-and-error enterprise—as much a global system of thought and technology as it is a localized and improvised practice. Livingston's own work seeks to wield ethnography as a species of salve through which to socialize pain and enact care. Her descriptions—vivid, difficult, and often also funny—dramatize the physical suffering of cancer patients and their caregivers' efforts to provide relief. They draw the reader into this network of care, demanding our empathy as a prerequisite to analysis. Empathy alone, certainly, offers no guarantee of any improvements, but it is an alternative to raising our hands in defeat, dismissing the pain of others as epistemologically inaccessible and impervious to action. By arguing that pain is itself a social language that must be learned, Livingston emphasizes the very human and humane ways in which people deal with anxiety and duress in the absence of painkillers, while at the same time signaling that the failures of palliation, both interpersonally and institutionally, are also failures in communication, flaws in our ability to see beyond the envelope of our own skin and imagine life in others.

* * *

Even the most magical of bullets can only succeed by taking into account the nuances of micropolitics and of local notions of disease causation. Technology adoption strategies are unruly. Understanding this on-the-ground unruliness requires acknowledging the "others" among and between us, as well as the importance of meaning-making in any intervention take-up. In her chapter, Amy Moran-Thomas takes the program for the eradication of the guinea worm in northern Ghana as a launching point from which to examine the different epistemologies at work in global health initiatives. The ethnographer teases out the ways in which the local landscape of health care is changed and imagined through such initiatives, and the ways in which people actively engage with them, transforming biology and magic into heuristics for one another.

Diseases have stories to tell. In Moran-Thomas's case, the eradication of guinea worm becomes the stage for the encounter (and confrontation) between multiple histories of medicine and the theories of causality and self, and beliefs in the power of things in which these histories are entrenched. In a social context where many understand themselves as inhabited and inhabitable by other selves, this understanding encompasses the guinea worm as well. Western epidemiology, on the other hand, posits a population as the subject and touchstone of health and views the guinea worm as a parasite that enters an individual body through the consumption of infected crustaceans living in shared bodies of water—that is, as an alien agent and harbinger of disease and economic collapse.

Internationally, the parasite has offered a political rallying point to organizations that seek to make their mark in the world of development. Because of its graphic visibility, the worm can be mustered as a powerful symbol of poverty and decay (even when there are other, far more fatal diseases in the region) and an objectifiable target for interventions. Here we see symptoms of a semiotics of medicine overtaking the pragmatics of care in global health policy: targeted people often do not use water filters, or use them in ways that were not originally intended; filters are introduced in the absence of a longstanding contact between doctors and their patients that could enable an understanding of biomedical explanations for the disease; doctors and campaign workers express their puzzlement at the locals' refusal to comply with their treatment, while the latter are often bewildered by and suspicious of the formers' intentions, their methods, and, certainly, their perplexity.

Here, as elsewhere, the metrics of delivery often eclipse people's own assessments of the value of interventions. As Moran-Thomas shows, the physical objects used in these interventions—these magic bullets—can become integrated into local structures of political and religious power. To possess a guinea worm filter or a malaria bednet is to be aligned with the privilege of the foreigners, a perceived status that can be reinforced and put to use by programs that seek to hire persons well positioned within villages, who often articulate their roles through the language of traditional authority. Thus, not only do such interventions reinforce existing power differences, but they can expand the language in which social distinctions are expressed or contested. Moreover, the requirement that locals comply with a treatment also opens the door for them to voice other needs and desires and to be recognized as other kinds of subjects.

Moran-Thomas's analysis casts a refractive light on the world of Western biomedicine and global health, exploring the myths that orient it and the ways in which local magic can sustain it. As the anthropologist tacks between one person's fictions and the other's realities, she sheds light on the ways in which discourses and actions are produced and transformed in a field that, despite its insistence on vertical approaches, is alive with voices and cosmologies that regularly collide with one another.

—*João Biehl and Adriana Petryna*

5

Therapeutic Clientship

Belonging in Uganda's Projectified Landscape of AIDS Care

SUSAN REYNOLDS WHYTE, MICHAEL A. WHYTE,
LOTTE MEINERT, AND JENIPHER TWEBAZE

When we first met Saddam in December 2005, he had come with another soldier, also on antiretroviral therapy (ART), to pick up antiretroviral medicines. In civilian clothes, they sat together on the bench waiting to see the clinical officer, chatting in Kiswahili and English. They shared lodgings in the barracks and sometimes made the 15-km journey together to Mukuju, where they were enrolled in an ART program at the government health center. Mukuju was not the nearest source of antiretroviral drugs (ARVs) for Saddam, but it was there he belonged as a client through the eighteen months we followed him.

Saddam was forty-five years old and had been a soldier ever since he dropped out of secondary school to join Amin's army. He was from Masindi, in northern central Uganda, but had formed ties (a wife, now ex-, and three children) in eastern Uganda after being sent there on army operations in 1988. It was in 2003 that he began to lose weight dramatically and spent almost a million shillings in vain, visiting "witch doctors," first with the help of a civilian comrade, and then with his mother back home in Masindi.

Finally a friend, a medical assistant in the army, advised him to go for an HIV test. He tried The AIDS Support Organization (TASO), one of the oldest and best-known NGOs in the country. But at their branch in the nearby town of Tororo, the machines were out of order. So he went further to the District Hospital, where tests were provided by the AIDS Information Center, another NGO. When they found him positive, they gave him some forms to take to TASO. In turn TASO gave him a card and some medicine, which, as he told us dismissively, was merely the same medicine they had at the barracks health unit. So he went back to his friend the medical assistant, who asked him if he had money to pay for real help. When Saddam affirmed that he did, the friend took him to the Joint Clinical Research Centre (JCRC) branch in Mbale, about 30 km to the north. There he started on ARVs and managed to pay for his treatment for two months.

Then something snapped. He told us that he had become angry and bitter about being infected, and annoyed at the "witch doctors" who ate his money for nothing. Perhaps he was also distressed at the high cost of ARVs. In any case, he simply left and went to his home in Masindi for seven months. His mother encouraged him to go back to the army so that he could earn money to buy his drugs and help his children. But when he did return, he was imprisoned as a deserter. After so long without drugs, his health had deteriorated, and the discipline committee released him for fear he would die in jail. His pay had been stopped, so he now had no money to buy drugs and had to turn to another source. As he explained, "They were always announcing on the radio about free drugs at the health units. So I went and talked to my friend the health worker and he advised me to start getting free drugs at Mukuju Health Centre."

Saddam joined the Mukuju program in 2004, when JCRC was establishing ART clinics in collaboration with government health centers. Saddam was a faithful client, it seems, even though he sometimes had to walk the long distance. He spoke warmly of his health worker, Henry, who supplied him with quinine and other medicines, in addition to enough ARVs to cover his needs when he was deployed on operations in remote places to pick up dead and injured soldiers. In fact, Saddam liked Henry so much that he did not want to be seen by anyone else. Once when we visited Saddam, he was having terrible pain in his legs, a common side effect of his ARV medicine Triomune, but had not sought help because Henry was on leave.

The health center actually had three different ART programs: the JCRC TREAT collaboration, supported by the US President's Emergency Plan for AIDS Relief (PEPFAR); the Prevention of Mother-to-Child Transmission Program funded by PLAN Uganda/International; and the Ministry of Health (MOH) roll-out program, financed by the Global Fund. We had assumed that Saddam was on the JCRC program, since that is where he originally started when he was buying drugs. Saddam was not sure himself, but he had noticed the letters MOH written on his file. When we asked Henry, the clinical officer, he confirmed that Saddam was on the MOH program. It seemed illogical to us that three ART programs, with all their paperwork, should be run out of the same rural health center, but the health workers let us understand one advantage to this arrangement— that it was sometimes possible to borrow drugs from one if another ran out.

Once when we visited Saddam, we asked him to take us round to the military hospital in the barracks. It turned out that they had been supplying ARVs for the past five months. They had enrolled forty people, soldiers and their families, and even provided Septrin for soldiers who were getting their ARVs from TASO. The nursing officer in charge, after mentioning pointedly that Saddam was one of those who insisted on continuing his treatment elsewhere, explained that many went to Mukuju because some of the ART programs there distributed food items, which the Ministry of Defense could not afford to offer. Others went to TASO because it provided medicines for opportunistic infections and skin rashes, which the military hospital did not. As we walked away from the hospital, Saddam muttered that he would not want to receive his medicine there, because they only gave enough ARVs for one week at a time.

The next time we saw him, Saddam looked thinner. We asked about his health and he said his CD4 count had increased from 213 to over 300. He realized that he did not look well, but insisted that he was very fine and challenged us to go to Mukuju Health Centre and check his CD4 results in his file—file number MOH/72. He added that he was now getting drugs for two months at a time.

As our study came to a close, Saddam received a military transfer to Masindi. He was pleased that he and his three children, who lived with him in the barracks, would be close to his family there. And despite his loyalty to Mukuju and to his health worker Henry, it turned out that he could enroll in the ART clinic at a hospital near Masindi and receive the very same medicine and treatment from which he had benefited at Mukuju.

The Projectification of AIDS Care

Saddam's story was one of many we followed through a Ugandan landscape that can best be described as *projectified*. The list of acronyms for programs providing ART is long, and to that can be added many projects providing other kinds of support for HIV-positive people. The proliferation of ART programs in Uganda came about because of three factors that worked together.

First, the country's policy of openness about HIV/AIDS was coupled with hospitality to donors and a willingness to acknowledge that support for the fight against AIDS could be provided by many different organizations (Parkhurst 2002; Parkhurst and Lush 2004). From the time he took power in 1986, President Museveni not only assumed leadership in the campaign against AIDS, he used it, consciously or not, to legitimate leadership of the nation: "In part, one might say, the state-building strategy of Museveni's National Resistance Movement, after a devastating civil war, was to mobilize around the AIDS epidemic in order to bring more of society under its purview" (Swidler 2009b:141). Far from being a sign of weakness, donor dependence (or donor mobilization) became a strategy to strengthen the state.

Second, donors responded with unprecedented generosity. Funding came from many sources and supported a plethora of different treatment programs both within and outside of government health facilities. The rollout of ART was made possible by a huge influx of funding that began in 2004 and 2005. PEPFAR was by far the biggest single donor, but even within PEPFAR there was no homogeneity, because PEPFAR's policy was to support many different projects, some faith-based, some secular NGOs, some parastatal. Donors have played a major role in Ugandan public health care since the present government came to power. Immunization, essential drugs, safe motherhood, malaria control, and many other programs depended on outside funding. ART was different, however, because of the nature of the treatment.

The requirements of AIDS therapy constitute the third factor. Biomedical experts emphasized the overwhelming importance of adherence to a lifelong regimen of medication and regular examination. The nightmare they feared was treatment chaos and the development of drug resistance. Second- or third-line drugs would be even more expensive. Their strongest argument for tight control was one that patients and their families readily took to heart: those who did not follow the regimen would soon die. Salvation, or at least control, would come with faithful participation in programs. The need for continuing treatment meant that ART projects had to take root and persist, enroll members and sustain them.

For all these reasons, the landscape of health care blossomed with an array of programs instead of just one standard package of care provided through the existing government health care system, as was the case, for example, in Botswana. Each program recruited its members, monitored their medication and health status, and kept their files. The result was a new pattern in Ugandan health care. The change was marked in discourse by a shift that occurred around the turn of the millennium in the way health workers spoke of their patients. They began to refer to them as "clients." To be a client of an ART program is to belong to an organization that registers your information, provides you with regular services at a treatment site, and has certain expectations of you. It is a kind of contractual relationship that differs significantly from the usual encounter that patients have with health workers, or that customers have with the attendants in the drugshops and small private clinics that provide the lion's share of health care in Uganda. As one patient, Robinah, said of her Home-Based AIDS Care program, "I am their person."

In this chapter we want to examine clientship as an innovation in Ugandan health care. We will suggest that the idea of therapeutic clientship is heuristic in that it marks out a field of social relations and a set of research questions. We think of the term neither as constitutive nor descriptive: not "this is clientship," but rather, "in what sense might we think about this as clientship?" What interests us are the links through which people connect to programs, the nature of clientship as expectation and obligation, and the "transactables" that are exchanged in such a relationship. Empirically it is clientship—joining and belonging to a particular program—that has given so many people in Uganda a second chance to live. Yet, because the projects on which they depend address only one disease and because they differ in terms of the benefits provided (the kinds of medicines, tests, and material support), inequities have arisen in an already unequal landscape of health care. To put it bluntly, public health in this setting does not mean rights and equal opportunities for all citizens of Uganda. Rather, it means building patron-client relationships locally, nationally, and internationally.

At Home with ART

Leaving aside the quantitative biomedical research that focuses on adherence and effect, qualitative research on the social and political aspects of ART relies on methodologies that address different perspectives and positions. Some analyze the media or rely on interviews with politicians and program implementers. Others observe interactions in clinics and have discussions with health workers. Of those researchers oriented to patients, many interview people in one treatment program or contact members of support groups. Often they talk to people only once. Given the composite nature of the ART landscape in Uganda, the historical changes that have occurred, and the fact that many ART clients are not active members of support groups, we adopted another strategy. We were four Danish and four Ugandan anthropologists who had been working together on health care for some years.[1] After a preliminary exploration of access to ART (Whyte et al. 2004; Meinert et al. 2004) and ART challenges to health workers (Whyte et al. 2010), we decided to study the experiences of people living with ART. Our focus was what we call the "first generation," those who benefitted from the rollout in 2004–5 that made ARVs widely available and nominally free. We made contacts through seven different treatment programs, in Kampala and rural eastern Uganda, with forty-eight people who were willing to tell us about their lives and current situations. Among them were twenty-three who agreed that we might visit them seven more times over the following year and a half, that is, from late 2005 until mid-2007.

While about half of the first "life story" interviews took place at clinics, none of the follow-up visits did. We visited people at home or, in a few cases, at work; almost always we met family, friends, and neighbors. This method had the effect of de-centering illness and treatment, or at least of putting them into the context of everyday life, and of foregrounding sociality (Whyte 2009). The combination of life histories and visits that stretched over eighteen months ensured that attention would be paid to time and change. This data is rich in itself, but our interpretations draw as well on our earlier work on the composite health care system, family patterns, and the social dimension of therapy-seeking.

Our material is not only "experience near"; it also reflects interactions over time in the course of which we investigators became socially positioned; that is, we became participants to some extent in the social worlds of our subjects. We are dealing with extended cases. Our goal is not to generalize across cases, for doing that would violate the individuality of our interlocutors and their circumstances. Rather, we hope to discover through our cases new implications and insights (Mitchell 1983; Kapferer 2005).

Achieving Treatment with Support from Others

In principle—from a policy perspective—AIDS programs offer services to the population at large on an equal basis. But in practice, people hear about and access these services through other people. They "achieve" services with the help of others; they are not simply caught up as individuals in a net thrown out by providers. Many people learn of testing and treatment options through various official channels and media, just as Saddam did. Yet the actual move to test or to join a program is almost always mediated through a trusted social connection. Saddam talked with his friend about what he had heard on the radio. This emphasis on the sociality of decision-making and action featured in most of the stories we heard about how members of the first generation came to take an HIV test and in time found their way into a treatment program.

In Saddam's telling of why he first tested and how he got onto treatment, his friend the medical assistant played a key role. It may be that this man was simply performing his duties as a health professional in the military, but Saddam always spoke of him as his friend. And he actually took Saddam to the clinic in another town when he started ART, which was certainly beyond the call of duty. He was part of what John Janzen (1978) has named the "therapy managing group," the network of relatives and friends that advises and forms contacts with treatment sources. Reading through our material on how members of the first generation decided to test and, more important, how they got into treatment programs, we are struck by how many included health workers in their advisory networks. Either they knew someone who had some kind of position at a biomedical institution (one woman had a daughter who worked as a stores assistant at a health center) or they knew someone who knew someone. The informal practices of health workers in making connections for relatives and friends are significant. But they point to a more general pattern of seeking and providing advice—the vernacular and informal counterpart to counseling, a practice that has been standardized and widely institutionalized in the response to HIV/AIDS.

Mediated access to AIDS programs through social connections is sympathetic and underlines the importance of human agency and sociality. Official structures and programs cannot create action on their own; they need human actors. All of the stories about using connections give a picture of positive people acting as socially embedded seekers of health, not passive recipients of donor beneficence. But the importance of connections reveals and reinforces inequalities in the population as well. Some people are better connected than others; some have large networks, some know important "big" people, while others have smaller and less influential social networks. The other downside of depending on social connections is its contingency. Overall, better-educated people have more useful connections, but for any individual there is an element of luck and chance to knowing a person in a strategic position. It is also possible that one might lose touch with such contacts. Being dependent on persons rather than institutions introduces an element of fragility. Uneducated Robinah was fortunate to have a sister, Joyce, who was a teacher, knowledgeable about treatment possibilities, and a leader in the local Post Test Club. She and her sister quarreled, however, and she moved back to Kumi after the end of our study. She was able to continue with her ART program, but she lost her connections to all the AIDS projects that came through Joyce and the Post Test Club.

By definition the people we interviewed and followed were people with enough resources—social, cultural, economic—to achieve and maintain treatment. Over half of them had, like Saddam, started their treatment by paying for their drugs. They had more wherewithal than most Ugandans, which is not to say that they were in comfortable circumstances; many, again like Saddam, were not able to continue ART on a fee basis. They were also better educated. Thirty-seven of our original forty-eight interviewees had managed to get beyond primary school at a time when only about a quarter of the national population between the ages of fifteen and forty-nine had done so (UBOS 2007:35). In late 2005, when we initiated this work, estimates were that less than half of those who needed ART were receiving it. There were not enough drugs and human resources to get all the people who needed it into treatment (and this is still true today). Those who did achieve treatment were those who had support and contacts to help realize their own motivation. We cannot say much about those who did not achieve treatment. But considering how connections function illuminates the workings of advantage and inequity. It also shows how people have to work at connections, and how those links are sometimes marked by contingency and fragility.

The point we are making has been put forward by other researchers. Feierman and Feierman, working in northeastern Tanzania, found that the most vulnerable children were those whose mothers lived alone, as widows or divorcées (S. Feierman 1985:83). The children at risk were not those who were taken to traditional healers, but those whose therapy-managing network was so limited that they did not receive any kind of treatment. "Those who continue to search for therapy together with a managing group, and continually change therapies, do better than those who fare alone. It is the seeking of medical care until the desired effects are attained that results in the healthy patient. . . ." (E. K. Feierman 1981:402–403). The broader the therapy-managing group, the more chance that a variety of treatments will be tried. Another group of medical researchers, epidemiologists working in Guinea-Bissau, has demonstrated the effects on health outcomes of personally knowing a physician. Among children admitted to the pediatric ward in Bissau, those whose mothers knew a doctor had a risk of dying within thirty days that was 48 percent smaller than those whose mothers did not count a doctor among their acquaintances (Sodemann et al. 2006).

Connections are important when it comes to deciding to test and to join a treatment program. They continue to be important even after one becomes a client of an ART program. Through her sister, Robinah not only started treatment; she was also able to link up to other projects and groups that might provide extra support. Sometimes, the way people react to researchers reveals key features of the situation the researchers are trying to understand. Both our own informants and other people we met in the process of doing this study seemed to see us as potential connections, or at least as resource-full contacts who might be useful. On our last visit to Juma's home, his wife, who had also tested positive, seemed worried and unhappy. "By the way," she asked, "how do I access the porridge provided by TASO?" Once, while we were waiting at the hospital AIDS clinic for Jessica to pick up her drugs, another client, thin and with a sickly looking baby, asked one of us if we were from TASO. "I really want to talk to someone from TASO," she said, "I need to join in order to get food." On one occasion, we realized that a client named Bernard had been hoping that being interviewed by us might help him get into a research project on discordant couples that he had heard about at the Infectious Diseases Institute. Benjamin, a client who was paying for his drugs, asked us if we could connect him to someone who could help subsidize his treatment. When we said we did not think so, he replied, "You never know, keep trying." This phrase seemed to capture perfectly the sense of possibility with which people explored potential connections.

What we have learned from our interlocutors is that networking is not just having a set of connections that can be worked. Terms like "technical know-who" summon to mind the Soviet *blat* or the Chinese *guanxi*, suggesting already-existing personalized webs of influence that can be set in motion to get things done. While these certainly exist in Uganda and are mobilized by those with resources, there is also a disposition of openness toward making contacts that is found across the social spectrum. There is a kind of gambling element at play, a hoping for luck ("you never know") that makes much support-seeking more like a lottery than a systematic investigation of available possibilities.

Unpacking Clientship

A client is a user of professional services such as those of a lawyer or social worker, and no doubt it was this connotation of service with the patient as user or consumer that led to the introduction of the term. While patients should be passive and quiet (in fact, "patient"), clients are interlocutors who have expectations about services. There is a neoliberal tinge to "client" in this sense, which suggests enlightened consumerism and user friendliness. Moreover, the term "client" implies a more enduring relationship, unlike an exchange with a customer or even a patient, which might be a one-off affair. In the context of the Ugandan health care that actually exists, this notion of clientship sounded ironic, if not utopian. Public health care is notorious for poor service, understaffing, stock-outs of medicines, inadequate equipment, and indifference or rudeness to patients—at least for those who were not known to the staff or willing to supply "tea" in the form of a little cash. For many Ugandans, "health care" has long meant buying medicines from a drugshop manned by someone without sufficient professional credentials. Proper examination, diagnosis, and monitoring over time does not really figure. By comparison, ART programs are exceptional indeed, offering the patient a markedly higher standard of service that includes dialogue and a long-term relationship as a client.

In social science, "clientship" has another meaning as well. A client is the dependent of a patron. The relationship is hierarchical in that the patron provides access to scarce material resources needed by the client in exchange for less tangible prestations, such as loyalty (Wolf 1966:16–17). There is in the relationship a tendency to personalization and a certain emotional charge; Wolf (ibid:16) cites Pitt-Rivers's description of the patron-client bond as a "lop-sided friendship." Patronage, or patrimonialism, has a special resonance among scholars of governance in Africa. Drawing on Max Weber's distinction between systems based on impersonal rational bureaucracy bound by law and family-like personal systems of redistribution to dependents, they argue that in many African states, patrimonialism in politics and governance is tightly woven into rational-legal bureaucratic systems established during the colonial period to form a system of neo-patrimonialism that somehow *works* despite appearances to the contrary (Chabal and Daloz 1999). Researchers have been intrigued by the ways in which donor-funded projects fit into this pattern of neo-patrimonialism. They point out that project resources such as cash, contracts, equipment, jobs, the location of new infrastructure, and even the perks of workshops and transport allowances flow through relationships of patronage and clientship. At the same time, the projects are logically frameworked, benchmarked, quality assured, and evaluated through standardized mechanisms that belong to the realm of rational legal bureaucratic authority.

The patterns of patronage traceable in donor-funded projects are evident in HIV/AIDS endeavors as well. Ann Swidler (2009a) argues that international NGOs working with AIDS are inserted into personalistic patron-client systems in Africa. She is interested in this interface and in whether those NGO interventions make patronage systems more accountable and responsive. Our own concern with AIDS interventions and clientship is somewhat different, because we focus on clients while she focuses on patronage as an institutional logic. We are concerned with treatment while she studies other kinds of AIDS projects. But our material also shows traces of the interplay between the rational-bureaucratic principles espoused by donors and biomedical experts, and the personalistic patronage tendencies that can be found nearly everywhere but are especially strong in African societies.

"Therapeutic clientship" is a term we find useful in exploring the field of relationships through which people on ART find their ways. It affirms the new quality of service-mindedness in patient–health worker interaction, flagged by the term "client," which policymakers wish to realize. At the same time, it points to essential aspects of the Ugandan world of personal interdependence. Resources are accessed through and invested in social relationships. Technical know-*who* is often considered necessary for getting anything done that involves bureaucracy. The ideal of kinship amity that sustains orphans and helps pay school fees extends, hopefully and by analogy, to those health workers who might be kind enough to make an extra effort.

Therapeutic clientship may call to mind another analytical concept used in social science studies of the response to the AIDS epidemic: therapeutic citizenship. Vinh-Kim Nguyen and colleagues (2007:S34) used that term in relation to the rights and claims of HIV-positive individuals in a wider global community, as well as the personal obligation that requires self-transformation. They recognize the existence of "local moral economies" where "individuals call on networks of obligation and reciprocity to negotiate access to therapeutic resources" (Nguyen 2004:126). But the notion of therapeutic citizenship does not encourage the examination of those relations on their own terms. With its emphasis on individual rights in a polity, it is perhaps more useful for understanding the positions of the donors, activists, advocates, policymakers, and, to some extent, providers. They are the ones offering inclusion; they feel they have an obligation to help; they make claims on (or at least appeals to) the state or the international community on behalf of the hundreds of thousands in need of ARVs. Peter Mugyenyi, Director of Uganda's JCRC, exemplifies this position in his advocacy in relation to PEPFAR (Mugyenyi 2008, 2009). Most people on ART in Uganda are not talking about their rights and claims in the abstract sense. They are worried about their chances of obtaining much more immediate benefits, favors, and assistance from people they know or would like to know.

Paperwork and Belonging

Saddam's remark that we could just go to the health center and check his CD4 test results in his file—number MOH/72—marks the radical change in Ugandan health care we are underlining. It indexes membership in a treatment program that keeps records and follows people over time. The association between paperwork and health care is not new in itself. In government health units, the health worker writes down the diagnosis and prescription on a "Medical Form 5," or in a school exercise book brought by the patient. The act of writing is an appreciated form of acknowledgment (Whyte 2011), which is part of what constitutes the higher quality of care in a professional bureaucratic facility. (The contrast sometimes noted between a public health unit and a small private clinic or drugshop is that no record is made in the latter.) The main use of papers in ordinary health care is to show the dispenser or a drugshop attendant which medicines are needed. Patients are supposed to keep them and bring them next time, but the papers tend to get lost and are not usually treated with great care. For people on ART programs, paperwork is more comprehensive and precious. Not only do they keep the papers documenting their registration, treatment history, and appointment dates but, exceptionally, the treatment facility keeps a file on them as well, as Saddam so clearly knew.

The significance of the file staying at the facility is that it indicates a kind of contractual obligation, or at least an intention, to provide treatment. In a related study, Jenipher Twebaze was present when a client was being scolded for drunkenness and for generally living as he pleased rather than as he had been advised to do. That is to say, he was a bad client, one who did not keep his side of the exchange agreement. One health worker suggested, "Punish him—let us chase him away because he does not care about his life and he is wasting our time and drugs." At this, the clinical officer dealing with him said, "Mmm, mmm, I don't know what to do to you. Get your file and go home. When you settle and make up your mind to live a healthy and happy life, you come back and we start treatment." And she handed over the file to him. The drunken client pleaded not to be sent away until finally the health worker took the file back again.

In principle, if someone wants to switch programs, that person's file should be transferred. In recognition of the fact that membership in an ART program is exclusive, switching should be formalized by the conveyance of papers. But when Dorothy and her husband were angered at the way the doctor in her program treated her, and her husband decided to take her to a friend who had close contacts at TASO, things took a different course. At TASO the couple wanted Dorothy's file, but her husband did not want to confront the doctor in charge of her program to ask for it. So he waited until the doctor was out and then connived with another health worker to get the file, which he photocopied and returned to its place. This suggests that belonging to a program, being "their person," as indicated by their maintenance of your file, is a status taken very seriously by others as well as by the client.

The paperwork of clientship is far more comprehensive than the treatment file kept at the facility. It starts with the HIV test. People who have tested positive ("reactive") receive a card on which is written "for continuing care," code for "HIV-positive and eligible to join AIDS programs." Such a card is a ticket to various kinds of support programs, which help with food rations, blankets, income-generating projects, and various kinds of medical care. The oldest and best known of these is TASO. Many of our interlocutors, like Saddam, were enrolled in TASO after testing positive. Ivan told us, "They immediately gave me TASO forms to fill—also for my wife—and we registered as members. . . ." TASO was particularly active in eastern Uganda; during the time of our study, it was re-registering its members and some of our informants were impressed with this bureaucratic process. Hassan, living in Tororo, told how he used to have only a number at TASO but had been recently issued a card. He had been called to have his photo taken and was told that one copy of his picture would be retained by the Ministry of Health. "The computers that took the photos were from Entebbe." He showed his new health card, with his number, and his TASO membership card, with another number. Interestingly, the list of "membership benefits" on the TASO card did not mention the material support that figured so prominently in most people's talk about TASO. But the paper itself was a valued token of belonging, just like the file kept at the treatment facility.

Cards, forms, and files were mentioned by all of the people we followed. It was not uncommon that people brought out their papers to underline something they were telling us about their treatment. Harriet got out her card to confirm for us that she first tested for HIV on May 26, 2005. Others pulled out cards or papers to check on their next appointment or the details about medicine doses. Registration papers and cards were part of the first, more bureaucratic, meaning of "clientship": being entitled to services. Yet getting those papers was often described as a process that involved going through someone else, being instructed how to go about it by someone you know. And having the papers did not always guarantee realizing the benefits that were supposed to accrue; that was thought to depend on the individuals administering them.

Exchange between Unequal Parties

Patron-client relations are ways of structuring exchange between unequal parties (Lemarchand and Legg 1972; Eisenstadt and Roniger 1980). Even though ART clientship differs fundamentally from the patron-client relations described in the older ethnographic literature (Mair 1961; Lemarchand and Legg 1972), using the framework of clientship encourages us to consider the nature and "stuff" of exchange. Those who paid for their drugs were engaged in a more specific, limited, or direct exchange. They gave money for medicine, and received only that medicine for which they had sufficient cash. But even they sometimes expressed an expectation of more than drugs and an appreciation of what they took to be personal concern and advice. The free programs involve more generalized reciprocity; what is given and received does not have to balance out in the short term, but should involve mutuality over time. While the personal relationship between a client and a health worker is often important, exchange may extend as well to other staff, fellow clients, potential clients, and other programs providing other kinds of support.

The most important item of exchange is, of course, the antiretroviral medicine. In all of the free programs, receiving these required preliminary educational and counseling sessions, "studying ARVs," as some called it. A client exchanges time for drugs, in that he or she has to keep appointments and wait, sometimes for hours. Moreover, a client must submit to monitoring by showing the remaining drugs before getting a refill, so that a health worker can check for adherence. "If you don't do it right, they will stop you," one man said. In fact they may not even start you if you do not seem capable of punctuality and compliance. Since most people begin a daily regime of the antibiotic cotrimoxazole (Septrin) before being put on ARVs, health workers can assess their abilities to live up to their side of the bargain.

Discipline, shown by putting your body on the line by coming to get refills and to be checked for health problems, is the basic requirement for getting drugs. After some time it may be possible to negotiate an arrangement for a family member to fetch the drugs, but not before responsible clientship has been demonstrated. What this discipline provides to the program are numbers and documentation, which it, in turn, exchanges with its donors for more drugs, equipment, salaries, and further opportunities.

Whether clients also receive medicines for opportunistic infections and other health problems depends upon which program they have joined. As we have already seen, clientship can be more or less comprehensive. Moreover, some programs provide regular testing of CD4 counts and viral loads, so that the effects of the drugs can be measured. Where this is done, clients learn to quantify changes in their bodies, as they also do with respect to weight (knowing your kilos). But other programs do not provide these expensive tests, and people must either pay for them or, more commonly, do without (Meinert et al. 2009). At the Ministry of Health facilities funded only by the Global Fund, most clients had never had their CD4 counts measured.

Beyond discipline, what else do people give in exchange for drugs? They give openness in return for advice and reassurance—ideally at least. They offer their narratives or fragments of stories in return for moral support. To be a good client and to realize the benefits of clientship one must talk, tell about one's bodily and social situation. It is expected that people will enter into dialogue with their health worker and their counselor or home visitor if they have one, sharing problems in order to receive advice and assistance. Openness is especially valued if it extends to discussing HIV and the benefits of treatment with others. The clinical officer who took a personal interest in Hassan told us with warm approval of how Hassan spread the word about ARVs, comparing them to *ebigwasi,* the blessed sacramental millet balls consumed at offerings to the ancestors in their part of eastern Uganda. Hassan was not an activist, but his efforts at public relations for his ART program were a part of his exchange with the patron he liked so much. Joseph, a client of Mbuya Reach Out, was quite explicit that such efforts were a kind of exchange: "For us, we don't pay anything. Instead the only reward we give back is to encourage others, also telling them about the program and asking them to join."

Openness and talking about problems can also bring material support in the form of referral to programs that distribute food supplies, blankets, loans, school fees, training, and other goods. These were the negotiable aspects of clientship. Whether or not people gain access to these benefits is often interpreted as depending on personal goodwill. Dorothy was disappointed with her counselor at TASO: "He is not helping me at all. I knew that in TASO they were giving blankets, food, and many other things, but when I asked him why I was not getting them, he said that it depended on the patient! . . . He is a difficult man. I don't know why they cannot change [counselors] for me. I asked in TASO why they were not helping me. That hurts me so much."

For a minority, but an important and high-profile minority, openness and storytelling lead to other kinds of return. These are the AIDS stars, clients who have returned from the very brink of the grave after terrible suffering to enjoy a second chance at health and life. Their stories are told and retold by fellow clients and by their program patrons. One man working for the Home-Based AIDS Care (HBAC) program explained that Brenda was their success story because she was really on her deathbed and no one expected that she would make it, but she is now very fine and studying at Uganda College of Commerce in Tororo. When the American ambassador came to visit the program in Tororo, he was brought to Brenda's home to meet a living example of what USAID support meant (Meinert et al. 2004). She thus gave to her patrons in the treatment program the stuff that they could pass on to *their* patrons.

Joyce and her sister Robinah were both positive, but Robinah's was the more dramatic account of rescue and resurrection. As chair of the Post

Test Club, Joyce promoted her sister: "Members such as Robinah are the testimonies of the Post Test Club, and each time she goes there and people see her, aware of how she was close to her death, people don't hesitate to come out." When Robinah's winning drawing about her life earned her a trip to Kampala, she remarked to us that being in treatment had given her opportunities and widened her horizons. She got to meet people, they came to visit her home, and she even got to travel. "How would I ever have gone to Kampala?" she reflected. The widening of horizons was an important part of being an active client. Ivan's wife, also HIV-positive, had been given a job as a nursery school teacher by an NGO working with AIDS. At first she was paid, but later the salary stopped. Even so, her husband remarked, "It has helped her because she doesn't stay at home to quarrel with my mother as they used to do. She is even looking better now because of being busy." To be occupied, to travel, and to meet new people, including visiting donors, were among the benefits of clientship for more active program members.

Being an AIDS leader and spokesperson put Joyce in a position to play the part of patron herself, just as Kaler and Watkins (2001) have shown for community-based distributors of family planning in nearby western Kenya. Joyce told how she became popular and well known for her campaigning about HIV. "Oh, here people like me, and I am known as the AIDS doctor. This is because of what I do for them, especially in the Post Test Club." She explained that when NGOs came to help needy HIV-positive people, they asked her to identify those needing assistance. In this way she had been able to facilitate access to projects distributing seed and providing pigs or goats or cash for investment. On one occasion, we found the two sisters at a Post Test Club meeting. Robinah was pleased that she had been selected for a drama group but was aware that other members envied her. Joyce explained how being the chairperson exposed her to accusations of unfairness in choosing who should get opportunities and assistance. Sometimes she feared taking the lead or including her sister for that reason.

For a few of our interlocutors, being a client opened the possibility of becoming an employee. The chances were best for those who were better educated. Jolly told us with delight at our final visit that her program had chosen her to be a peer counselor. "They looked for people who had some level of education and could speak English . . . we shall be starting training in two weeks time." As is often the case, she was taken on as a volunteer. "But they will be providing us with transport so I don't know," she said hopefully. Although she was to work without salary, she would have the chance to receive allowances and to position herself in case a proper job opened up. Ivan's wife later quit her volunteer job as a nursery school teacher because it offered neither pay nor prospects. A colleague of hers came by to try to persuade her to come back, urging, "I want us this time to teach and we do not request for any money because Plan International thought that for us we just want money without teaching. So let us not pull out, we will teach those children until they realize that we need to be paid."

All of this may sound calculating and opportunistic. In part it is. People short of resources have to keep an eye on possibilities, and most people in Uganda are short of resources, as are the people in Malawi who position themselves in relation to "sustainable" donor interventions (Swidler and Watkins 2009). This general disposition of hopefulness was even more pronounced for people who had to find ways to live what is called the Second Chance. What we want to emphasize is that expectations were oriented toward programs and very much toward the individual people who might have it in their power to provide help.

Yet clientship was more than the exchange of drugs, compliance, dramatic stories, and job opportunities. What struck us was that something else was being reciprocated as well, something in the nature of acknowledgment or respect or regard. To have a file at the program office, to have your photo with the Ministry of Health, was to be made visible to a powerful organization. To belong to a program was to be noticed, to be recognized as a person with needs, and to have some expectation of benefit. Not that people always felt they were treated with sufficient respect, or that they always received everything they might have hoped for. But the contrast with the typical experience of health care seekers in Uganda was enormous.

Projectification, Inequities, and Uncertainties

The first generation came on to ART in a time when Uganda's policy was to welcome donors and "to let a thousand projects bloom." The funding sources and supply lines are extremely complicated, as tracking research by Sung-Joon Park reveals. He points out that the data is so scattered that it is difficult to produce a comprehensive picture of free ART (personal communication). Nevertheless, his diagram (figure 5.1) gives a good idea of the situation, showing the supply of ARVs from sources of funding at the top, through supply organizations, to the treatment providers at the bottom.[2]

Given the complexity of the landscape, it is not surprising that most people have little idea of who in the world it is that has made their medicine possible and how it reaches their treatment site. As one interlocutor put it, "I thank God or Museveni or whoever brought these medicines." However, people on ART are aware that there are different sites of treatment offering different kinds of service. Unlike countries such as Botswana or Mozambique, Uganda does not have a standard ART package that is available primarily through the national health system. Being a client in a program like Mbuya Reach Out is very different from being one at the large impersonal Infectious Diseases Institute in Kampala or at a rural health center like Mukuju. The projectification of AIDS care means that much depends on who is your service provider (patron). Inequity is inevitable when there are so many different models of care.

Awareness of the inequalities in therapeutic clientship came in two ways. Some people knew someone on another program, which they reckoned to be better or worse than their own—like Saddam, who did not want to switch to the program at the military hospital. In a few cases, people in the same household were clients of different programs. Robinah and Joyce lived together, but Robinah was a client of the "deluxe" Home-Based AIDS Care program, while Joyce received her medicine from TASO. At the time when HBAC was recruiting clients, Joyce's CD4 count was not low enough to qualify her for the program. They agreed that Robinah was fortunate in that HBAC staff visited her every week, while Joyce only saw her counselor every two months. Another pair of clients, Mama Girl and Mama Boy, were both on HBAC, but Mama Girl was also a member of TASO, which provided food rations for a period, while Mama Boy was not. Benjamin thought JCRC superior to TASO, where his sister was a client. Martha also preferred JCRC, which allowed discretion about HIV status and did not have such long lines. However, she noted that TASO helped its clients to form clubs and recreation groups where they shared problems and helped each other to handle them. Moreover, TASO clients had first priority if any job opportunity opened in TASO, "which is a good practice and lacking here at JCRC."

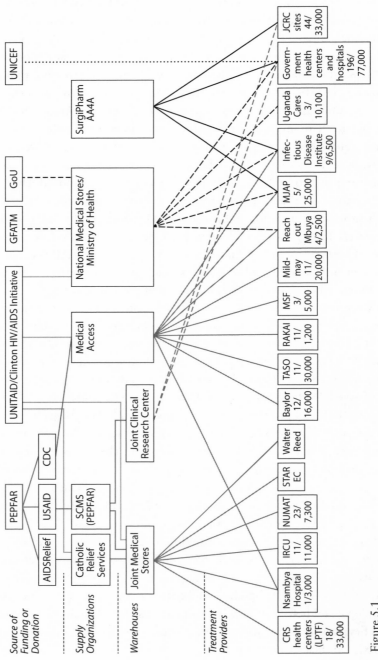

Figure 5.1

Others actually switched programs, and so could compare on the basis of firsthand experience. Those who switched were almost all people who had started on a fee program and moved over to one that was nominally free. The differences were partly medical, in that different drugs were provided, but there were other considerations as well. An important cost of free treatment was time. Those who had moved from fee to free programs frequently mentioned the hours spent waiting their turn to see the health worker and get their medicines. Dorothy had started paying for her drugs, then moved to free treatment at TASO, but she opted to go back to fee treatment: "There are long queues at TASO and sometimes you do not get all the drugs." Godfrey remarked, "I would like to be on free drugs but the problem is time. I hear those who go there spend the whole day in long queues, but at JCRC you don't spend more than ten minutes." James said that he spent an average of five hours waiting at Infectious Diseases Institute (IDI) at Mulago Hospital, even though he had friends there who tried to help him get through the process faster. First you had to wait for your consultation, then you had to wait at the pharmacy to pick up your drugs.

A few people mentioned a cost of free treatment that is taken for granted, even promoted: the loss of privacy. Martha, a paying client of JCRC, was critical of free programs: "Well, yes, they give free drugs, but you know there is always a queue and time wasting. But here I just come, pay, get my drugs, and go to work. Here nobody would ever see you coming to pick up drugs, but in TASO, everybody would know because they make you sit there, read files, then call you to pick drugs even after so many hours! It is tiresome and unnecessary revealing someone's health status as far as HIV is concerned." She did not agree with TASO's policy of involving other members of the family in a client's treatment. As the breadwinner she wanted to keep her secret and not let her health problems be "paraded" before her dependents.

Different programs involved different kinds of exchange: money, time, contact frequency, discretion, and opportunities were being given and received, as well as drugs and discipline. Worries about the future often revolved around the fate of the particular treatment program of which one was a member. Ivan, a client of the HBAC program, had heard rumors that it was going to close and that clients would be moved over to TASO. When a CDC employee discounted them, Ivan seemed relieved: "At least there is hope for us that we shall live longer, otherwise we were worried of going to join TASO." (In 2010, the closure and transfer came to pass, and a newspaper account [*New Vision* September 6, 2010] reported that former HBAC clients were complaining about the poorer standard of care they were receiving from TASO.) Hanifa had read newspaper reports that the IDI would run out of ARVs in three months, but she said that she still had her file with JCRC and TASO and that she would try to continue at one of those treatment sources if things got bad at IDI. The larger debate about the sustainability of ART treatment in Uganda, which is almost 100 percent donor dependent, did not seem to preoccupy our interlocutors. They were much more concerned about their own immediate position as clients of a particular program, with its particular exchanges and particular expectations.

Conclusion

In our study of the first generation, we have adopted a methodology that puts people first almost to a fault. Our forty-eight life stories and twenty-three extended cases are all accounts of personal situations. But in the spirit of the extended case method, we have tried to analyze *social* situations by moving back and forth between case details and what we know about the changing landscape of AIDS responses in Uganda. The term "client," for example, is not one the people we worked with used themselves. But when we picked it up from talking with health workers and put it together with the way our interlocutors spoke of belonging, of their relations to health workers, and of their obligations and expectations, it opened our eyes to a whole set of research questions. When we reviewed the history of AIDS policies and of ART availability, we saw how projectification shaped the topography in which our interviewees had to find their way. Our task now is to consider what more general implications this approach and these findings might have for the study of innovation in global health.

We have suggested that the term "therapeutic clientship" has heuristic value in that it draws our attention to a field of sociality rather than to a set of claims and entitlements in an abstract global arena. The specificities of joining and belonging and the qualities of social relations are amenable to ethnographic study, not least because they can be contextualized in relation to other aspects of social life. The clientship perspective leads us to an examination of expectations and transactions between parties, rather than to a focus on individual subjectivity. The discipline of self-care, for example, becomes a practice encouraged by others who inspect your medicines and to whom you can display virtue. The details of interaction between the social self and specific others are what produce, reproduce, and transform dispositions and values.

"Clientship" is a productive double entendre when applied to the field of ART in Uganda. The patients receiving ARVs through AIDS clinics are clients in the "user-of-services" sense; that is, they are people utilizing the professional expertise provided to them by rational bureaucratic organizations. They are also dependent for their lives on access to ARVs dispensed by donor-funded projects, and they are drawn into exchange relationships with the projects and people controlling access to those vital resources. In the classic pattern of patron-client relations, they tend to personalize their interactions with health workers and other project personnel. Accepting this double meaning of clientship allows us to explore differences among programs and situations. The big anonymous institutions in Kampala are more service providers than personal patrons, while smaller rural clinics have a more intimate flavor. The difference between being a user of services and a dependent of a patron is not merely an academic matter. The familiarity and friendships that develop over regular consultations in smaller settings build clients' loyalty to their treatment sites and health workers. They can motivate clinicians to live up to a patron ideal. But on the other hand, the greater bureaucratic efficiency of a large service provider can facilitate the transfer of patients between treatment sites and can enhance confidence in institutions rather than individuals, as seems to have happened for Saddam by the end of our study.

Burawoy (1998) has argued that extended cases provide the basis for testing and refining theoretical positions. ART has been interpreted within the framework of biocitizenship, drawing on inspiration from Foucault. Our cases suggest that the concept of "clientship" rather than "citizenship" may point toward an explanation that is more productive, more capable of capturing the diversity that characterizes our social field, where different programs involve different kinds of sociality. "Clientship" can, for example, facilitate exploration of the diverse nested levels of relationships. An AIDS activist who is a client of an ART project can herself function as a kind of patron when she takes on "volunteer" roles and funnels access to benefits to others. Likewise, an ART clinic is dependent on a higher-level organization that controls the clinic's access to medicines, training, allowances, and other resources. Hierarchies of access extend from local treatment sites to regional or national offices to funders overseas. Exactly how these links work in practice can be studied ethnographically; in fact, Sung-Joon Park, the creator of the supply chain diagram, is doing just that. The work of Swidler and Watkins (2009) on the consequences of donor-funded AIDS programs beautifully demonstrates the concerns and expectations held by different strata of Malawian society as they enter into hierarchical relations of exchange.

The concept of "citizenship," by contrast, points to more abstract considerations about the nature of people's relations to a polity, and the rights and obligations they hold. In the case of Uganda, the government has recognized the needs (rights?) of its HIV-positive citizens and has facilitated their access, as clients, to organizations providing for those needs. The state does not directly control access to ART resources, nor can it guarantee the rights and entitlements of those who meet the biological criteria for treatment. For that matter, even international agencies cannot pretend to provide entitlements to all who would claim them. The prospects of their being able to meet the increasing need for ARTs are, in fact, dim. Realistically, most HIV-positive people in Uganda are not so much claiming rights as hoping for help from a "patron" with resources to distribute. What remains to be seen is whether the client-patron variant of ART distribution will raise expectations and lead to claims on, not just appeals to, the government and international donors.

Finally, we wish to emphasize again that the social organization of ART clientship is a substantial innovation in Ugandan health care from the point of view of patients. They find themselves in a landscape of different service providers; even the government health facilities are just one possibility among many. They must join an ART clinic and submit to the restrictions and inconveniences of following rules and being monitored. Yet joining and belonging to a treatment program that monitors their therapy is not generally seen as unwelcome surveillance; rather, it is a demonstration of acknowledgment and continuing concern. Many people on ART experience a standard of health care well above what they had in the past.

What significance might ART projects have for the health care system more generally? Thus far, the focus of health systems researchers has been on the distortions brought on by a "fixation" on AIDS that diverts human resources away from other areas of health care and mobilizes external funds for only one disease. Realizing the potential of the innovations that ART has brought would mean carrying over the model of belonging, with its features of counseling, a regular supply of drugs, and follow-up, to other chronic diseases that require lifelong treatment.

Notes

1. Phoebe Kajubi, David Kyaddondo, Lotte Meinert, Hanne O. Mogensen, Godfrey Siu, Jenipher Twebaze, Michael Whyte, and Susan Whyte had worked together for ten years under an Enhancement of Research Capacity Grant from Danida that linked departments at two Danish universities with the Child Health and Development Centre, Makerere University.

2. Treatment programs can have many different sites: for example CRS (Christian Relief Services) has 18 sites treating 33,000 people (shown as 18/33,000). Park used the diagram to open discussions with people supplying and providing ARVs, who had many comments and additional information. He does not consider it a final authoritative document, but rather an indication of how difficult it is to map the field. The Uganda AIDS Control Programme has compiled a list of 19 treatment providers with 436 sites, and numbers treated as of the first quarter of 2010. This list comes the closest to being a detailed overview of anything we have been able to find; however, there are many questions about the list. (Some programs we know about are not included, and some of the facilities listed as ART service outlets have never provided ART.) Many facilities are supplied by more than one program, as was the case at Mukuju Health Centre.

6

The Struggle for a Public Sector

PEPFAR in Mozambique

JAMES PFEIFFER

The President's Emergency Program for AIDS Relief (PEPFAR) has significantly transformed the global health landscape by injecting US$15 billion into HIV/AIDS care and treatment programs in twenty countries between 2004–2010. In Mozambique, PEPFAR funds constituted nearly 60 percent of all health sector planned spending by 2008 (HPG 2007). While debates about PEPFAR's restrictions on condom promotion, sex worker education programs, and abortion/reproductive health have dominated critiques of the program, perhaps the single most important aspect of PEPFAR's rollout has largely escaped scrutiny in the wider global discussion: PEPFAR funding, by design, does not directly flow through the public sector. While there are occasional exceptions, this massive injection of new funds is mostly being channeled to international nongovernmental organizations (NGOs) rather than to public sector health systems. While the funding is certainly welcomed by the public health community, the sheer scale of PEPFAR financing, which is set to jump to over US$60 billion in the next five years, means that the choice to bypass public sector players and to support foreign NGOs instead has major consequences for African self-determination, for the future of public sector health systems, and for human rights–based approaches to citizenship and health.

The diversion of such a large-scale resource away from a national health system and into transitory and unsustainable NGO projects represents a potentially tragic missed opportunity to build lasting local public-sector health institutions, unless this approach can be corrected in the next five-year phase of the initiative. I will argue here that developing the kind of "people-centered" and rights-based approaches to the AIDS epidemic that we as anthropologists attentive to the social and physical suffering of patients and communities might propose can only be realistically imagined in the context of an at least minimally functional and effective public sector—and this holds true not for health care alone, but also for education, agricultural support, transport, social action, and other social safety nets. However, PEPFAR has been rolled out within the constraints imposed by structural adjustment programs (SAPs) and the broader neoliberal shift in Africa. As Jean Comaroff (2007:197) points out, "In retrospect, the timing of its [AIDS'] onset was uncanny: the disease appeared like a *memento mori* in a world high on the hype of Reaganomics, deregulation, and the end of the Cold War." Likewise, the response to the epidemic has been determined and constrained by its coincidence with the neoliberal assault on the public sector, that is, with the radical scaling back and defunding of government programs that has been operationalized through SAPs (now euphemistically relabeled Poverty Reduction Strategy Papers, or PRSPs; see also Pfeiffer and Chapman 2010). The political economy of the PEPFAR phenomenon, its entanglement with the broader neoliberal project (especially with structural adjustment), its dominant position in the flow of resources from rich to poor countries, and its impact on health care for the poor can be no more poignantly illustrated than in Mozambique where the organization I work for, Health Alliance International (HAI, a US-based NGO), has been engaged in support for primary health care for over twenty years. HAI had been the designated PEPFAR "partner" for central Mozambique for the first five-year period in three central provinces, its mission being to help scale up HIV/AIDS care and treatment. I worked for HAI Mozambique in the 1990s as its country director, and in 2004 I returned to HAI as the director of Mozambique projects, based at the University of Washington, Seattle. In that position I have helped coordinate the development and implementation of HAI's programs funded by PEPFAR, the Global Fund to Fight AIDS, Tuberculosis and Malaria, the World Bank, the William J. Clinton Presidential Foundation, the Doris Duke Charitable Foundation, and other major grants supporting HIV/AIDS treatment scale-up and primary health care. As a global health practitioner and anthropologist deeply involved in the pragmatics of service delivery, I will draw on this firsthand experience in Mozambique to describe the tension, conflict, and potentials created by these new major aid flows to Africa.

Scaling up Antiretroviral Treatment in Mozambique: A Brief History

Mozambique's HIV epidemic is especially alarming as it is unfolding in one of the poorest and largest countries in southern Africa, a region that is characterized by extraordinarily high prevalence rates—in Botswana, Swaziland, South Africa, Zimbabwe, Malawi, and Zambia, as well as in Mozambique. While Mozambique's national HIV prevalence is currently about 11.5 percent, provincial rates in the center and south of the country range between 15 and 25 percent. In the city of Beira, prevalence may be as high as 35 percent (Mozambique Ministry of Health 2009). Mozambique remains one of the poorest countries in the world, with one of the lowest healthworker-to-population ratios and most inadequate local resources to combat the epidemic (WHO 2006).

Concerted HIV testing efforts were only initiated in 2001, while prevention of mother-to-child transmission (PMTCT) services began in 2002. The scale-up of antiretroviral treatment (ART) in Mozambique finally began in 2004, using the WHO "public health" approach, with support from PEPFAR, the Clinton Foundation, the World Bank, and the Global Fund, among numerous other donors. A "business plan" was drawn up by the MOH with technical support from outside agencies, including HAI. As in other African settings, the eventual embrace of an ART scale-up strategy resulted from a struggle between those in the development community who argued that it was simply not "cost-effective" and would fail, and those who fought for ART in Africa as a moral commitment and human rights issue (cf. Farmer 2001). The Clinton Foundation's success in negotiating lower drug prices from generic producers provided a final impetus for Mozambique to sign on—a decision politically promoted by then Prime Minister Pascoal Mocumbi and then Minister of Health Francisco Songane. The scale-up was to be implemented primarily through the public-sector National Health System and would be provided for free, since Mozambique has very few commercial private providers (a legacy of its recent socialist past). Mozambique had quickly embraced the Alma Ata primary health care concept after achieving independence in the late 1970s and constructed a national health system that brought basic services to its poor majority throughout the country for the first time (Walt and Melamed 1983). However, PEPFAR funding for Mozambique would not flow directly to the government health system but rather would be provided primarily to NGO partners and charities, which would manage the resources in presumed collaboration with local health authorities.

While other bilateral donors tended to contribute to "basket funding" jointly managed with the Ministry, PEPFAR had been the outlier among donors, insisting on nongovernment targets for support. PEPFAR could not completely avoid the public system, since the vast majority of services are provided by the Ministry, but its projects and partners have been awkwardly grafted onto the public system—especially in the provision of drugs. The initial PEPFAR approach was also highly "verticalized"; it focused narrowly on the scale-up of HIV services only and avoided addressing either the larger needs of the health system or the broader social concerns of the hundreds of thousands of extremely poor patients targeted for treatment. (See discussions of the limits of vertical approaches in Frenk 2006; England 2007; Maeseneer et al. 2008; Coetzee et al. 2004.) This resulted in the creation of parallel medical supply, data collection, and management systems dedicated only to HIV. These shortcomings notwithstanding, the initial scale-up success—tens of thousands were placed on treatment in the first year and nearly 180,000 (40 percent of those eligible for treatment) were on ART nationwide as of March 2010—was viewed accurately as a major public health success. Several years earlier, when drug prices were still high and political commitment questionable, few had imagined so many Mozambicans successfully initiating ART; indeed, by 2008 the number of Mozambicans on ART exceeded even the most optimistic official projections in the 2004 business plan. PEPFAR clearly provided vital political impetus and resources to make treatment a reality in Mozambique and much of Africa.

In spite of the initial success, drawbacks to the vertical/technical NGO approach became apparent very quickly in Mozambique (Pfeiffer and Chapman 2010). Most visibly and dramatically, the vertical approach managed primarily by NGOs resulted in twenty-three new ART-focused "day hospitals" constructed beside crumbling primary health care infrastructure in existing public urban health system compounds. The imbalances were disruptive. Day hospital staff were often paid better than other health workers, NGOs often used expatriate doctors to provide clinical care, and basic materials and equipment were plentiful compared to the other sections of the health system. Additional data gathering tools and systems to collect information for PEPFAR were set up in parallel to the struggling and under-resourced Ministry Health Information System. Extensive specialized HIV trainings were conducted with health staff, who were taken away from other basic duties. Other HIV-related services were also vertically organized, with freestanding VCT (Volunteer Counseling and Testing) sites in communities and vertical PMTCT programs awkwardly imposed on pre-existing and struggling antenatal care services in the public system.

In principle, the ART scale-up was being grafted onto the public-sector national health system, but in practice each NGO partner tasked with the scale-up in their region had a different approach to collaborating with the Ministry, staffing clinics, collecting data, selecting a geographical focus, and providing services. The result was a fragmented approach that has been typical of PEPFAR countries across Africa. In response to these challenges, the Ministry began in 2006 to promote "integration" of HIV testing and ART into other primary health care services in Mozambique (Pfeiffer and Chapman 2010). This meant moving away from the larger day hospital model and instead training and equipping staff at smaller health centers and posts to provide HIV care and ART. Staff in TB wards and Antenatal Care (ANC) services were to be trained in HIV testing and counseling, CD4 testing, and initiating ART. Staff in other inpatient and outpatient services were trained in testing and referrals to ART services, and in the recognition of opportunistic infections. The provinces in the center of the country, where HAI works, were among the first to initiate the integration process. HAI's model is to collaborate very closely at the provincial level with the Ministry of Health to strengthen rather than substitute for their systems, and this allowed HAI to use PEPFAR funds to help expand ART access at dozens of smaller health units distributed across each province (see figure 6.1).

Mozambique's ten provinces are the key organizational divisions through which primary health care (PHC) services are managed, coordinated, and brought to scale. Transport, drug and material distribution, supervision, and data collection systems are organized administratively and logistically by the province and must also be strengthened and harmonized at that level if integration is to succeed. If limited to isolated sites or districts, integration would be ineffective and unsustainable, since it would be disconnected from provincial system strengthening. The vertical or NGO-led approaches that focused narrowly on single sites or small geographic areas had great difficulty in broadening access geographically and expanding to many new sites, since the administrative logic of the public system had been ignored.

Even though PEPFAR funds were being used to help integrate and decentralize ART and HIV care, the fundamentals of the system remained unsupported. The health workforce stayed small, training institutions were expanded much too slowly, and the transport and basic administrative systems were inadequate to accommodate hundreds of thousands of new patients. Even more concerning, many PEPFAR-funded NGOs recruited clinical staff, including doctors, directly out of the public service, further weakening that system and creating an internal brain drain of staff from the public to the private sphere (Mussa 2009). Mozambique, at the time of writing, was at a crossroads after five years of ART scale-up, while new five-year tranches of PEPFAR funding were being allocated under a new US administration.

PEPFAR, AIDS, and Structural Adjustment

The dilemmas Mozambique now faces in addressing its AIDS epidemic can only be understood if one appreciates how twenty years of structural adjustment policies have intersected with PEPFAR initiatives. During a lengthy war (that ended in 1992) with an apartheid South Africa–backed insurgency known as RENAMO that began after the struggle for inde-

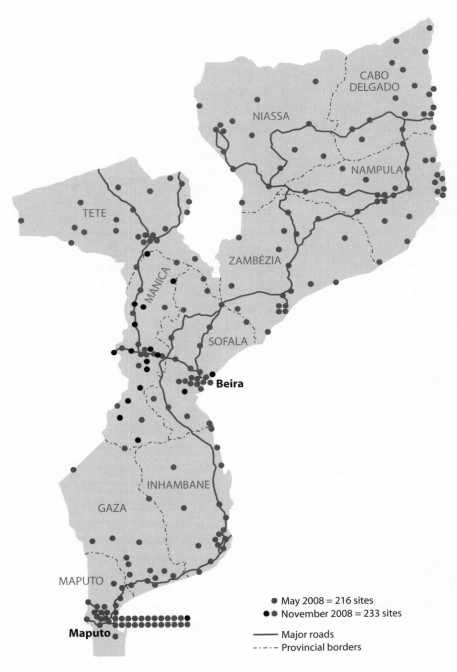

Figure 6.1

pendence from Portugal in 1975, sweeping changes in social and economic life were introduced through a World Bank/IMF structural adjustment program initiated in 1987. Rapid class differentiation (in contrast to the postindependence socialist period), glaring economic disparities, and growing corruption emerged over a very brief period, as the SAP (Structural Adjustment Program) pressed for privatization of public services and industries, cuts in the budgets for health and education, removal of price subsidies for food and fuel, the scaling back of other social safety nets, and cutbacks in social services (Cliff 1991; Fauvet 2000; Hanlon 1996; Pitcher 2002). These initiatives were accelerated after the ceasefire in 1992, as the society returned to life without war. However, with the loss of aid from socialist countries, the government's turn away from socialism to the IMF's market fundamentalism, and budget cuts in the health sector, increasing numbers of foreign aid agencies and NGOs began to descend on Mozambique in the late 1980s and early 1990s.

A large proportion of health-sector aid from donors was being redirected to NGOs as state services contracted under the SAP. Much of the foreign funding that was still channeled to the National Health Service (NHS) came in the form of project aid directed toward specific donor-identified objectives rather than broader health system strengthening. By the early 1990s, nearly 100 agencies were spread throughout the country supporting the health sector (Hanlon 1996). By 1996, there were 405 individual projects managed by these agencies within the NHS. While many projects were integrated into NHS programs, Mozambicans often did not have genuine control over budgets or project development (Cliff 1993; Hanlon 1996; Pfeiffer 2003).

By the late 1990s, the NHS was dependent on international donors for about 50 percent of its recurrent expenditures and 90 percent of capital expenditures from international donors (Pavignani and Durão 1999), but IMF conditionalities prevented the flow of aid to "on-budget" needs. Perhaps most concerning, these conditionalities, and specifically the hiring caps they imposed on the public sector, prevented the training and hiring of significant numbers of new health staff (see Rowden 2009 for additional explanation of IMF practices around wage-bill ceilings). The Mozambique health system still has one of the lowest healthworker-to-population ratios in the world. With only three doctors and twenty-one nurses per 100,000 population (WHO 2006), the capacity to scale up

ART effectively has been severely constrained. The MOH budget for recurrent costs and training institutions remains anemic, starving the dilapidated infrastructure, logistics, and transport systems of desperately needed support and human resources. Ministry program directors struggle to coordinate and plan around the chaotic donor and NGO pet projects whose funds and resources bypass Mozambican control. While the level of PEPFAR funding is unprecedented, it has done little to alleviate the basic constraints on the national health system itself.

Over the postwar period Mozambique has been slowly rebuilding, and by the end of the 1990s it was hailed for its relatively robust economic growth, attributed in part to the impact of the SAP (cf. World Bank 2002). However, the Bank's triumphalist claims over the national GDP figures have concealed a growing inequality that has left most Mozambicans mired in poverty (Ministry of Planning and Finance 1998; Hanlon 1996; INE 1998). Recently published data from the national Rural Income Survey (Hanlon 2010; Ministry of Planning and Development 2010) confirmed what many observers have suspected. From 2002 to 2008, mean total income increased while median total income fell. In other words, most people became poorer, but the best off became richer. The total income of the richest 10 percent is forty-four times that of the poorest 10 percent (up from only twenty-three times in 2002 and thirty-five times in 2005). Child malnutrition rates have remained the same since the end of the war in spite of a decade of economic growth.

Over this same period, international aid, mostly for health and HIV through PEPFAR, has quadrupled. The initiation of new programs as complex and resource intensive as HIV care has of course created huge new stresses on the system, as hundreds of thousands of chronically ill patients stream through. However, even with this surge of resources from PEPFAR and other donors, IMF conditionalities on debt relief continue and are operationalized through the blandly named Medium Term Expenditure Framework (MTEF). The MTEF is the instrument through which caps on civil service hiring are imposed, as well as limits on recurrent budget spending and training institution investment (see Rowden 2009). The result is an ART scale-up with millions of new dollars flowing into the health sector but little support for the building blocks of the health system that make the scale-up possible: most glaringly human resources, but also laboratories, supply chains, data collection systems, transport, and bricks and mortar. The health system at the time of this writing had over 180,000 patients on ART cycling through it on a regular basis, creating a patient volume and flow that is unprecedented. The numbers are projected to increase since an additional 200,000 are estimated to be ART eligible.

Figure 6.1 shows the distribution of ART sites across the country; it is impressive but does not reveal the striking differences in how the services are provided and by whom. In some provinces, various NGOs support different clinics with widely disparate linkages to the national system. Some districts and clinics continue to receive ten to twenty times the support that others of similar patient volume receive. At HAI-supported sites, HIV-positive ART activists had worked closely with clinics to follow up with patients in the community, but the Ministry was unable to absorb these workers because of funding restrictions. At some clinics comanaged by other NGOs, some higher-level clinical staff are expatriates, while other partners focus on clinical mentoring of Mozambican health system staff. In some provinces, provincial supply systems are so weak that NGOs simply substitute for them. In several instances, NGOs or donors had chosen to create showcase clinics in remote areas with large-scale investments, while clinics in neighboring districts atrophied.

Ethnography of ART and the Public Sector: A View from the Community and the Patient

While adherence rates were initially impressive, they now appear to be deteriorating in many regions as stresses on the system become increasingly apparent. The most troubling problem so far from a health systems perspective has been the stubbornly high "lost to follow-up" (LTFU) rate of patients who test positive. Up to 50 percent of those testing positive at VCT sites did not follow up with referrals for HIV care. The problem has been especially acute among pregnant women. At some antenatal care sites where HIV testing is routine, up to 70 percent of HIV-positive mothers either do not register for care and treatment or are lost further along the treatment "cascade." Disentangling the systemic versus community-based factors that influence LTFU and patient flow has been a challenge in the sites where HAI worked in central Mozambique. The best answers would likely come from a closer ethnographic look at the lives and experiences of HIV-positive Mozambicans so that implementation of "people-centered" approaches could strengthen public services and enable them to become more responsive to the extraordinary struggles of their beneficiaries. But more broadly, how has the NGO-centered vertical approach taken by PEPFAR influenced LTFU, access, and adherence challenges? The first qualitative and ethnographic accounts from the three provinces where HAI worked are just now being completed as a result of several qualitative and exploratory studies on adherence and PMTCT. What emerges is that LTFU is, in part, a product of both a struggling, understaffed, and fragmented public-sector health system, and an undermined public sector for other services and safety nets.

High lost to follow-up rates remind us of critical influences on the epidemic that lie beyond the health care sector and now stand out in high relief after five years of treatment scale-up. As in much of Africa, LTFU among pregnant women continues to be perhaps the major concern. Mozambique recently embraced an integrated antenatal services approach in which, in addition to routine ANC services, women receive opt-out HIV testing, CD4 counts, and ART at some sites. HAI, working together with its provincial health system partners, was among the first to roll out this approach at Ministry sites. As a result LTFU has been greatly reduced at those facilities, but it remains unacceptably high. A qualitative study recently completed by HAI has begun to give some clues as to why pregnant women disappear from the system at such high rates (Thome 2010). Certain predictable "usual suspects" emerged from interviews, such as distance and transport problems and migration out of catchment areas. However, the transport challenge seems to be a more nuanced barrier than was previously thought. Most poor women in Mozambique have virtually no access to cash, so getting transport often requires asking others for money, usually spouses, while concealing the reason for the need. Money had to be provided to pay for private minibus fare in most cases. But even with cash in hand, many women still confronted the terrible dilemma of deciding whether to use the money to pay for transport or to buy food for themselves or their children. Making it to follow-up appointments often involved trade-offs between potential disclosure to others to obtain cash for transport or foregoing a meal. If transport was secured, women complained of long waiting periods and rude treatment by overworked health staff. Our interviews, combined with other ethnographies of pregnancy in Mozambique (Chapman 2003), remind us that pregnancy is a time of great physical and social vulnerability for poor women, and many choose to hide their pregnancies to protect themselves from perceived social threats, HIV-positive or not. Adding the stigma of HIV into the mix leads at least some women to disappear even more quickly from the system than they otherwise might. Given these circumstances, it is not difficult to understand why transport expenses, long waiting periods, poor treatment by staff, and a fear of spousal rebuke or violence might lead to a decision to drop out.

Among other adults testing positive, the long series of visits needed to initiate treatment (it takes an average of three months from testing to treatment initiation) requires money for transport, involves regular threats of disclosure, and is difficult to comply with since migration in and out of catchment areas heavily influences decisions to follow up. Once treatment is begun, new challenges emerge that point to perhaps the single biggest shortfall in the global response to the African AIDS crisis: food security. Some have called the hunger caused by AIDS a "new variant famine" (de Waal and Whiteside 2003). In HAI's recent qualitative adherence study based on interviews with over 100 patients, access to food emerged as the single greatest challenge faced in staying on treatment (Lara 2009). The problem is especially severe for women, who are often responsible for daily meals in their households. Once treatment starts, the body rebounds and has additional nutritional requirements. Patients describe an almost intolerable hunger that develops. For many, the medications cause severe side effects if taken without food, especially after several days without a meal. But many ART patients have lost their incomes or source of food because of their illness, which compounds the trauma of the experience. Because of extreme poverty, the skipping of meals is common in Mozambique, and patients describe dropping out of treatment because it is so difficult to obtain the food necessary to make the treatment tolerable. Trade-offs between paying for transport to appointments, medications at pharmacies, and food are also a perennial dilemma for many of these patients.

To be sure, efforts at nutritional support for patients have been funded by PEPFAR and other donors, but these remain strikingly inadequate. In provinces where HAI works, the World Food Programme had partnered with HAI to provide food through a handful of warehouses where food supplies, mostly from the United States, are delivered by a system modeled on emergency response. Patients in towns who meet social criteria were provided with a voucher that entitled them to visit the local warehouse to pick up a sack of flour or other limited goods. Patients only received these benefits for three months, however, and the system was dysfunctional from the start, with myriad logistical challenges and late deliveries of rotten or inappropriate food. As the depths of the food security problem became more evident nationally, a new voucher system was rolled out by the MOH in some areas, in which eligible patients receive a coupon that can be used at local participating stores to purchase a nutritious and diverse "food basket." The approach represents a modest attempt at a type of safety net and is supported by major donors, but it has yet to be evaluated and the rollout has been slow because of difficulties in arranging trainings for health staff, recruiting local merchants to participate, and challenges in the logistics required for setting up the voucher system itself.

Innovative Solutions

The delivery of ART and other HIV-care services requiring complex and multiple interactions with patients in extreme poverty over long periods presents novel challenges to African primary health care systems, challenges that can only be met by reconstituting the public services and public programs that have been dismantled by structural adjustment over the last several decades. We cannot hope for a more humane and responsive health workforce as long as it is understaffed, underpaid, and overworked. New innovative programs and initiatives will be unsustainable unless there are workers to implement them, and the workforce can only be expanded through major investment in training institutions and increases in salaries. Long waits and poor service will continue as long as basic administrative systems are not supported. Community health workers are essential to provide community-based outreach and to promote the social support needed for patients to remain on treatment, and they should be trained and paid through a public system that is prepared to manage them in order to guarantee coverage, equity, and sustainability (Mukherjee and Eustache 2007).

Outside the health care system itself, food insecurity is the norm in poor populations, and it is especially severe for those with AIDS. While the new food voucher system is a helpful though modest form of social protection, it is hardly a solution to the wider hunger crisis, a crisis that has deepened with AIDS even while Mozambique's economy has grown briskly. The AIDS "new variant famine" underscores the urgent need for public food subsidy systems and price protections that were eliminated decades earlier by structural adjustment. Local farming cooperatives and home garden collectives, also eliminated by adjustment, should be reconstituted with public-sector support to provide local food safety nets. Clearly the public education system requires massive additional investment throughout Africa, if the rich world's commitment to fight AIDS is to be taken seriously.

This list of remedies may not be innovative, but it identifies elements necessary for a foundation on which further innovation in social approaches to health and new technologies may be built. There is a risk that as the global health and international aid communities recognize challenges to expanding and maintaining AIDS treatment in Africa, the call will be for new innovative technologies and new innovative approaches that can cope with severe "resource constraints." (Lack of resources is still asserted by many as an a priori assumption, even in the age of a $60 billion PEPFAR AIDS package.) A call for innovation has, in fact, been the focus of global health agenda-setters such as the Gates Foundation and others (Birn 2005b). But is it possible that a focus on innovation might distract us from the more fundamental challenge at hand? The basic strengthening of public institutions, services, and safety nets requires a reinvestment in well-known fundamentals, not necessarily new innovations in programs, and it requires, specifically, a rejection of structural adjustment such as is now happening in much of Latin America (Paluzzi and Garcia 2008).

An NGO Code of Conduct?

Meaningful improvements do not have to wait for large-scale political change. There are smaller, more immediately possible interim steps and actions that can be taken to make AIDS treatment more "people-centered" under prevailing conditions. Innovation is most badly needed in approaches to advocacy for strengthening public systems and promoting a health commons in the current environment. A recently proposed "NGO Code of Conduct for Health System Strengthening" advanced by a consortium of NGOs is one modest example of such an advocacy strategy (Pfeiffer et al. 2008). The proposed code calls for foreign NGOs to adopt practices that 1) avoid luring the local staff of public-sector health systems to their projects, 2) support local Ministry priority setting and close coordination with public-sector providers, 3) avoid creation of parallel services and systems of health care delivery, and 4) advocate for debt relief and increased public-sector spending. Well-funded NGOs can be pressed to avoid the temptation to go it alone so as to achieve quick but unsustainable results, and to commit instead to working collaboratively with local ministries to strengthen their systems on their terms. These efforts may involve finding innovative ways to channel NGO funds into ministry budgets and pay for additional health staff. NGOs can learn how to negotiate with their donors around results and expectations that square with longer-term support for the public sector. NGO workers and other advocates can have meaningful impact in the local donor country offices of, say, the World Bank or USAID, pressuring them to work more collaboratively with local public sectors. HAI's experience in Mozambique has shown that thoughtful in-country PEPFAR staff often have the authority and insight to support the public option within their policy constraints. Local coalitions among NGOs and like-minded donors in Mozambique successfully forced the initial PEPFAR program in 2004 to back down from their preconceived approach to drug supply and to follow instead the previously developed Ministry plan. Innovative approaches to working with local communities to mobilize for greater government service accountability have the potential to pressure governments and international donors to improve public programs. (South Africa provides a more recent example of this kind of activism.)

Anthropologists have a potentially valuable role to play in moving donors and PEPFAR toward a more public focus and a people-centered approach. The gulf between those with experience of PEPFAR programs on the ground and higher-level donors and policymakers is vast. The recent emphasis in global health circles on "operations research" and "implementation science" (Madon et al. 2007), methods adapted primarily from industrial engineering, will help focus on system strengthening. But the continued domination of "behavior change" and "social marketing" approaches to community engagement suggests again a technocratic and top-down approach that may obscure the view from below that is vital to reorienting the current narrow focus of most ART scale-up efforts. Engaged anthropologists, in our roles as interlocutors, are needed to gather the stories of those on treatment and strategically relay them to the global health community in language that is accessible to a wider audience. Anthropologists should not shy away from an advocacy role, but could and should develop innovative ways to convey their insights both to policymakers and to the emerging social movements pressing for more accountable public services in many African countries. Bottom-up and longitudinal ethnographic studies of AIDS treatment in Africa can provide a badly needed corrective to the current dominant ART narrative that ignores the public-private funding dilemma and that does not address concerns about food, education, and social safety nets so crucial to treatment efforts.

Anthropologists can help relay the stories of African health workers who carry the weight of the AIDS treatment project without the systemic support they need and deserve. A recent HAI-supported qualitative study of health worker attitudes toward foreign aid in Mozambique revealed a surprisingly deep resentment and frustration with NGO and foreign technical assistance that ignores day-to-day work needs (Mussa 2009). A greater appreciation for the struggles of these frontline public-sector health workers in Africa, whose voices and wisdom are rarely appreciated by global health leaders, would help underscore the urgency of donor support for basic systems.

Anthropologists can continue to lead in exploring notions of therapeutic citizenship, human rights, and health that highlight the central importance of a health commons and public sector. The surge of resources for health brought about by PEPFAR has dramatically altered the calculus and sense of possibility in global health broadly, and in Africa specifically. The experience so far brings into high relief the choices and dilemmas the public health community faces—and some of those choices are stark in their consequences. Increased funding has mobilized many vested interests, such as pharmaceutical companies, NGOs, universities, and foundations, while belying the "resource constraint" claims that have justified the "cost-effectiveness" approaches that guided public health in the era of adjustment. In this state of high agitation in global health, major progress and innovation are possible—but only if we maintain a focus on the resurrection of a public-sector health commons as the pathway to human rights and health for all.

7

The Next Epidemic

Pain and the Politics of Relief in Botswana's Cancer Ward

JULIE LIVINGSTON

This chapter looks closely at some of the more fine-grained processes of clinical care in order to suggest how cancer, as an emergent issue in African public health, forces longstanding questions of palliation to the foreground and highlights the intensely social nature of pain.[1] I will explore the conditions that facilitate the marginalization of pain and palliation in African clinical practice and in global health more widely, and I will examine the contemporary clinical dynamics that engender this marginalization in the specific context of oncology, where many patients suffer severe and intractable pain, as a result either of their illness or the effects of biomedical therapies. In other words, this essay is an exploration of how and why biomedicine proceeds in Africa with so little palliation and so much compliance.

The context for this ethnography is Botswana's lone cancer ward, where I have been researching conditions of care since 2006. The ward opened in late 2001 in Princess Marina Hospital (PMH), Botswana's central referral hospital, in anticipation of the cancer that would follow the scaling up of the national antiretroviral (ARV) program. At the time Botswana had the highest reported prevalence of HIV in the world and was initiating what would become the first public ARV program in Africa.

Pain is a capacious category of experience, and in what follows I will remain tightly focused around cancer-associated pain. I will not make claims about any other forms of pain, which may have different moral valences, engender different phenomenological experiences, and carry different social effects. In any event, cancer pain is quite a worthy site of investigation in contemporary Botswana. A cancer epidemic is emerging rapidly in the country, and this appears to be a trend across the continent.[2] Botswana now boasts higher reported incidence rates of certain cancers (e.g., cancers of the esophagus, cancers of the cervix, and Kaposi's sarcoma) than the United States, and in 2003 *Lancet Oncology* reported a projected rise in cancer rates across Africa of 400 percent over the next five decades.[3] A more recent study reports that "even leaving aside the huge load of AIDS-related Kaposi's sarcoma, a woman living in present-day Uganda (Kampala) or Zimbabwe (Harare) has a chance of developing a cancer by the age of sixty-five that is only about 30 percent lower than that of a woman in Western Europe, and her probability of dying from a cancer by this age is almost twice as high."[4]

Thanks to the widespread public provision of antiretroviral drugs, many patients in Botswana are now surviving their HIV disease only to find themselves grappling with viral-associated cancers facilitated by their history of immunosuppression.[5] This unfortunate by-product of the otherwise marked success of Africa's first national antiretroviral program couples with the significant burden of other cancers already prevalent in the population to create a situation of overwhelming proportions. The biological and clinical challenges of oncology in the face of HIV are tremendous, as are the technical challenges of providing meaningful cancer care in an essentially ad hoc clinical setting, and the public health challenges that an emerging epidemic of cancer poses for a health system with extremely limited screening capacities.[6] Profound pain highlights one critical aspect of these difficulties. Many of Botswana's cancer patients have aggressive and advanced disease. Such cancers are often relentlessly painful, and clinicians may respond to them with therapies that are deeply aversive.[7] At the same time, because such patients are understood to be very sick, and because many of them become known to clinical staff through cyclical visits and hospitalizations, the ethic of palliation that holds in the cancer ward is unique in the hospital and in the broader health system.

A focus on pain in such a ward suggests how ethnography at the coal-face of clinical care helps to sharpen and contextualize the complexities of drug policy, while also reminding us that biomedicine is localized practice as much as it is a global system of thought and technology.[8] While the chemical tools of palliation are standard, the circulation of drugs and the politics and logics of palliation vary tremendously across clinical contexts. For example, in the modern United States, the issue of doubt is at the center of the long and thorny history of pain politics and often hinges on fears of malingering and/or opiate addiction.[9] Botswana's oncology ward points us in other directions, suggesting the need for a very different sort of pain politics than one that focuses on gate-keeping individual access to an assumed supply of palliative technologies, or on developing new analgesics. As Human Rights Watch has documented, though cancer rates are rising, widespread shortages, and in many cases the outright absence of strong pain relief are the norm across Botswana and much of the global south, and it is on this issue that African pain politics should focus.[10]

This focus on doubt that drives American pain politics is also at the center of Elaine Scarry's now famous proposition that pain is an individually held experience, one that "shatters language."[11] Scarry found that pain simultaneously produces certainty in the person in pain and doubt in the onlooker, a dynamic of witnessing (and even inflicting) from which a series of ethical problems around what to do about pain cascades. She goes on to examine these ethical problems of *doing* in part through an examination of a wide variety of texts, including writings on torture and war, scripture, memoirs, and Marx, all the while rendering pain as an object located in an individually bounded body.

Yet this conceptualization is ill suited to capture the logics of pain and the processes of palliation on Botswana's oncology ward, and I suspect in many other places as well. In conversations with Tswana healers I found that it was nearly impossible to talk about pain as pain—to imbue it with ontological import, to construct it as an object. Pain, it seemed, could not be separated out. Invariably, it collapsed back into its underlying pathology, which in Tswana medicine is necessarily a social pathology. This total situatedness of pain, its refusal to be separated from the flow of pathological social experience, is meaningful and helps us move from the problem that doubt presents to the social effects of certainty.[12]

The oncology ward is an intensely social space, one where doubt is simply not at the center of the problem around "doing" that pain presents. As we will see in what follows, everyone knows with certainty that drilling into a patient's bone marrow or sawing off a patient's leg produces pain, and yet this pain, which is caused in order to heal, is often seemingly ignored as it is being inflicted. In taking a social approach to pain I am in sympathy with anthropologist Talal Asad's ideas about the body, agency, and pain, which contrast with Scarry's proposition. In moving from text to experience, from the specificity of torture to broader categories of social interaction, Asad does not see pain as an object to be overcome by an agentive individual. Instead, he argues that pain is a relationship. Asad acknowledges that the somatic experiences of injured persons cannot be fully accessed by observers, but he reminds us that this is not all there is to pain. He writes, "Sufferers are also social persons (animals) and their suffering is partly constituted by the way they inhabit, or are constrained to inhabit, their relationship with others."[13] In other words, pain begs a response. In order to take a close-up view of these social dynamics of pain and palliation, I am going to offer an unfortunately somewhat grisly excerpt from my ethnographic field notes.

After the Amputation

Field Notes: January 25, 2007

A Kaposi's sarcoma patient, M. This man is in his 30s—he was amputated above the knee on the 15th. We are on ward rounds visiting cancer patients in men's surgical and he requests to see Dr P. Dr P asks for him to be brought to the oncology clinic after rounds. I remember the meeting before the amputation, and how M (accompanied by his sister) willingly agreed to rid himself of the swollen, rotting, and now useless leg. Later in the morning M arrives in oncology from the men's surgical ward in a wheelchair with an orderly. He is in CRAZY pain. His eyes are bulging and rolling and he is pouring sweat. He is in agony. (I looked later at his medical card—he was originally given pethidine 100 mgs then tapering to

50 mgs, and then codeine for a few days, and now for about a week he has been given ibuprofen only).[14]

He is anxious and he tells Dr P, they want to push me out—to send me home! But I can't manage. There is a problem with the leg. You can even smell it. Dr P tries to touch up high on the stump and M cringes in agony. Silent—but in agony nonetheless. I am on the edge of my seat, cringing, and wondering if I should say something about the obvious pain. Dr P seems cognizant of the pain, but not particularly interested in it. Intense. At one point he absently places his hand on M's thigh as a sign of compassion, and M recoils with force. Dr P has him unwind the bandage and show the wound—M is squirming in pain as he does it and as he gets down to the last layer of gauze he is really crying out short breathy sounds. Eesh! Tjo Tjo Tjo!! With force. It is unbearable and it is just coming out of his mouth involuntarily. Then as he gets to the point of exposing the wound it is too much and he can't go on. I fear he will pass out. I can see that Dr P is a bit impatient, and I know why. There is a tremendous queue of patients waiting for him (the only oncologist), many of them are very ill, and this is taking a long time. Besides, it is a surgical problem not the KS that is causing this.

So Dr P calls for a nurse and Mma L comes. Dr P asks her to take M to the treatment room across the hall and take off the bandage with water, because it is stuck to the wound. And please give 75 mgs pethidine first. As you can see it is very painful. Mma L glances over at M and protests that she is covering the ward and she can't also be here. Dr P asks where is Mma M who should be here? Mma M has gone on tea break. A little debate and then Mma L agrees to do it. But she wants Dr P to put the pethidine order in the hospital card. He says he will do it later. No, you must do it first. All the while I am squirming, feeling like I am the only one with a sense of urgency about the pain here. I also feel like M must be SO freaked out to see his leg like this. He is only 10 days after the surgery. Who knows how he is currently making sense of the trauma of profound disfigurement.

We leave and go to the private ward to see another patient. When we return Dr P is about to eat a peach for his impromptu tea when Mma T says No, don't eat that. You need to go and look at the leg in the treatment room first. What? It will make me vomit—I won't want to eat afterwards. So we have some joking. Dr P quickly finishes his peach and washes his hands.

We enter the treatment room and M's stump is covered with a piece of gauze just resting on it. M is still sweating and his eyes are still bulging, but he is calmer after the pethidine. Dr P lifts the gauze and exposes the wound. It has completely burst the sutures—the jagged end of the bone is jutting out like a roast beef and it is all totally infected, swollen, white rotting meat. They failed to disarticulate the bone during the surgery.[15] He can't possibly be discharged. Nor should he be transferred to oncology—he needs to be re-amputated immediately—and as Dr A later says, the remainder of the femur removed and the wound closed. I am appalled! Dr P less so. Dr A comes in and is a bit dazed by it—asking if we've seen it (did he say "it"? Or did he say "the guy with the KS amputation"? Or did he say "M"?) and then commenting on how dangerous this is. I remember this patient—I remember M—he had accepted the need for amputation and was almost cheerful about it—now this. If I were his relative I would be through the roof. *Go ferosa sebete.*

Pain Management in Botswana

My purpose in presenting this very visceral incident is not to exploit poor M for theatrical purposes, and I confess that I feel a bit uncomfortable about exposing the intimacies of his vulnerability. Yet given how abstract (and in doubt, cf. Scarry) the pain of others can be, I fear that ethnography of this sort is necessary here in order that you might begin to imagine what it would be like to be in extreme and serious bodily distress, groping for some sort of communicative possibility that will bring relief to you, and this in an institutional setting where the mechanisms of relief are closely controlled, and where the nearest thing to a relative or friend you have—someone actually invested in you—is (you hope) this German oncologist. And at the same time I am also asking you to imagine being a nurse or a doctor in a chronically overwhelmed hospital, a decade into an AIDS epidemic in which you have seen untold suffering and death.

What are we to make of this decidedly African scene, with its German oncologist (Dr P) in a profoundly overcrowded urban hospital named for a European princess? Setting aside the clinical issue of how M's amputation went so wrong, we are left with his pain. Where were the pain charts of smiling and frowning faces, and the 1-to-5 pain scales we see in contemporary American and European hospitals?[16] How is it possible that someone in such obvious distress was not given pain medicine sooner? Why was it that M drew attention to the smell of his leg, but did not complain of his substantial pain? Why did I (and perhaps you) feel such discomfort at M's obvious pain, while the clinical staff seemed significantly less affected, even though Dr P and the oncology nurses were caring people and passionate about their work? How and why did M manage to stay so relatively calm and quiet in the face of such agony? Why is it that almost every patient leaves the hospital or clinic with a packet of paracetamol or ibuprofen—whether he or she needs it or not—yet many clinical staff are reluctant to use opioids even for patients who are dying, despite longstanding WHO protocols encouraging their use? How could we be joking and laughing about this human leg of rotting meat while enjoying a peach?

It is ironic that biomedicine proceeds in Africa with so little palliation, given that pain is what propels many patients into clinics and (often iatrogenic) hospital spaces. Health planners go to great lengths to encourage patients to go to biomedical sites rather than "traditional" healers, yet they seem generally (there are exceptions) to ignore the role of pain, this fundamental bodily experience, as a motivation for seeking help. The sheer force of pain has many swimming upstream in an overwrought health system. True, there is now an African palliative care movement. The Botswana Ministry of Health has been developing palliative care guidelines, as have other governments that are following WHO recommendations. But so much has been pushed under the palliative care rubric—from the writing of wills to the provision of soap and basic nutrition—that the imperative of pain has been greatly diluted.[17] In such a configuration, attention to bodily pain may be compromised by the vast array of other problems in need of attention. But the fact of pain, the desire for relief, and the phenomenology and materiality of palliation are not to be underestimated, even though they largely seem to happen around the edges and in the interstitial spaces of African health care.

In Botswana there is a particular economy of expression, and an ethic of palliation, such that pain may be spoken of, but it is rarely screamed or cried over. This has critical consequences in contemporary clinical practice that are compounded by a nursing culture that has historically shied away from the use of strong painkillers.[18] But we should not romanticize patient silence. A national survey of terminally ill patients and their care-givers conducted in four districts of the country found that 64 percent of respondents listed "severe pain" as a crucial problem of the terminally ill, making it the most commonly reported issue.[19] Nor is the problem limited to Botswana. Another study that contrasted the experience of dying of cancer in Scotland and western Kenya found that "the emotional pain of facing death was the primary concern of Scottish patients and their carers, while physical pain and financial worries dominated the lives of Kenyan patients and their carers."[20]

There are many factors that contribute to the marginalization of concerns about pain in contemporary African clinical medicine. African medicine, even in a comparatively wealthy country like Botswana, as an out-growth of British colonial medicine and as a particular node in a broader international health logic, has historically operated as a grossly under-funded zero-sum enterprise. Its history of vertical health campaigns and strong focus on primary care and its politics of emergency do not favor robust attention to issues of pain and symptom control. In such a system meaningful pain relief is also invisible when it comes to the evaluation of care (which is structured to record statistically known mortality, fertility, and disease transmission outcomes). Thus pain management can appear to be something of a frill rather than an imperative in policy formulations, a status that manifests itself in the daily logics of clinical practice.

Though pharmaceutical interventions are only one aspect of pain relief, they are nonetheless suggestive of the wider problem. In 2004 the Inter-national Narcotics Control Board reported, "Developing countries, which represent about 80 per cent of the world's population, accounted for only about 6 per cent of global consumption of morphine."[21] Why and how is it that Botswana, with its relatively strong economy, progressive public health infrastructure and politics, public-private health partnerships, and profound AIDS and cancer epidemics (with all the attendant pain that im-plies), in 2004 had a per capita morphine consumption of .52 mgs, while in its former colonizer, the United Kingdom, per capita morphine consump-tion was more than thirty-fives times greater at 19.15 mgs per person?[22]

The challenges are complex. Maintaining adequate stocks of drugs (any drugs) in African health systems has long been problematic. Even when adequate national stocks of morphine are available, they are difficult for many nonhospitalized patients to access, due to barriers of travel, the need for a professional referral from a clinic to a hospital, and so on.[24] There is reluctance to allow nurses to prescribe opiates, and they are the ones who by and large staff rural health centers. This is certainly the case in Botswana, where opioids are available only in the pharmacies of referral hospitals, and where morphine and codeine are frequently out of stock (as are all medical supplies). Nurses, for their part, may limit the use of opiates for pain management, and thereby the demand they broker, on account of widespread anxieties about creating addiction. And of course the presence of opioids in a broader pharmacy network does potentially invite the development of a black market in highly addictive drugs—a dynamic the Ministry of Health quite understandably wishes to avoid. In addition, a lack of expectation around chemical palliation also shapes patient demands. In other words, if patients do not know that such relief is possible, then they are much less likely to demand it. M's agony was created out of a complex political, economic, technocratic, and cultural history.

In a place where the reliance on chemical analgesics is as greatly attenuated as it is in Botswana, efforts to socialize pain are particularly important, if subtle. Nowhere perhaps is this more important than in relation to cancer. In the PMH colposcopy clinic, Dr T, a central European gynecologist, diagnoses cervical cancers. He remarks to me that the women here endure pain *much* differently than in Europe—even the pain of stage-3 cervical cancer. He has to struggle to convince the nurses to give morphine, because the patients will tolerate the pain with just ibuprofen. In the cancer ward, there is now less hesitation to chemically palliate, evidence surely of the ease with which the culture of palliative care for the critically ill can be changed. The oncologist jokes that he beat it out of the nurses when he arrived, this reluctance to use strong painkillers. That is a good joke—pain is inflicted in some to ameliorate it in others. Hospitals are full of such jokes, and in Botswana there is a rich culture of joking about beating. It should be noted that nurses in oncology (all of whom are Batswana, except for one Cuban woman) do take note of pain and will advocate on behalf of patients for relief when they think it necessary.[24]

Cancer and palliative care share a history, and pain highlights the particular somatic predicament of Africa's cancer patients. Oncology in particular is a set of grueling and at times brutal and violent practices, albeit ones performed with great hope and determination. And cancers themselves are often extremely and relentlessly painful in their own right, especially in places like Botswana where so many patients are diagnosed when their disease is already advanced. What are we to make of the insults of oncology at its rawest when we realize that often in Botswana, chemotherapy, radiation, and amputative surgery are performed *as* palliative measures for terminally ill patients?

And yet, clinical oncology, like all public biomedical care in Botswana, proceeds with few of the niceties—the powerful antiemetics, the morphine pumps, the fentanyl patches, the sedatives, the informational literature, the counseling—that can smooth the rough edges of chemotherapy, radiation burns, severe mucositis, surgical wounds, nasal-gastric tubes, and invasive diagnostic procedures. Cost matters, but cost alone cannot explain how a health system could afford to irradiate Mma Pula Motswapele's cervical cancer, but could not properly palliate her when terminally ill. When I accompanied local clinic staff to her village home we found her in severe pain with profound wasting. She had developed an intense fear of the pain of defecation after the aforementioned costly radiation treatments had created an inoperable fistula so deep and painful that she tried by all measures to resist her own hunger.[25]

Striving for Silence

Most patients comply with painful diagnostic and therapeutic procedures with minimal complaint. Some of course simply fail to return for subsequent rounds of dreaded chemotherapy, and others reach a point in the advancement of metastatic disease and treatment complications where they are overwhelmed by the pain and so begin to cry out or to grip the nurse's (or visiting ethnographer's) arm in a silent plea for help. Over time, acute, prolonged agony has the ability to grind down even those highly practiced in the art of forbearance, such that eventually even the scratch of the sheets, the prick of the needle, and the grip of the blood pressure cuff become exquisite insults. Many do not mention their pain unless directly asked about it by the doctor, nurse, or ethnographer, but when asked what their problem is, these patients will readily report pain, with great firmness.

This is not to say that there is no complaining. In many ways the minor insult is easier to express than the major one. After exchanging greetings during social visits and clinical encounters alike, elderly women often re-cite a litany of places in their body where it hurts. Such are the privileges of old age. Cancer patients, or their relatives, protest the nausea of chemo-therapy, which for some can be overwhelming. But generally in Botswana, people from approximately age five up are expected to endure all but the worst pain in silence. The few who do cry excessively are sources of hilar-ity for onlookers (including medical staff), and even for themselves. This means that subtle calculations are continually being made by onlookers, who would never laugh at the cries of a patient they deemed to be in true agony or distress.

Silence

Field Notes: Achieving Silence in the Surgical Ward

JUNE 18, 2008

We are rounding in a female surgical ward, because we don't have a bed in oncology for Margaret, the woman with the massive Burkitt's lymphoma swelling in her thigh. While there we can visit our post-mastectomy pa-tients. At the far end of the cubicle, I see Dr Z, a senior surgeon from India who has been working at PMH for decades, with his team. The woman in bed 1 begins crying out in pain as he palpates her. We all turn to look. Dr Z is firm and a bit irritated. No, Mma. You may not do that! We see these problems all the time and I know it may hurt, but it is no reason to cry. He chastises her further and then continues with his exam. She is now quiet with maybe 7 or 8 people all looking at her.

Field Notes: Almost Achieving Silence in the Obstetrics and Gynecology Ward

MARCH 31, 2007

9:30 pm. I arrive at the Labor department for the night shift and meet Dr M, a Bangladeshi doctor in his early forties, who is currently assigned to Obs and Gynae. We go straight to Gynae. There is a patient—a woman age 41 moaning and writhing in pain. She is in the corridor on a narrow gurney. She has had pethidine in Accident and Emergency and is still in a good deal of pain. Dr M takes her case history. She's been bleeding and gets bad pain each period since 2001—but this time is by far the worst. Grava 5 para 2. Dr M examines and suspects fibroids—he can feel a large one. As he examines and she cries out he says each time firmly, but gently—NO. Try to tolerate. And she does. The crying stops, but she is still moaning. An obese woman in bra and panty. She's had 80 mgs pethidine already, but when we see her she is still writhing, putting her leg into the handle of the supply closet door to brace herself while on the exam table, clutching the table, etc. Dr M tells the nurse to give her 100 mg IM stat of pethidine. It is amazing that she was in so much pain—but when she had to climb from the stretcher onto the exam table she just was able to focus and get it done though I am sure it was a huge challenge for her. Dr M acknowledges to her that This is very painful!—but explains it is not life-threatening. But that it will have to come out.

Field Notes: Achieving Silence During a Bone Marrow Biopsy in Oncology

JANUARY 31, 2007

It is about 4:30 pm—nearing the end of a long day that began at 7:45 am in the incredible heat of Botswana's summer. This will be Dr A's very first bone marrow biopsy. He has watched Dr P perform many of these procedures—but now it is his turn to try himself. The patient, O, speaks good English. He has been waiting on one of the long benches outside the clinic for his turn. O is in his mid forties, and he has what looks like a hematological tumor in his abdomen of unknown origin. By sampling his bone marrow, Dr P [the German hematologist/oncologist, and head of Botswana's cancer ward] hopes to identify the precise nature of the tumor and to learn if the tumor is a metastasis that actually originated in O's bone marrow. This is explained to O: We are to do a test so that we can help you with your cancer. You will need to lie still.

Kitso, one of the nursing sisters (a really excellent nurse) in her early 30s, sets up a sterile surgical pack on the small cart next to the high narrow exam table. We pull the exam table away from the wall so that Dr P can fit alongside Dr A, a medical officer ("resident" in American terms) from Egypt who has been assigned to the oncology ward, though his specialty is actually anesthesia. Kitso, a student nurse, and I are all on the other side. After being instructed to do so, O takes his shoes off, pulls his trousers off, folds them and places them on an empty chair, pulls up his t-shirt a bit, to expose his buttocks. He lies face down, head tilted towards Kitso and me on the table, the student a bit behind us. You must remain still. Drs P and A both put on sterile gloves from the packs over the regular latex exam gloves.

Dr A wipes the area with Betadine (a rust-colored antiseptic). They give O a shot of local anesthetic first. This will numb the flesh on his buttock and make it possible for them to go through the flesh with the big boring needle. But it will not numb the bone itself. The needle is very large, and hollow. O is lying on his stomach, and so he cannot see how big the needle is. Dr A guides it in until he hits the bone, then he pulls the needle guide out. Now comes the painful part, the anesthetic we use does nothing for the pain of extraction, Dr P explains to me, knowing my interest in pain.

Keep still, they tell O, and I keep my hand on O's upper back in what I hope is a gesture of comfort and solidarity. Dr A starts drilling into the bone, twisting the boring needle in a mechanical way that requires deep pressure, and hard physical labor. Turning and turning the needle with effort. At one point Dr P has to step in, because Dr A is not hitting the bone quickly enough. He lays his hands over Dr A's and guides him, showing him how the bone runs in one direction and it will be easier to run with the bone. O's eyes are open. He is still. Dr A keeps drilling. Dr P explains to me—you see as you drill in, it pushes the material further in—so in extracting the sample you have to wiggle the drill back out while holding a finger over the opening in the needle where you removed the guide—this will make a vacuum. It has been at least 15 minutes. Kitso turns to me and says BOTLHOKO! (Setswana: PAIN!). I almost don't dare look at poor O—but there he is still as can be, his face pouring sweat. My only job was to open the specimen container of formalin and pour a bit out to make room for the sample and even this small thing I was having a hard time managing. The last thing I wanted was to be the reason this procedure needed to be repeated.

Dr A pulls out the core sample and drops slices of it into my jar of formalin. He too is sweating. Dr P puts the lid on the container and then, not trusting the pathologist entirely, presses a few pieces between glass slides to examine personally, taking care not to crush the cells. Dr A presses a piece of Betadine-soaked gauze over the wound, and then we hand him strips of tape to cover it. He and Dr P pull off their gloves and step out of the clinic and across the breezeway to the lab to take the slides for staining. Kitso folds up the used surgical packs and goes with the student nurse to deposit the used instruments.

O pulls up his trousers and comes and sits down next to me on one of the other empty chairs in the clinic room. He turns to me and quite calmly says in a combination of Setswana and English—Well, that was certainly the worst pain I have ever experienced in my life. Please tell me that they don't ever do that to children. I can't even imagine what would happen if they did that to a child. He looks a bit dazed. I say, OK, I won't tell you, but yes it is done to children and it takes several adults holding them down to accomplish. Tell me again, why exactly they did that to me? I try to give him a more detailed explanation of the biomedical logic behind the procedure. It is hard to express in Setswana, and I stick mostly to English. But I too am dazed—even though Kitso had said "BOTLHOKO!" I hadn't fully realized the extent I think, since O had lain there so calmly until I talked to him afterwards. O wants to leave to catch his bus, he needs to squeeze into a crowded minibus taxi to the bus rank, from which he will catch a bumpy bus ride to a stop in his village, and then walk the path to his house. I check with the doctors and let O go, he will return next week for the results.[27]

In the oncology ward, an open ward of twenty beds, there was pain as far as the eye can see, yet it was rarely given voice. But even pain that remains unvocalized is nonetheless meant to be actively heard, anticipated, and negotiated. The social nature of pain and of embodiment in Botswana places a grave burden upon both patient and practitioner. Unlike the individuated patient encased in her envelope of skin as envisioned by contemporary clinical practice, here patients' surgical and other anxieties are as much about maintaining composure in front of others as they are about the potentially isolating, individuated experience of bodily pain.

Kitso did her job well by announcing BOTLHOKO! She did it so that O would not have to. Effective nurses here often announce the pain of patients. *Botlhoko!* they will say during a bone marrow biopsy. *Botlhoko, sorry my dear, botlhoko!*—while cleaning a necrotic wound. Of course not all nurses are so effective. The entire bone marrow biopsy is enacted as a drama of few words, but of many meaningful glances, looks, gestures. Bodily contact keeps participants linked in a silent network of social connection, and this socialization is an inherent part of palliation and healing. As the procedure ends, O speaks to me, drawing me into his experience, seeking to socialize his pain. In an inpatient ward, with minimal and highly regulated visiting hours, with patients drawn from a catchment stretching hundreds of kilometers, socializing pain is one of the most significant tasks facing the oncology team, where the ward as a social space must do some of the proxy work of the family.

Botswana's cancer patients come to the ward usually after some months or even years of debilitating pain, fearful for their children, parents, siblings, and lovers as much as for themselves, uncertain of the outcome. The anxiety of pain in oncology is also the anxiety of death, of orphaning one's children, of abandoning one's parents, one's siblings, one's lover. They learn of cancer mainly through experience, and through a lengthy quest for relief, but they are almost entirely disempowered by rituals of communication and process that seek to shield and protect them from knowledge of their fate. Though they embrace biomedical practice, it is within a context where its hegemony is far from certain. And lastly, of necessity, they bear these procedures with minimal expectation of chemical palliation.

I think there is a way in which a particular institutional culture in the hospital and clinics meets a particular patient culture of complaint to complicate the problem of pain. In the clinic patients rarely announce their pain unasked. This job is left to the relatives who accompany them, or else it is left up to the doctor to ask them. In interviews and clinic visits, relatives often revealed a tremendous depth of concern for the pain of their loved ones. In private homes mothers, aunts, daughters, brothers, fathers, and even entire families might wake in the night to stay with and provide solidarity and comfort to relatives whose pain was intense enough to prevent or interrupt their sleep (though not every patient is fortunate enough to have such a family). Young men in their twenties would pause in interviews with me to reflect on how loved and well cared for they were by a favorite aunt or mother who massaged them and sat with them through endless nights of wakeful pain. Such patients knew that their relatives, motivated by care and love, read them closely, noticing when they became too quiet by day, or too restless or mournful at night, seeking out and affirming their pain. In clinic visits when patients failed to mention their own suffering, accompanying relatives would often raise the issue, requesting assistance for their patient. For those like M, whose relatives were far away, it fell to the clinical staff, or a patient in a neighboring bed, to announce his pain, as Dr P had done in telling Mma L, "As you can see it is quite painful."

Pain begs a response. In 2006 my friend Boitumelo and her sister-in-law Glorious held down Glorious's twenty-three-year-old son and forced morphine down his throat. D, Glorious's son, was dying of a head and neck tumor that had already resulted in the surgical removal of a quarter of his jaw. The tumor was now pushing his eye out of its socket. Profoundly disfigured, perpetually nauseous, and in serious agony, D "just wanted to let the pain kill him," but his mother and aunt felt differently. Unfortunately, by this stage in his disease the maximum dose of oral morphine was only providing him with thirty minutes of relief.

While patients like O usually sat calmly and quietly for bone marrow biopsies and aspirates, and even lung biopsies performed with only a superficial local anesthetic, when asked directly, they would report intense burning or crushing pain. Some writhed or moaned or wept as the nurse painted gentian violet into open sores in their anus or mouth, the sores themselves products of palliative radiation treatments. Others sat with teeth clenched as I drove them to the private hospital across town to get a radiological consult—carrying back to PMH X-rays riddled with the clear white circles of bone metastases that explained why they winced every time I hit a bump in the road. Pain, after all, was what had pushed so many of them through the health referral system and into the ward and clinic. But expressions of pain were highly constrained.

There is a complex logic to this disposition. Bodily reserve and continence in the face of pain is in and of itself a technique of autopalliation. Women learn during labor, and children during the scrapes and accidents of childhood, that becoming overwrought only intensifies their pain. In the past, this knowledge was further concretized during painful initiation rituals. This is a cultivated disposition, one that is respected as much for its rationality as because it is a mark of self-discipline and control. Unfortunately, this logic, which is never recognized as the product of an intellectual effort to grapple with the dilemma of pain, produces contradictory effects in contemporary biomedical settings.

Pain and Laughter

There is also, sometimes, absolute hilarity in the face of pain. Patients will laugh in interviews when talking about their pain or the pain of others. Women reference labor pains and laugh at the image and the memory. And in the oncology ward and clinic, somewhat to my surprise, I have found (and deeply enjoyed) that laughter is ubiquitous: elderly women perform outrageous, hysterical pantomimes of the predicament of simultaneous nausea and diarrhea after chemo; middle-aged men mock the very German mannerisms of the oncologist; young men and women make deadpan humor out of their hair loss; women with breast cancer joke about their own fear of death. There was one truly funny fifty-year-old woman who would joke about hooking herself for tamoxifen. And then there is the black humor that sometimes follows death, when an oncologist strides into the ward and asks the nurses, "Which of you killed my patient?" In the final section I will explore the way in which this laughter begins to open up a social phenomenology of pain in Botswana's cancer ward.

DECEMBER 19, 2006

A woman patient, in her 50s(?), who is also a nurse, is lying on the narrow table in the clinic office. She is getting a bone marrow aspirate—but she doesn't want it. She had one in 2003, and she doesn't want it again. But it takes only two minutes, Dr P insists. They negotiate as she tries to wheedle out, but then he does it, quickly, plunging the needle into her sternum. She whimpers, he talks her through—there is a small wail, and then it is over. Now everyone is laughing. The other nurse in the room kept saying sorry, sorry as the procedure went on. They know each other. "Sorry, my dear." But then she burst out laughing at the wail. In the end, even the patient laughed when told by her friend that she had cried like a baby. Even ten minutes later another small bout of laughter at the memory sends us all up again.

JANUARY 8, 2007

A young woman, 19, with breast lumps. Probably not cancer— she needs an aspirate and there is much struggle. She keeps wriggling away. Her aunt is laughing so hard at the spectacle, and then she says she needs to leave the room. Dr P asks the aunt to hold the patient's hand—he is doing it very quickly, but the aunt starts laughing and leaves. We all laugh—all of us. She struggles more and 2 nursing assistants and the nurse all now are holding her and laughing—it is very comical and Dr P is chuckling. Chasing her across the table. Just a small prick. It is nothing. You must sit still. Why all this fuss? This is not painful really. Afterwards she finally has it done, lying down and three people helping hold her in place—Dr P jabs the needle in, pushing it in and out several times to collect any possible calcius material in the lump. She is crying and the nurse is starting to look a bit annoyed (a young nurse—L, she is only in her early 20s) and Dr P asks what is wrong? It's over. But she says *botlhoko* (pain) in a quiet voice and looks injured and angry.

MARCH 13, 2007

Dr P needs to do a fine-needle aspiration on a 3-and-a-half-year-old boy. He gives him a banana first, trying to make friends. Then, at the nurse's instruction, the boy hands his mother the banana and lies on the table as Dr P says—"small prick"—and then jabs the needle into the swollen lymph node on the boy's neck. The kid is screaming and writhing, so the whole thing is chaotic, but the procedure is over in a minute and the nurse, myself, and the nursing assistant have successfully held the boy still enough to get the needle in and out. Afterwards he is crying and screaming and lying on the table demanding his banana—*ke kopa banana ya me, banana, banana*! His mother gets up and brings it to him. Dr P is happy that he wants to eat his banana now, feeling certain this will calm him down, and terribly proud that he has thought to give him a piece of fruit. As Dr P turns his back to empty the syringe onto the slides, the boy comes up behind him and throws the banana at Dr P's bum with all his might. Everyone collapses to the ground in laughter.

Missionaries, expatriate clinicians, and other observers from the nineteenth century through to the present often took such examples of laughter in the face of the pain of others as a troubling comment on the nature of care and compassion in Botswana, or as a curious cultural artifact.[28] And yet upon closer examination it appears to be something other than just insensitivity or some feature of an exotic culture at play. In fact, the banana-throwing boy became a favorite memory in the clinic, affirming as he did that the procedure *was* painful, though we all (including the patient) were meant to pretend that it wasn't. The laughter was particularly cathartic for the oncologist, who spent his days inflicting pain in the name of care.

Laughter, it seems, has long been a social strategy for shaping particular forms of autopalliation. Laughter, when it works, as in the case of the nurse/patient above, is meant to socialize and redirect patient anxiety into the disposition of calm forbearance that lies at the heart of autopalliation. It is followed by patting or stroking and the repetition of "sorry, sorry," a common way of soothing babies and small children. When laughter doesn't work, as in the case of the young woman with the breast aspiration, it is put down to the dramatic excesses and foolishness of the young, and this too is comical. In the same way, women often laugh and openly mock the screams of young women in labor—their cries are seen as a sign that these girls, who thought they were ready for sex, are not yet ready for motherhood.

This is certainly not to suggest that the laughter is disingenuous, or an explicit and conscious strategy, but rather to remark on its social effects. If pain with its potential for isolating embodiment threatens social rupture, laughter offers the prospect of reestablishing an embodied sociality. I do not intend to be overly functionalist here. Laughter is often an overwhelming experience that comes on suddenly, not a practice that emerges out of purpose and forethought. We know that laughter, like all emotional experiences and expressions, has a cultural logic, and that it is possible to decode this logic, though at the risk of taking all the fun out of the laughter itself. Some of its joy, no doubt, derives from its irreverence. Laughter in the oncology ward often acted to acknowledge the absolute absurdity of misfortune. This, as we well know, is not unique to Botswana, and while there I was often reminded not only of Bakhtin, but also of keeping my friend Matthew company while he sat receiving the chemo drip for the liver cancer that killed him back in 1994 at age twenty-eight. When the nurse would check in and ask if he was OK, he would reply, "Nothing to worry about here, just a little cancer," and somehow it was absolutely hilarious to us. Laughter often comes in moments when a cultural norm fails to be enacted—the patient fails to keep silent, the doctor fails to maintain his authority—and in its recognition of the absurd, laughter reinforces the norm, by socializing it. In none of these scenarios does anyone laugh alone!

Of course laughter can be cruel, as when R, a long-standing KS patient, cried all the way back to her bed from the toilet, where defecation had been painful. Her overwrought cries, so out of place on the ward, were met with cynical laughter by the nurses. But R had a long history in oncology, and though she could be wickedly funny in her own right, cracking jokes that would have us howling with laughter, she was also "naughty," as one fellow patient put it, drinking to excess, sleeping with many men, and even joking about making a sexual advance on her own brother. "She likes this hospital too much," a nursing assistant commented, meaning that R was not taking enough responsibility for her own well-being. Pain and laughter, as fundamental and at times overwhelming bodily experiences, point to the potential for both positive social connection *and* profoundly isolating social alienation, and they often bundle together for just this reason. They can counteract and balance or accelerate one another—and in tandem they reveal something of the strength of social embodiment.

In Tswana medicine and popular thought, pathological experience is at least in one key sense the outcome of social rupture and antagonism. In this configuration pain is a fundamentally social phenomenon, and palliation, like healing, an attempt to resocialize through the benign intimacy of companionship, physical touch, and, of course, laughter. This socialization and intimacy that laughter provides is especially critical in the face of cancer. Because of the constraints of the health system, many cancer patients are not only suffering from pain but must also endure the disfigurement of tumors or amputations. There are some whose throats overflow with saliva because they are entirely blocked by an esophageal tumor; others stink because necrotic tumors have broken through their skin, exposing rotting flesh.[29] Sociality is potentially tenuous for these patients, and laughter all the more powerful for its potential not only to facilitate autopalliation, but also to strengthen and animate benign social connectivity, which *is* healing and care for the Batswana.

Laughter, of course, is not the only popular response to pain in this culture of silent expression. Nor did callousness seem to be at issue when S, a woman with stage-4 metastatic breast cancer, began crying out in terrific pain in the ward. In my field notes I wrote, "After lunch in the ward, S—

the woman with metastatic cancer of the breast, who got chemo in a lumbar puncture on Friday, is really crying out in pain. This is such an unusual sound in the oncology ward. Drs A and P and Mma M all hurry over. She has a crushing pain in the head and wants to vomit. Dr A doubles her dose of pethidine and then there is a question—Does she have meningitis? She will get antibiotics just in case, etc. But there is a deep and swift reaction to her crying out in pain. I am impressed." Though pain threatens to isolate an individual in his or her body, ideally (if not always in practice) every effort is made to socialize it through active affirmation of its presence, through palliation, through laughter, through bodily contact.

Many patients, when I asked them if they thought their pain had a purpose, remarked on its ability to deepen their empathetic and perceptive capacities. They replied that it had given them new insight into their fellow citizens in the "country of the sick," as Susan Sontag would have put it. Some remarked that the purpose of pain was to cause them to remember God, and to recognize and care for others in times of suffering. And yet, for many veteran patients, the experience of traumatic pain opens them to perceiving pain in others without any need for words. Doubt was no longer an issue, for they *knew* pain. Some felt that they had to turn away when they now witnessed the pain of others. It was simply too exquisite, too intense of a mnemonic for their own agony, now that they had such a clearly embodied sense of what a grimace, a cringe, a tightly held brow indexed. Some found themselves comparing their pain to that of others they met on the ward or while waiting in the clinic, measuring their own pain against the presumed suffering of others, "placing it on the scale to weigh." In this way they either consoled themselves, openly acknowledging the pain of a fellow patient, or affirmed their sense that their own suffering was indeed extreme. Maybe pain doesn't shatter language, maybe instead it *is* a language, one that needs to be learned.[30]

Conclusion

I have tried to suggest that pain is a fundamental social experience in Botswana's cancer ward. Pain drives patients into the institution, and pain is also created by the practices of the institution itself. Yet despite the fact that pain is one of the central animating forces of biomedical care in Africa, of which Botswana's cancer ward is but one instantiation, the biomedical technologies of palliation are in short supply and put to often uneven and uncertain use. Pain reveals the intensely social nature of the ward, and the ward the intensely social nature of pain. But, in this context, the mechanisms and semantics of acceptable expression are particular, and often difficult to achieve. There may be problems of expression and access, but they do not center around doubt. Into the breach of expression comes laughter, a social experience for re-instantiating and reestablishing community in moments of terrible anxiety and duress.

Coda on a Failed Learning Curve

JANUARY 20, 2007

In the bed opposite Michael's in men's surgical lies M, the man with the botched amputation, which is now scheduled to be cleaned up, the bone removed, etc. He is still here. M sees Dr P and beckons him—then, after Dr P leaves, he grabs the male nurse who is with me and asks him for pain meds—the pain is too much—"I need an injection." The nurse says no, he can't have an overdose of pethidine. But the nurse hasn't looked at the file, I am not sure if he knows when the last dose was. The patient says maybe I can take it at noon—and the nurse agrees. I am not sure why he is still on pethidine and not on morphine. The nurse doesn't seem concerned about this. He wants to ask me instead about job opportunities in the US. M, empowered by my presence in this context where my white skin and moniker ("Dr Livingston"—as Dr P insists everyone call me) causes this nurse to mistake me for an American doctor, is learning to ask for relief. Yet, the effort comes up short.

Notes

1. A version of this chapter was previously published as "Creating and Embedding Cancer in Botswana's Oncology Ward," in *Improvising Medicine*, Julie Livingston, pp. 52–84. Copyright, 2012, Duke University Press. All rights reserved. Reprinted by permission of the publisher. www.dukeupress.edu.
2. See, for example, Travis (2007); Morris (2003); Botswana National Cancer Registry (2006).

3. For comparative rates, see the International Agency for Research on Cancer (IARC) global fact sheets at http://globocan.iarc.fr/ (consulted on June 14, 2010). Note also that there is much more likely to be serious underreporting of cancers in Botswana, where the registry is new, diagnostic sites are few, and screening is nonexistent except for a new and still-developing Pap-smear program for HIV-positive women. See Morris (2003).

4. Parkin et al. (2008).

5. I say "public provision" because the drugs are provided free of charge to all citizens who require them. But the program itself is provided through a public-private partnership in which Botswana pays 80 percent of the bill. Anthropologist Betsey Brada is currently researching these partnerships in Botswana (Brada 2011).

6. Many of these ideas and analytic frameworks around improvised medicine come out of conversations with Steve Feierman about an ongoing collaborative project. I am grateful to Steve for sharing his ideas about how biological, technical, and social challenges combine to shape clinical uncertainties in Africa. On oncology, see the excellent work of Kenyan anthropologist Benson A. Mulemi (2010).

7. Because of the lack of screening capabilities, a majority of Botswana's cancer patients are diagnosed after their disease is already advanced. Such cancers are widely recognized to cause moderate to severe pain in the vast majority of patients. See Cleland et al. (1996); Daut and Cleland (1982); Portenoy and Lesage (1999); Foley (1979).

8. Long et al. (2008); van der Geest and Finkler (2004); Finkler et al. (2008).

9. Keith Wailoo is currently writing a book that hinges on this question in American medical policy. See Wailoo (2010); Rouse (2009); DelVecchio Good et al. (1992); Jackson (1999).

10. Human Rights Watch (2009).

11. Scarry (1985).

12. Pain medicines, however, do have a thingy-ness. Patients are clear that some medicines are "pain-killers," separating pain from pathology. This dynamic of separation and attendant individuation around pain (in dentistry) has been beautifully articulated by historian Paul Landau in relation to early twentieth-century mission practice (Landau 1996).

13. Asad (2003); Das (1997).

14. Pethidine is strong synthetic opioid. American readers may be familiar with its brand name, Demerol.

15. Later there would be some debate as to why, with the surgeons arguing that M himself had requested to keep as much of his thigh as possible, balking at the loss of the femur. My point here is not to showcase surgical failure. I am not qualified to judge who, if anyone was at fault in this case of amputation gone wrong, and I have the utmost respect for the skill and commitment of the hospital's orthopedic surgeon. Advanced Kaposi's sarcoma often necessitates amputation, but surgeons are faced with a difficult challenge since the skin above the amputation site is often unhealthy, thus making it difficult to close the wound safely.

16. Pain assessment has been part of nursing training in Botswana since the mid-1970s, but is not integral to daily practice in the hospitals and clinics. See Manyere (1996).

17. McNeil (2007); Logie and Leng (2007); World Health Organization (2003).

18. See, for example, Mosweunyane (1994); Moyo (1994).

19. World Health Organization (2003).

20. Murray et al. (2003).

21. International Narcotics Control Board (2005), cited in University of Wisconsin Pain and Policy Studies Group, *Availability of Morphine and Pethidine in the World and Africa*, 2006, 4.

22. University of Wisconsin Pain and Policy Studies Group, *Availability of Morphine and Pethidine in the World and Africa*, 2006, table 1. These statistics need to be taken with a grain of salt. Some necessary figures appear to be missing, and there are some dramatic and unexplained spikes. Distribution through Central Medical Stores (the national centralized pharmaceutical procurement system) has been a problem in Botswana, as it scales up the quantity and array of drugs available in the face of changing epidemiological norms, the AIDS epidemic in particular, and as attempts to localize purchasing and distribution continue. It is not my aim to pin down exact figures, but rather to make the general point (which can be supported by the statistics) that in this place with a lot of sick people, strong painkillers are not widely used.

23. Koshy et al. (1998).

24. Yet upon occasion I also found myself—an ethnographer with a public health background but no medical training—being the one who suggested or requested that a patient receive pethidine before wound cleaning, or a prescription for morphine tablets for use at home. This, I think, was the result of the pressures of work in this setting where the clinical staff were extremely busy. The attitude of nurses on the oncology ward, where they were usually fairly attentive to pain, was quite different from that on the medical and surgical wards, where some doctors (mainly European or American expatriates) and one Motswana nursing professor complained about the reluctance of nurses to administer strong pain relief. And yet when I rounded with staff in these other wards, I found that often these same doctors did not explicitly ask patients about pain. Nurses in Botswana are shifted among posts every two years, so the explanation is not that oncology nurses had special training in oncology or were otherwise different from the other nurses in the hospital. Rather, the strong personality of the oncologist, his emphasis on palliation as a critical element of cancer care, and the oncology training and ethos of compassion of the nursing matron in charge of the ward were responsible for this marked difference from other domains in the hospital. Once the doctor and nursing matron emphasized palliation as an important practice, nurses in the ward did so as well.

25. Interview with Mma Pula Motswapele, January 12, 2007. Pseudonyms are used throughout.

26. Field notes: I have seen Dr P do bone marrow biopsies already, and I understand the purpose. But after my conversation with O, I want to double

check my understanding of the procedure, so I get on the Internet. Web MD and the Mayo Clinic both describe the procedure and advise their presumably middle class (Internet accessing) American patients who learn they may receive a sedative, and who will presumably be provided with a hospital gown to wear during the procedure. The contrast between the description provided online and what I witnessed is instructive. http://www.mayoclinic.com/health/bone -marrow-biopsy/CA00068. http://www.webmd.com/a-to-z-guides/bone-marrow -aspiration-and-biopsy?page=3.

27. Landau (1996).

28. For more about disgust and its effects in the cancer ward, see Livingston (2008).

29. I think these patients were trying to convey a sensibility quite like that described by Veena Das in her meditations on Wittgenstein and pain, a rumination perhaps best explicated by her interlocutor Stanley Cavell (1997). Or, as Carolyn Nordstrom (1997) puts it, "There are many 'languages' in any social setting, some competing, even contradictory, but nonetheless true. Pain both undermines communication and communicates throughout a society at large."

8

A Salvage Ethnography of the Guinea Worm

Witchcraft, Oracles and Magic in a Disease Eradication Program

AMY MORAN-THOMAS

This is a story about a hard-fought health campaign against a centuries-old pathogen, a program now nearing its final goal of global eradication. Yet it is also a story full of conflicting priorities and values, and the laden paradoxes of humanitarianism at play as medicine breaches boundaries not normally thought of as permeable.[1]

Or at least, that is one way of saying that on the morning when the Ghana Guinea Worm Eradication Program sent two team members to a small dam in the village of Taha to put treatment chemicals in the community's drinking water—hoping to interrupt the plague of three-foot-long guinea worms that for centuries had emerged from farmers' legs and bodies every harvest season—they were met at the waterside by an angry crowd of local men armed with cutlasses and knives.

"They believed the worms were in their blood already, that people were just born with them there," a longtime Ministry of Health official explained to me in 2009. We were walking slowly through the September heat as he recounted the event, weaving between reckless goats on the dirt road that cut through Taha's clusters of earthen homes. "They thought it was witchcraft that made the worms come out. The guinea worm mainly comes during harvest season, you understand, and so a lot of people believed that someone had sent them this worm as a curse to keep them from their fields." He shook his head. "That year, there was an issue of timing . . . and then people thought it was the ABATE chemical itself that woke up the guinea worm. They thought the water treatment chemical was causing the worm instead of killing it."

The Ghana Health Services expert nodded, adjusting the top button on his official program shirt. It was made of beige cloth patterned with images of a turbaned woman filtering her drinking water for guinea worm alongside circular icons of the program's supporters, set against blue background tessellations of gently curling worms and their tiny crustacean vectors. "So that is why they threatened the lives of the program team who came to their village to put ABATE chemical in the water," he recalled distractedly, scanning his cell phone contact list for the local guinea worm volunteer's number so that he could be summoned for my interview.

When discussing African histories of magic and witchcraft, anthropologists tend to automatically think back to E. E. Evans-Pritchard's classic 1937 monograph, *Witchcraft, Oracles and Magic Among the Azande*. From a wealth of ethnographic detail, Evans-Pritchard extracts a famous observation: that when the Azande spoke of causality they were not trying to figure out *how* something happened (in his example, how a granary house collapses on a person); rather, they were appealing to unseen forces to figure out *why* it happened to that person specifically. Indeed, throughout my fieldwork in Northern Ghana, local people's understandings of accountability, causation, and fate were often permeated by a similar logic;[2] it was common to hear questions like "But if it comes from water, then why did *I* get guinea worm when the others drinking from the same dam did not?" Seeking answers to such questions of "why," many people in the past—and some even after twenty years of worldwide eradication efforts—would visit oracles to determine whether the worms were messages from "the ghosts," usually meaning their ancestors, or sent through witchcraft by an evil person wishing them harm. But perhaps more unexpectedly altogether, on that day in Taha, the villagers' answer to the question "why" suddenly shifted to the eradication campaign's own treatments instead.

I want to use this emblematic moment in Northern Ghana as a point of departure for this essay, to address the knotted social, political, and medical understandings that collided on that day. We begin with a question buried at the heart of this conflict. In the minds of these Dagomba farmers, what fields of meaning were in play to allow scientific chemicals to take the place of supernatural explanations for guinea worm with such ease?

I observed that these colliding fields—humanitarian interventions for guinea worms, on the one hand, and local understandings of them in the rural West African communities where this public health campaign is unfolding, on the other—at times also give way to unexpected but deeply meaningful resonances. Such unlikely congruencies, alongside the more obvious conflicts over the meaning of these worms, demand to be explored side by side—perhaps shedding light on the political forces, intricate ecologies, and cultural histories that have shaped the tensions surrounding guinea worm eradication, even as the parasite itself may finally disappear from this earth.

Ghana recently celebrated a tentative victory over guinea worm: not a single case was reported in the country in 2011. There were only 1,060 remaining guinea worm cases in the entire world in 2011, spread across just four countries: 8 in Ethiopia, 12 in Mali, 10 in Chad, and 1,030 in South Sudan (Carter Center 2011). This progress suggests that guinea worm is now firmly poised to be the second disease (and first parasite) to ever be eradicated from the world. There are already numerous articles and even a forthcoming documentary film that depict this pending historic moment as a celebration of inspirational success. Yet, as an anthropologist, my aims here are somewhat different. I examine the campaign's progress from a premise perhaps more attuned to the way Ghanaian moral philosopher Kwame Anthony Appiah summarizes his own work: "Everything is more complicated than you thought" (2008:198). There are entangled social relations and challenging questions within this unfolding story that often fall outside the clean lines of policy agendas or headlines, what historian Nancy Leys Stepan might call "useful ambiguities" of eradication policy (2011). It is in the democratic spirit of critical inquiry and probing debate that I sketch some of these multiple sides and perspectives, attending also to the tough questions being asked by people on the ground and the ethical ambiguities of technological tools. In this way, this chapter unfolds at uneasy interstices, trying to offer an ethnographic snapshot that lets messy situations remain messy: showing thought-provoking setbacks occurring side by side with equally thought-provoking successes. It considers the complexities of biology in relation to local environments, as well as the shifting rationales and difficult choices of prioritization that face both international and state actors with limited budgets—and it maintains that dissonance within local communities evinces not "cultural barriers" or "superstitions" to be overcome, but deep-seated questions and critical insights that require careful listening.

Salvage ethnography has been a bad expression in anthropology for decades, associated with heartbreaking legacies of colonialism and the extinction of entire peoples. Such anthropologists once documented and "salvaged" whatever remaining bits of information they could about a culture before it faded forever. But this particular opportunity for salvage ethnography presents us with a rare celebratory moment—it signals the end of a parasitic disease, rather than a dying people perched on the brink of extinction. By collecting remnants of worm stories, traditions still remembered but no longer believed, fading memories, or scrap-chance moments, I am in part seeking to critically document a seminal moment in public health—a field with a notoriously short memory—in hopes that the experiences gained from this historical eradication program may hold lessons for future policy efforts. But I also mean to create a record of the living guinea worm itself, the human struggles it has crystallized and fragments of stories from the people, politics, and places it traveled through for centuries. For there are certain knowledges and societal practices that will die along with this worm, a signifier whose deep and even conflicted social meanings deserve to be remembered in all their complexity.

Guinea Worm in the History of West Africa

Some information about the parasite itself will help set the epidemiological stage for the struggles that follow. For people unaccustomed to seeing it, guinea worm is a visually spectacular disease. Its life cycle in humans begins when a person drinks water containing microscopic *Cyclops*[3] crustaceans, known as copepods or "water fleas," which have themselves ingested tiny guinea worm larvae. Inside the human stomach, gastric acid dissolves the water flea's exoskeleton and liberates the captive guinea worm larvae, which then penetrate the human intestinal wall. Over a slow two-week migration, the nascent filament-thin larvae travel beyond the peritoneal cavity and into the thorax or abdominal muscles, where they remain until reaching adulthood, nourished in their growth by the bodily fluids they ingest.

When the male and female worms reach sexual maturity about one hundred days after they are first swallowed, they seek each other out to mate in a strange subcutaneous romance: neither of them will survive the ordeal. The male worms usually die not long after mating,[4] their boneless corpses eventually encapsulated by the soft muscle tissues surrounding them. Meanwhile the impregnated female worms continue their migration and gestation until they are a full year old, by which point they have developed into thin white worms about three feet in length. Before emerging from the body, these female parasites slowly move through the host's muscle planes, dissolving a pathway through human muscle and tissue. The entire body cavity of each female guinea worm is filled with her uterus, which contains up to three million embryos. Her pregnant body is literally on the verge of rupturing by the time she reaches the skin's surface. There, the female worm causes a break in the skin by provoking a blister, usually emerging from the host's feet or legs (boring out of lower limbs remains the worms' best chance of being submerged in a pond, which offers some slim chance of survival to their progeny). Guinea worms do, however, occasionally emerge instead from wayward locations such as tongues, ears, and eye sockets. The searing sensation that accompanies guinea worm blisters typically drives their victims to seek water to soothe the burning pain,[5] which is key to the parasite's evolutionary strategy—immersion in cooling water causes the blister to burst and leaves the female's anterior end extruding through the host's raw tissue, where contact with water induces a contraction in the waiting mother worm.[6] She spews hundreds of thousands of first-stage larvae from her ruptured uterus and through her head in her final act. Her pale body bursts like a popped balloon and she dies in the birthing process (Cairncross et al. 2002; Hopkins et al. 1993; Ruiz-Tiben and Hopkins 2006).

In a world where most sickness manifests via invisible pathogens and ambiguous symptoms, the dramatic appearance of this affliction has contributed greatly to the charged meanings ascribed to it. Certainly it allowed the worm to be understood as a distinct disease entity centuries before the advent of microscopes or germ theory. Guinea worms have been found in the bodies of Egyptian mummies, and scholars argue that the biblical "fiery serpents" that plagued the fleeing Israelites in the Old Testament book of Numbers were in fact guinea worms (Grove 1994:694). Historians have even theorized that the caduceus emblem of a snake wrapped around a rod, still a symbol of the medical profession today, originated from what remains the most effective treatment for an emerging worm: wrapping it around a stick to ensure it cannot retract back into the skin, and reeling it out inch by inch over a period of several days. (While commonly attributed to Asclepius, the renowned Greek doctor and patron deity of medicine, the caduceus symbol actually predates this demigod and can be traced back to ancient Mesopotamia).[7] These winding techniques remain important today, because it is critical not to break off the guinea worm before it fully emerges, which could cause a potentially lethal secondary infection. Although they often leave lasting exit scars and can cause great pain with their emergence, it is quite rare for guinea worms themselves to actually cause death.

The Guinea Worm Eradication Program still uses a version of this treatment today, in its specially designated "case containment centers," where people with emerging parasites are brought. The first time I witnessed a guinea worm emergence in person, it was coming out of an eight-year-old boy's foot. He looked as though he was trying not to cry in front of the other children waiting for their bandaging, but he still shrieked in pain when the Japanese volunteer tugged gently on the worm, adding the length of its body that she had pulled out to the glistening-wet coil resting near his toes. I had always pictured the guinea worm writhing, but it drooped out of his foot like a limp noodle.

Yet despite several weeks of intense discomfort and pain that the worm's emergence caused, many adults in Ghana took the experience in stride. Some even went about their daily work, coping with the worm secretly rather than following the treatment and isolation recommendations of the eradication program. "There are those who run away and hide on their farms when we try to give them treatment," explained Dr. Andrew Seidu Korkor, a deeply reflective man from Bole who heads Ghana's National Guinea Worm Eradication Program. "They do not think it is an emergency, because everyone knows it won't kill you. To them, it is just part of their lives." The worm even became such a naturalized fixture in the seasons that its *absence* from the body caused spiritual concern, as one Ghana health services program official told me with a laugh. "I remember when we went to Diare. One man said that for him, the guinea worm was in his blood and if every year it *doesn't* come out, that's when he knows something is wrong. So if it doesn't come one year, then he has to consult the ghosts to ask why."

Indeed, for many in Northern Ghana, guinea worm was once thought of not only as a common feature of people's lives, but as an intrinsic part of their anatomy. The long-standing belief that guinea worm lies latent in human blood from the time of birth—a perception common in many parts of West Africa (Bierliech 1995; Brieger et al. 1996)—made more sense to me after a field visit one day, when the program truck stopped in a small Gonja village called Kampong to check on a reported case of guinea worm. We walked past women reclining on the ground and stirring pots of shea butter with bare hands, to the house of the concerned man who had notified the program. He emerged from a nearby yam field wearing a prayer cap and Islamic robe, which he pulled up to reveal a thick worm-shaped bulge on his thigh. The Ministry of Health worker poked at it, and after some observation announced it was just a varicose vein.[8] "You can tell because it doesn't move when you touch it," he explained.

The fact that diagnostic ambiguity between human veins and worms continues today evokes older West African associations between the guinea worm and blood. But the recurring notion that the guinea worm can be an intrinsic part of a person also reveals deeper working ideologies of the body and self, which allow the physical resemblance between worms and veins to take on such layered meanings.

In his two-part series "Worms Are Our Life," anthropologist P. Wenzel Geissler explores outlooks on experience and the human body in a Luo community of rural Kenya, charting how local people's understandings of coexistence with worms are often dramatically different from the biomedical paradigms of elimination promoted in nearby schools and hospitals. Writing about intestinal parasites, Geissler describes his Luo acquaintances' efforts to placate the worms in their bodies and to read the parasites' actions as meaningful signs to be negotiated—a phenomenon, he points out, that is common in various local knowledge systems.[9] He then fits this recurring image into a broader understanding of social ties and life processes:

> In this view, 'lives' overlap, grow into each other. And the action of the worm in the stomach has its place in this overall process of life, as has the decay and disintegration of the corpse, decomposed by the worms, turning to soil . . . life and death are not analogous to order and disorder, but included into one orderly process. (Geissler 1998a:74–75)

His words contextualize the widespread Luo belief that worms are a latent and even intimate part of the human body as an element within a different way of understanding life's arc—one that sometimes blurs the distinction between inside and outside, and phenomenologies of self and other, just as the boundaries between the living and the dead can also become profoundly blurred.

In Ghana, those who once considered emerging guinea worms a sign from their ancestors did not fear the parasite as a symbol of death, but rather often respected it as an angry message from their honored dead, a white finger from another world searing through them in the flesh. A 2006 *New York Times* article described a similar situation in Nigeria, where former head of state General Yakubu Gowon (who led the Nigerian military in the Nigeria-Biafra civil war of 1967–1970) traveled with other dignitaries to a small village called Ogi to personally pour ABATE larvicide into a guinea-worm-infected local pond. But just past the tall grass that surrounded the water's edge, he met a group of village women who had formed a human wall around the sacred pond. " 'They had colors rubbed on their faces to show resistance, like Indian war paint,' a Carter Center field officer said. 'They were chanting songs of their refusal.' The women shouted, 'This disease is a curse from our ancestors, it has nothing to do with the pond water! If we let you touch anything, the ancestors will deal with us. We heard them crying all night' " (McNeil 2006:2).

The view of guinea worm as a potentially sacred ancestral message mingled and, at times, overlapped with other perceptions of the parasite in Northern Ghana. Another set of perceptions that persisted during the eradication campaign related to fears that the worms were sent as dark curses from a witch, wizard, or other ill-intentioned person who possessed a dangerous magic (like the guinea worm itself, such powers are sometimes said to run in families and to be inherited at birth through the intrinsic bodily matter of witchcraft substance).[10] There was not a systematic distinction between these dense repertoires, seemingly contradictory views of the worm as a messenger from ancestors, a consequence of drinking unclean water, or a curse from an ill-wisher; each case was interpreted according to many contingent factors, including the social background of the victim and the timing and context of the worm's emergence. For example, as a handsome young program worker from Accra told me, it was not surprising that local parents immediately suspected witchcraft when their daughter had twenty-eight worms emerging from her at once, their sinewy white bodies crawling out of her arms, legs, and face simultaneously. The majority of the guinea worm cases were much more subdued, however, and interpretation could be ambiguous. Uncertain cases could be brought to oracles in the hope that divination would reveal the worms' underlying cause.

People's continuous struggles to determine the reasons behind the guinea worms' appearance bring us back to Evans-Pritchard's legendary observation about Azande ascriptions of accountability, magic, and the logic of causality. But as Didier Fassin responds to humanitarian programs' expectations that he will give "'cultural keys' for interpreting 'resistance in the population'": "the analysis should encompass the entire intervention scene—not just aid recipients but the association and its members" (2010:40). In other words, in order to understand how the Guinea Worm Eradication Program's own biomedical treatments suddenly became enfolded in some Dagomba farmers' accusatory answer to this question of *why*, we must first turn to a reading of the health campaign's own history.

A Social History of the Guinea Worm Eradication Program

Guinea worm became a global health priority during the "International Drinking Water Supply and Sanitation Decade" of the 1980s, when the World Health Assembly's steering committee resolved that the worm's eradication would stand as a lasting legacy of their efforts. Since the guinea worm's survival depends on people first drinking infected "water flea" vectors, which are easily visible even to the naked eye and can be strained out with any common cloth, and then, later, submerging their blistering ulcers into a water source, the disease should be extraordinarily easy to interrupt with even the most basic standards of water sanitation. Guinea worm once existed in the Americas, but spontaneously died out as water supplies improved. For this reason the World Health Assembly assumed that eradicating the parasite would be a natural consequence of improved water supplies, and an index of their success toward achieving their primary goal to bring clean water to every village in the world (Brieger et al. 1997:354; see Yacoob et al. 1989). "The Water Decade provides a vehicle aimed already at insuring disease-free water," UN health expert Dr. Peter Bourne wrote in the early eighties (Bourne 1982:3). "[I]f the Decade is only 6–7 percent successful in achieving its overall goal it should still be sufficient to eliminate guinea worm" (Bourne 1982:2).

At the time, Bourne was both a top UN spokesman for the world water project and a former adviser to President Carter, then fresh out of his presidential term. When he met with Carter to discuss the possibility of collaborating on the effort, the former president was looking for a cause to which he might dedicate himself. Among the materials about world water problems that Dr. Bourne brought with him that day, "'He had slides of guinea worm to show me,' Mr. Carter [later] said. 'I was intrigued'" (McNeil 2006:3).

Another legendary figure in guinea worm eradication had also opened discussions with Jimmy Carter's White House as early as 1977. Public health expert and US Centers for Disease Control (CDC) veteran Dr. Donald R. Hopkins[11] was involved in the landmark smallpox campaign in the 1960s, the first (and, at the time this is being written, the only) campaign to ever successfully globally eradicate a disease. At a time when *dracunculiasis* was rarely mentioned in public health domains, Hopkins believed that it would be possible to make guinea worm the second disease to be eradicated from the world. With a reputation for quiet dedication and unassuming genius, Hopkins initially established a program for guinea worm at the CDC in 1980, and he remains a driving force and lead expert behind the eradication campaign today—in fact, many in public health circles associate his name with guinea worm eradication just as strongly as they do Carter's. By 1987, Hopkins and Carter had officially joined forces. Today, the powerful coalition against guinea worm led by the

Carter Center also includes key partners such as the CDC, WHO, UNICEF, and the Bill and Melinda Gates Foundation, alongside many national governments and agencies. Hopkins has become Vice President of Health Programs at the Carter Center, and Jimmy Carter refers to him as one of the "few heroes in my life" (Bristol 2008).

If the guinea worm cause found a champion in Carter and his colleagues, the nascent Carter Center also found a perfect totem in the guinea worm. This choice of focus forever politicized the worm and simultaneously solidified Carter's new foundation under its banner. Yet it also fundamentally changed the deepest premise of the original campaign, for the first time transforming the guinea worm into a primary policy target unto itself, rather than a secondary index of the underlying issue of water purity. This policy prioritization perhaps evinces a blurring between symbolism and epidemiology, for although guinea worms are strikingly monstrous in image, they do not actually cause death, in contrast to many other diseases in Northern Ghana that do. Indeed, local people quite frequently pointed this out, expressing confusion about the program's dedication of major resources to a disease that many did not consider among their most important health issues. The group of Nigerian women who drove General Gowon away from their guinea worm–infested pond also expressed such concerns, shouting at him, "Why don't you go treat AIDS instead?" (McNeil 2006:2).

In Northern Ghana, where I often waited for buses at the Tamale station, many surfaces were plastered with bright red–rimmed decals of the parasite emerging from someone's foot, edged with the words "GUINEA WORM IS A MEDICAL EMERGENCY." Such urgent messages were once printed on stickers, backpacks, and T-shirts distributed throughout the region, reminders of the fact that it took years for the campaign to convince many people with guinea worm that they needed treatment (Watts 1998). Publicity articles often refer to guinea worm as a "forgotten disease of forgotten people," but, interestingly, it was often the "forgotten people" themselves—rather than private donors or health institutions—who for long years remained unconvinced that their disease was urgent enough to require medical intervention. Indeed, in statistics tracking the leading causes of death and disability among the world's most marginalized poor, guinea worm would not make the list (World Health Organization 2009a). Yet parasites can be poignant symbols of death and danger even when they do not scientifically cause it, as anthropologist Mary Douglas notes: "worms belong in the realm of the grave, with death and chaos" (1966:56).

Extracting a worm from the human body has long represented the quintessential act of healing in medicine. Ethnographic accounts the world over—from New Guinea (Hoeppli 1959) to South Carolina (Hyatt 1978)—tell of witch doctors healing complex sicknesses as well as economic misfortunes by removing worms from their patients. Georges Canguilhem uses a similar example in the opening of his famous work *The Normal and the Pathological*: "Magic brings to drugs and incantation rites innumerable resources for generating a profoundly intense desire for cure. Sigerist has noted that Egyptian medicine probably universalized the Eastern experience of parasitic diseases by combining it with the idea of disease-possession: *throwing up worms means being restored to health*" (1991:39, emphasis added). This figure also appears in Claude Lévi-Strauss's essay "The Sorcerer and His Magic," where the more potent sorcerer marks his power precisely by his ability to produce "a bloody worm," and his approach is considered more efficacious than that of other healers because "he presents them with their sickness in a visible and tangible form" (Lévi-Strauss 1963:176). However unconsciously, this dramatic symbol of removing a living parasite from the body imagistically elevates the impact of such a health intervention in the eyes of observers. But at what point does the symbolism of a disease overtake other rationalities in establishing policy priorities?

Of course, few policymakers would be comfortable with the idea that symbolism impacts how they allocate funding. Their own powerful forms of cryptic evidence furnish other rationales and justifications. When institutional priorities began shifting away from the Water Decade's infrastructural projects and toward a "targeted" campaign that made eradication a goal unto itself, health economists argued that the guinea worm not only emblematized inequality through its link to disease-ridden water (a *symptom* of poverty), but directly contributed to its pathologies (as a significant *cause* of poverty). Through extrapolations and economic rate-of-return equations, they predicted that eradication of the parasite would make local agriculture significantly more productive and profitable (by eliminating the days or weeks when the worm kept farmers from their fields), thus shifting local economies and bringing rural poverty a key step closer to alleviation

(Belcher et al. 1975; Cairncross et al. 2002; Centers for Disease Control 2011a; Voelker 2007).[12] But poverty is a tangled and often-unresponsive condition. According to the World Bank, farming productivity in Northern Ghana remained painfully stagnant during the years that coincide with guinea worm eradication efforts, marked by low and inconsistent crop yields that experts believe are linked to holes in local infrastructure and to insecure markets for selling what food products are grown (World Bank 2011:52–53). In fact, the number of people living on less than a dollar a day in Northern Ghana has actually *increased* by 0.9 million since 1992 (World Bank 2011:7), when the guinea worm campaign was in its first years of outreach there. Whatever profoundly complex factors are now sharpening the inequalities that have long marked the region, these recent figures suggest that the slow decline of the guinea worm—while clearly meaningful for other reasons—has not yet been able to make a statistically visible dent in the deep-rooted problem of poverty for the farmers of Northern Ghana.

Yet the parasite's evocative image of decay has undeniably captured the public imagination to a rare extent and has gathered major health policy momentum, propelling the guinea worm campaign into one of the most widely publicized and multipartnered eradication efforts in history. The program's long-standing international media popularity likely also derives in part from the broader biomedical ideas about worms that were already in play, a semiotic dimension that Wenzel Geissler also examines in his "Worms Are Our Life" series. After detailing Luo ethnomedical ideas of worms, Geissler then probes and denaturalizes biomedical understandings of parasites to reveal them as equally culturally laden:

> [B]iomedical concepts identify order with the maintenance of borders, which protect the vulnerable inside and the identity of the person and externalize and exclude other living things. The relationship to creatures transgressing these borders is conflict, in which both health and the order of life is at stake, and in which moral constructs of "good" and the fight against "evil" are evoked. . . . Worms are conceptualized as the enemies of order and a threat to bodily functioning . . . they have to be fought and possibly eradicated. (Geissler 1998a:75, 70)

Surely the eradication campaign drew strength from these sorts of preexisting biomedical conceptions of worms, as well as from the international publicity generated by such a grotesquely photogenic nemesis.

The Carter Center's first active tallies of guinea worm showed hundreds of thousands of unreported infections in some of the poorest corners of Africa. In light of how shockingly hidden the disease had formerly been during eras of passive surveillance, the guinea worm was also transformed into a potent symbol of neglect that could be remedied. There were almost 180,000 cases of guinea worm tallied in Ghana during the first official counts of 1989 (Hopkins and Hopkins 1992), the year that the national program launched in partnership with Ghana Health Services. The Carter Center was still called "Global 2000" then, and their multimillion-dollar backing, coupled with numerous partners and donors, was essential to the program's extensive reach into every community in rural Ghana where the parasite was endemic. A dedicated rotation of program field officers canvassed cities, crossed rivers in dugout canoes, and set off down narrow dirt paths so rough they could be traveled only by motorbikes, gradually making contact with even the most remote communities. "Sometimes people would tell us it was the first time they had ever seen a government vehicle in their village," Dr. Seidu said of the program's four-wheel-drive trucks, which have small black and blue emblems of the guinea worm emblazoned on their doors.

Going after the guinea worm as a single-target issue meant a dramatic change of tactics from the World Health Assembly's original vision. Instead of funding expensive clean water projects, the new program would focus on distributing straws that filtered only guinea worm larvae, and on establishing an unprecedented network of community volunteers to monitor and report developing cases. Yet after nearly fifteen years of applying these tactics, an explosion of guinea worm in a northern village called Sang still qualified this Ghanaian community as the most guinea-worm-ridden place in the world, and program workers began to consider integrating more comprehensive water-purification methods there. Although the Carter Center typically does not fund water projects directly, they had strong partnerships with other NGOs that did.[13] With the Guinea Worm Eradication Program helping to coordinate advocacy, a mechanized borehole well system was finally built in Sang. "You used to see everyone in this village sitting under trees with their worms coming out. But we got the well and cases fell to nothing, nothing," a community volunteer from Sang told me. Dr. Seidu was also impressed with the dramatic results that clean water provision produced in the long-problematic village. "I have seen the worst guinea worm villages turn on a dime once they have good water," he told me firmly. "It is something to think about." A similar view has been expressed by people who received cloth water filters from the guinea worm eradication campaign in Nigeria, as William Brieger and his colleagues at the University of Ibadan (1997) reported in the article "Eradicating Guinea Worm Without Wells: Unrealized Hopes of the Water Decade." They documented the campaign's success at reducing guinea worm in Nigeria, but also discussed the persistent human health risks of a backdrop where only 14 percent of rural citizens at the time had access to safe water (74 percent of residents in hamlets drank only unclean pond water, and another 11 percent had wells that had become dysfunctional). In this context, "people accept the filters reluctantly and continue to ask when the government will provide them with wells" (Brieger et al. 1997:359).

Indeed, in contrast to the widespread enthusiasm that borehole wells and other clean water projects have generated, the reception of the program's individual water filters has been ambivalent in Ghana as well, and their success at times markedly uneven. I will always remember the first time that I saw a guinea worm filter in its local context. It was in the town of Savelugu. I was sitting on a bench under an acacia tree, talking to some men with the help of a translator. When I mentioned my interest in the guinea worm, a tall, wiry young man signaled to his wife and said something enthusiastically in Dagbani. She disappeared behind half of a green fence, and returned holding some small objects in her extended palms.

It took me a minute to recognize the Carter Center's signature guinea worm straw, with their stylized eagle logo imprinted on the shiny black plastic tube. The nylon cord—which in theory could be strung around a farmer's neck as he worked in the fields, with the attached filter at the ready if he needed to take a sip from a nearby pool—was deeply folded at regular intervals, in that factory-fresh way that made it clear this cord was being unfurled for the first time. Eagerly scanning the faces of the older men as he explained how to use the straw, its owner theatrically demonstrated how to put the filter in his mouth, using a wriggling finger to represent the guinea worm that could not fit through its mesh. After a few minutes he gently passed the straw to me for inspection, then shook open the larger cloth filter with a dramatic flourish.

The second filter was edged with shiny cloth surrounding a wide mesh square made of synthetic fabric once donated by Dupont Corporation.

The nylon mesh was so clean and new that its white weave gleamed almost silver in the hot midday sun, still deeply creased in perfect, fresh rectangles after months (or years?) of storage. Such cloth filters were designed to be permanently stretched over the tops of the clay vessels in which a family's water was stored, to catch the tiny crustaceans that, if swallowed, might infect the drinker with guinea worm. I was puzzled as I watched the man's elaborate pantomime of how to employ devices that he himself had clearly never used. This technology had some significant value to him, I thought, but it wasn't a use-value.

The demonstration over, he carefully refolded the cloth filter and tucked the pipe filter's necklace cord back into neat loops and handed them both to his wife, who returned them to their designated hook on the earthen wall of their home. The unused filters hanging by the door reminded me of the placement of protective medicines in Dagomba households, which are carefully collected only to be positioned strategically in the house (usually hung in the doorway or buried in a corner of the room), other times worn on the body (often around the neck, along with herbal bundles or Qur'anic-verse-inscribed scrolls tucked in slender leather tubes only slightly smaller than the guinea worm tube filter hanging from its lanyard). In Northern Ghana, the efficacy of such traditional protective medicines is not understood to derive from their daily use; instead, it is the simple fact of their possession that matters (Bierlich 2007). Looking at the unused guinea worm filters draped with such care in a Dagomba family's doorway, I began to wonder: Were these biomedical artifacts the talismans of a new century?

An informal questionnaire administered by Ghanaian leadership in the eradication program in 2009 found that 55 percent of people kept their guinea worm filters in the bedroom. A head Ghanaian program administrator, who had helped to organize the unofficial mini-survey in a few villages of the Northern Region and cared deeply about figuring out why local people acted in ways he could not understand, shook his head as he read the survey results to me. "The bedroom!" he repeated. "That doesn't make sense. Why would they keep the filter in their bedroom?" The second most popular storage place, favored by 26 percent, was hanging on the wall. Another 11 percent declined to answer. Less than 3 percent reported actually keeping it on their water pot, where guinea worm filters are supposed to remain stretched for daily use.

At the time the survey was taken, individual water filters and education about them had been a centerpiece of the guinea worm eradication campaign in Ghana for exactly twenty years. But when asked *why* they used the filters, 54 percent of people had no answer.

A Case of Competing Magics

The familiar term "magic bullet" in public health discussions refers to an intervention's reliance on single-target medical technologies (such as chemical formulas, mosquito nets, or guinea worm filters), without focus on integrating these biomedical objects into more contextual, ecological, or holistic health care interventions (cf. Biehl 2007; Cueto 2007). In the public health seminars and policy lectures I attend at the Woodrow Wilson School, this phrase is bandied about frequently, often with air quotes and usually with critical implications.

But for a moment, I want to take this terminology seriously at face value. After all, the label "magic bullet" comes startling close to the "magic ammunition" (Evans-Pritchard 1937:180) that Azande witch doctors use to symbolically control danger and sickness. This is not to deny that public health's "magic bullets" do have obvious biomedical applications and technological capacities, but rather to question why they are sometimes treated by health officials as having value and efficacy beyond their observable worth, as if their distribution alone somehow taps into a distant all-protective power regardless of how they are used in practice. Such uncanny resonance with ritual manipulation deserves to be taken seriously. An Azande witch doctor shoots a magic "missile" and extracts a beetle from his patient's forehead (Evans-Pritchard 1937:179). Under what social conditions or political constellations can a health campaign distribute a "magic bullet" and expect to remove a worm?

Of course, this is a question that extends far beyond the realm of guinea worm and reverberates throughout the global health arena today. Elsewhere in Ghana, a study of river blindness showed that rates of the disease were not going down despite a major "vertical" campaign there. For unknown reasons, 75 percent of the people given ivermectin drugs by the campaign were not taking them, even though the pills would have prevented this crippling blindness, caused by the tiny microfilarial parasites of a larger parasitic worm (Kutin et al. 2004). During a visit to Princeton in winter 2009, another top Ghanaian medical doctor and health researcher spoke eloquently about the "cultural barriers" he has seen during his decades of applied research. He told us that the malaria bednets distributed to be draped protectively around pregnant mothers and their newborn children were occasionally reallocated within the household, noting particularly that they were sometimes rolled up and tied around the head of a husband as he slept. (Interestingly, this style of male headdress is uncommon but highly symbolic in Northern Ghana. Or at least, the only man I ever met who had a rolled cloth circled like a crown around his head was the paramount chief of Kumbungu, who presided over his court of attendant chiefs in a red La-Z-Boy-style recliner.)

Yet such status-steeped and sometimes supernaturally meaningful applications were hardly the only instances of biomedical objects being used in ways that their public health creators had not intended. There were also some cases where they were simply not used at all, as when polio vaccines were rejected by parents who feared rumors of sterilization, or mosquito nets were found tightly rolled in the corners of huts where children died tragically of malarial convulsions. Other times these health devices were put to highly functional sideways purposes; off the banks of Lake Bosumtwi, I once saw two small boys wading in waist-deep water with a mosquito net, trying to catch tilapia.

These divergent local uses of biomedical objects ranged from the profoundly tragic to the dazzlingly creative, but they all had one thing in common. The objects all came from "magic bullet" campaigns, where the seemingly misused devices were distributed in a vacuum of ongoing infrastructural development (usually by outsiders who departed from the village shortly afterward), leaving the health technologies to circulate unmoored in the intricate capillaries of preexisting knowledges and meanings.

It is therefore no coincidence that these magic bullets at times become embedded precisely in local magical systems, traveling in sideways directions. While donors and public health officials are perpetually puzzled by local people's "noncompliance" with such potentially lifesaving technologies, the recipients of these devices were often equally perplexed by the strangers who arrived abruptly in their villages and disappeared within hours, leaving behind the manufactured traces of their concern: fogs of insecticides, the banal lace of synthetic bednets, or plastic filters subtly etched with corporate logos, like illegible glyphs on artifacts from some distant world. It is no wonder such objects sometimes came to be imbued with meanings of power and danger, even when unused and simply *possessed*.

Interestingly, Carter Center officials and other proponents of guinea worm eradication often speak of the program's interventions as "a low-tech venture" (Bristol 2008), because the disease is now on the cusp of eradication without a drug or vaccine (Barry 2007). (There has never yet been a vaccine developed to prevent a known parasitic disease, a fact that marks a major tactical difference between guinea worm and the smallpox virus eradication campaign.) In fact, I imagine that some guinea worm program members might be taken aback that I consider some of their campaign cornerstones as "magic bullets." Yet I want to suggest that a closer look at these objects begins to complicate taken-for-granted notions that such intervention tools are simply "low" technologies, assumptions that become part of a rhetoric that forecloses deeper questions. The copepods that carry guinea worm are unusually large for a water-borne disease vector, measuring more than one millimeter in length (Muller 2005:522). This means that any cloth, even an ordinary T-shirt, can serve as an effective water filter against guinea worm larvae, a preventative measure long known in many parts of the world. As far back as 1666, one author in Beirut wrote of guinea worm: "The way to avoid this worm is to drink only wine or, if water is used, only such as has been carefully filtered through linen" (Grove 1994:713).

Guinea worm thus has the rare distinction of being a tropical disease that the majority of people living in extreme poverty already had the technical tools to prevent—most any piece of cloth would do. I wondered what it meant that the Carter Center's guinea worm filters looked distinctly like a piece of more specialized technology, when they had more or less the same medical efficacy as a T-shirt would. (DuPont scientists had developed a tough nylon mesh for the cloth guinea worm filters [Barry 2007], which would last longer and drain faster than cotton—fine enough to catch copepods, but too porous to strain out any other pathogens, such as microscopic vectors of fatal water-borne diseases.) Yet the novelty of the specialized-looking device may have served a double purpose. Perhaps it created a space for new behaviors, helping community health education to take root in the minds of both policy officials and program recipients—almost as a kind of branding. Certainly the sleek, logo-imprinted guinea worm filters carry with them an *aesthetic* of science. But for all the tremendous efforts and resources entailed in developing and manufacturing the synthetic filters in an American laboratory, and in hiring campaign staff to distribute them to remote villages around the world and spend years educating people about their use, it remains a somewhat painful fact that the filter's wide mesh can protect against only a single disease, and one that rarely ever threatens human life. A different type of water filter—ceramic, for example—distributed through the same channels to the same households could have prevented guinea worm and at the same time protected against the many other, far more deadly pathogens that often inhabit guinea-worm-infected waters (Brieger et al. 1997). Among these are polio, cholera, typhoid, hepatitis A, various intestinal worm infections, and the common diarrheal diseases that kill 1.5 million children in the world each year. Given this context, the eradication campaign's choice to develop specialized water filters that protect only against a single waterborne disease might be viewed as a downright iconic example of "magic bullet" technology.

A similarly complex story could be told about the ABATE chemical formula widely applied to dams and ponds, which kills guinea worm larvae but is not designed to purify the unclean water that local people then must continue drinking. The larvicide is now donated to guinea worm eradication efforts by the BASF chemical group, a corporation which (among its many diverse products) sells active ingredients to the pharmaceutical industry (BASF 2012). ABATE is BASF's particular brand-name of the generic drug temephos, an organophosphate larvicide; competing corporations have also produced versions of the compound under the trade names Abat, Abathion, Biothion, Bithion, Difennthos, Ecopro, Nimitox, and Swebate. By inhibiting cholinesterase enzymes in the brain, blood, and nervous system, temephos interferes with the functioning of the central nervous system and causes insect vectors to die before reaching adulthood. At much higher exposures (via accidents or spills, for example), temephos can produce the same effects in humans, overstimulating the nervous system and causing difficulty breathing, nausea, incontinence, convulsions, coma, respiratory failure, and death (National Library of

Medicine 2011). Indeed, it was not always easy for campaign workers to estimate the liquid volume of an irregularly shaped body of pond or dam, an important step in mathematically calculating the precise dose of ABATE needed. I was told of a case in Northern Ghana where many fish in a particular village's pond died after an application of ABATE, suggesting that the water was accidentally treated with a significantly higher dose than that needed to kill copepods. The local community was deeply and understandably concerned by this incident. Temephos has also been widely used in other global health campaigns over time, such as efforts to eradicate malaria and river blindness, and several insect vectors have already developed drug resistance (Polson et al. 2010; Rodríguez et al. 2002; Tikar et al. 2009). One study in Ghana found that the *S. sancti-pauli* blackflies (which carry river blindness) in a body of water that had never even been directly treated with the formula already had a fivefold drug resistance to temephos (Osei-Atweneboana et al. 2001). These flies had genetically mutated and developed inverted chromosomes that allowed them to survive the larvicide's neurological effects—an evolution suggesting heavy levels of temephos saturation in the environment over generations. In this light, the guinea worm campaign's focus on applying ABATE to local dams and ponds is perhaps not a case of a "low-tech" getting-away from drugs, but instead a displacement of the "magic bullet" chemical's entry point: in the absence of an effective pharmaceutical treatment, the environment itself becomes medicated.

In addition to the scattered threats that villagers occasionally addressed to health workers administering larvicide to their drinking water (as in the situation in Taha where this story began), the guinea worm's sheer persistence over the years testifies to the fact that many people did not use their painstakingly distributed household filters as instructed. Despite continuing campaign efforts and a consistently high demand for the program's fashionable filters, the guinea worm in Ghana actually *increased* from 1994 to 1995, from 1998 to 1999, from 2001 to 2002, from 2002 to 2003,[14] from 2005 to 2006, and from May of 2006 to May of 2007 (World Health Organization 2005:6; Centers for Disease Control 2007: 4). In a 2007 trip report, former president Carter even stated that "in our Guinea worm eradication effort, Ghana has been our worst disappointment" (Carter 2007). But in the face of mounting proof that the technological tools at their disposal had limitations on the ground when it came to comprehensively addressing guinea worm disease without funding to build clean water projects, the Ghanaian program was faced with an exceptionally challenging task: to make the available tools work anyway.

This required constant and creative negotiations, careful surveillance networks, and most of all a renewed attention to the underlying social contexts and community relations through which the program's distributed objects inevitably made their way. For example, ABATE chemicals usually rested at the center of the few more menacing conflicts that the program experienced—such as the rare but significant occasions when people came out and actively resisted attempts to apply ABATE to their water, or kept the locations of their ponds hidden from the campaign workers trying to treat them. Over time, the eradication program learned that the best way to quell such fears was to organize a community demonstration in which murky water collected from a local source would be combined with clear water in a glass jar and shaken, allowing people to see for themselves the white copepod vectors bobbing and swimming in the jar (Hopkins and Ruiz-Tiben 2011). If ABATE larvicide could be called a "magic bullet" solution on account of its vertical emphasis and chemical technology, then perhaps such demonstrations could be likened to showing people how a magic trick works. After such evidence-based demonstrations, community trust and lines of communication were generally much improved, and local people were less suspicious of the chemicals poured into their water. (After all, the *Oxford English Dictionary*'s [2010] definition of "magic" specifies that it usually involves "the use of an occult or secret body of knowledge." What better definition could there be of technology when it is left unexplained and enigmatic?)

Conflicts over the guinea worm program's technological tools were not always of this nature. At times they reified existing social differences, and even made new ways of addressing them possible. Bierlich reports that senior wives in Northern Ghana sometimes hoarded the household guinea worm filter as an object of prestige, forbidding junior wives to use it to prepare the family's drinking water in their absence (1995:506). Even in the case of Taha's conflict, it is notable that most of the farmers who stormed the water's edge with cutlasses that afternoon were younger men, who by voicing their suspicions of the ABATE chemical's dark purpose were also posing a challenge to their elders who had consented to its application. At work here are basic human motivations and power struggles, old as time, which technology made negotiable in surprising new ways.

But there is still the underlying fact that somehow, when ABATE chemicals were first applied to the dam in Taha with secrecy reminiscent of a sorcerer mixing a potion, the local villagers themselves embraced this observation. They enfolded ABATE (perhaps already a vehicle for symbolic authority) into their preexisting beliefs about the paranormal causes of guinea worm as another interchangeable unit of magic. In this sense, perhaps it is these Dagomba farmers' assumption that their own systems of magical causation were so plainly permeable to the eradication campaign's paraphernalia that ultimately attests most loudly to the existence—and the potential risk—of the campaign's magic bullets. Although devices such as guinea worm filters were designed as a quick fix to eliminate the parasite without costly infrastructural development, in Ghana "the programme stagnated for a decade" (Cairncross et al. 2012) and spanned more than twenty years. In this *longue durée*, supernatural suspicions and other very meaningful community concerns began to accumulate around the magic bullet technologies that were designed to eradicate a water-borne disease without providing clean water.

Yet to their great credit, program workers recognized the need to step outside this volatile overlap in order to move the campaign onto firmer shared ground. During my visits in 2008 and 2009, I observed government actors fight for clean water systems for communities even though usual Carter Center policy did not directly fund this strategy, painstaking national negotiations that resulted in a major new addition to the program staff in Northern Ghana: an "emergency response team" to assess water conditions and repair broken-down borehole wells. I was also impressed by many of the daily ins and outs of community relations (jokes, translations, compromises, return visits, village soccer games, and non-Muslim campaign workers who fasted during Ramadan as a mark of solidarity with coworkers, for example). I sometimes wondered to myself whether the campaign seemed to be making headway not because of its vertical blueprint but rather in spite of it, as behind-the-scenes swerves and human ties fiddled with the vertical model at its edges and remade its meanings on the ground—processes of trial and error that economist Angus Deaton might call "endless tinkering."

Reflections in the Twilight of the Guinea Worm

The office walls of the guinea worm program's headquarters in Tamale were plastered with worm "forecasts" for the year. Side-by-side poster boards painstakingly charted each parasite that emerged in black or red marker, month by month and district by district. These charts documented the gradual effects of program workers' persevering outreach as, one pond at a time, one village at a time, guinea worm slowly began to disappear from Northern Ghana. When I first visited the office in 2008, alternating ones and zeros dominated the forecasts, the hand-drawn binary code of guinea worm's last stand. But by the following summer, most of the cells in the chart's grid were filled with zeros.

In a back room of the air-conditioned office, a young Carter Center consultant spoke surprisingly fluent Dagbani for a twenty-eight-year-old from the American Midwest. For almost seven years he had worked tirelessly for guinea worm eradication efforts. Behind the desk where his laptop rested, there were numerous plastic vials, each filled with a single, long white worm suspended in clear liquid. "They are waiting to be sent to Atlanta for DNA testing," he explained, adjusting his glasses.

At the weekly staff meeting later that day, ambiguity over the identification of various parasitic worms became a major point of discussion. Now that Ghana was down to its last cases, it was important to differentiate the actual guinea worm from any look-alike that might emerge, such as the white "mother worm" of onchocerciasis that can grow over a foot in length, nestled in a hard nodule under its host's skin. Looking at the picture one program worker displayed on his laptop of a recently emerged false guinea worm, an example of the parasites that should not ultimately be tallied on the program charts, I thought fleetingly of the villagers with guinea worm who once used oracles to tell them whether they were responsible for the worms because of their own wrongdoings. With genetic sequencing and its digital divinations, the eradication program workers also needed to discern whether or not certain worms were their own responsibility to be counted.

Perhaps one might see in this a poetic analogy in which bioscience relies on its own secret knowledge. But meanwhile, the surrounding villages' traditional markers of occult magic had been equally reconfigured by the biomedical logic of guinea worm prevention. Where village elders had once guarded sacred oracles and shrines (Bierlich 2007), now locally respected villagers were hired as guinea worm "dam guards" by Ghana Health Services and paid a monthly salary to sit by the water's edge and make sure that no one stepped into the water—or, in cases where a borehole well existed, that no one drew drinking water from the dam. The punishment for doing so was a fine payable at the chief's palace, the dam guard I met one afternoon told me sternly, leaning heavily on his gnarled wooden staff. Yet even those villagers who had initially resisted such program efforts were increasingly grateful to be rid of the guinea worms that many had believed were painful but inevitable parts of their lives (and indeed of their bodies) for so long. "Once I had guinea worms coming out of me for a whole year, one after one after one," a man in Diare told me. "I could not farm, and weeds killed all of my corn. It was so hard to feed my family. Now," he shrugged as he shelled peanuts onto the cement floor, "I am free."

But even when the worm's life cycle is biomedically understood and locally reframed as itself the culprit, its intimacy *and even its absence* remained layered with other social meanings for such villagers. False or suspiciously unverifiable reports of guinea worm sprang up in places thought to have eliminated the parasite—247 such false reports were logged in Ghana in 2011 alone (World Health Organization 2012:185). People learned that they could use the politicized worm to make claims for long-needed clean water supplies. Missing worms became a sign that sickness of all kinds was not inevitable, and eventually might be eliminated from their lives—but also that it took certain channels of foreign partnerships and funding to do it. "I hope the Carter Center cures malaria next," one village volunteer told me. "That's the only way it will be fixed, if the Carter Center does it." He also credited the Carter Center for giving him a blue bicycle that, it turned out, had actually been donated by UNICEF.

In August and September of 2009, the last months I spent in Ghana conducting this fieldwork,[15] the country reported only one case of guinea worm each month—for the first time in history. The last known case in Ghana to date was reported the next year, in May of 2010 (Richards et al. 2011). A Carter Center 2011 "Guinea Worm Wrap-Up" newsletter reported that "after . . . over four million cloth filters, more than one million pipe filters, 72,000 liters of ABATE® Larvicide; at least nine ministers of health and nine missed target dates, we are confident that Ghana's Guinea Worm Eradication Program has finally achieved the demise of the worm" (2011). With the hard work of the program, the gradual incorporation of water projects, and long-term community relationships finally paying off, the worldwide eradication of guinea worm has been predicted for 2013—a date certainly to be taken as a hopeful estimate, given that eradication was also predicted in 1990, 1993, 1995, 1998, 2000, 2005, 2008, 2009, and 2011. Yet eradication does seem imminent, with only 542 cases reported worldwide in 2012 (despite an unexpected outbreak in Mali), down from an estimated 3.5 million cases in 1986 when the Carter Center first began its campaign.[16] Most of the remaining cases of guinea worm are found in postconflict South Sudan, where Carter once managed to use his diplomatic sway to negotiate a "guinea worm cease fire" so that nylon filters could be delivered safely. An experimental barter system there now encourages local peddlers to deliver guinea worm water filters and larvicide in exchange for gum arabic, a hardened tree sap they can use to make sale items such as watercolor paints, cosmetics, and shoe polish (Voelker 2007:1857). A feature film about guinea worm eradication, *Foul Water, Fiery Serpent*, was recently released, narrated by Sigourney Weaver. The movie poster depicts three African women balancing water vessels on their heads against a glaring red sunset, with a tagline reading, "IT'S NOT OVER UNTIL THE LAST WORM IS GONE." "Weaver's narration, given her role in *Alien*, seems oddly appropriate," eminent parasitologist David Molyneux wrote in a recent *Lancet* article (2010:947), adding that guinea worm eradication, in his view, means removing one of "the true 'alien monsters' from planet earth" (948). There is even a "Save the Guinea Worm Foundation" that has sprung up online with the mission statement of protecting the parasite against extinction. It purportedly seeks elite members known as "the Preservers" to volunteer themselves as guinea worm hosts and give the "world's most endangered species" a chance to continue its life cycle within their own bodies (2009).

But as this ancient disease nears the end of its time on earth, there is also cause for reflection. Parasitic worms by their very nature breach intimate human boundaries (Douglas 1966; Gardenour and Tadd 2012), which is exactly what makes the ways people struggle to understand them such a revealing microcosm of health cultures and local histories—and so it is not surprising that the guinea worms emerging from people's flesh became a battleground for much bigger social and political conflicts, raising questions of how to cure[17] and whose responsibility it is to heal, and even metaphysical issues about where life ends and death's parasitic hold begins.

As we drove away from Sang that day, it was not hard to believe that the village had once been the most heavily guinea worm–infected community in the entire world. I stared out the window at sights familiar in Northern Ghana, prayer calls echoing from the low plaster spires of neighborhood mosques, clusters of mud huts contrasting with the brilliant colors of women's head scarves. Mothers balanced enamel bowls of yams on their heads and stepped between burning piles of trash with babies slung on their backs; everywhere, beauty and decay folded into each other. A Brong Ahafo Region health student named Alfred sat next to me in the backseat of the Guinea Worm Program 4 × 4, writing in his notebook. He had accompanied us for the day as part of his summer rotation, and had helped me enormously that afternoon to translate my questions into a rephrased half-pidgin that my interviewees could better understand. Suddenly he tapped me on the shoulder and shyly handed me a crumpled paper where a poem was written in blue ink. When I asked if I could include parts of it in the essay I was writing, he smiled and painstakingly recopied it for me on a fresh sheet of notebook paper in the neatest handwriting he could manage as we bumped down the unpaved road back to Tamale.

> They say I am a blind old worm from Guinea
> But I say to them, look not unto my whitish nature
> And claim me holy
> You don't know me, I am not from the gods
> I can do much worse things to mankind.
> I bet you do not even try to memorize
> My Christian name when I mention to you
> I am called *Dracunculus medinensis*
> The ancient hero, I manifest myself in man,
> From drinking water containing my cyclops.
> There my ruling power begins internally.
> The rupturing of the blister releases
> My new generation into the world.

[Local] practitioners with their knowledge about me,
Have they not asked the oracles
How I managed to live successful with my victims?
I slaved them,
Made them unable to go to farm or work.
When man sees me at the shore of the body,
They maltreat me
By forcibly pulling me out with their hands.
Because they know who I am.
I only say to them, treat me gentle, gentle.
If you want to eliminate me,
Follow these rules of water sanitation:
Boil water before you drink
Never send blisters into streams
Treat all infected persons
Report any case of me to a health worker.
Then you won't see me again.
I say watch out.

—Alfred O. K., age twenty-two

(Kintampo Rural Health Training School)[18]

The worm's-eye view from which the poem is written—besides revealing the author's own imaginative force—also creatively reframes the guinea worm as the agent of disease, with the parasite itself denying all connections to local healers, oracles, and gods. Although the poem was ostensibly written as a teaching tool, by that afternoon in 2009 there were barely any cases of guinea worm left in Ghana. But in Alfred's school of rural health training, guinea worm seems to have become akin to a case study of how to overcome entrenched local beliefs about health.

More than that, the complex perspective that Alfred frames here with his own creative spark—a parasitic voice both scoffing and ancient, caught in the midst of a battle of human misunderstandings, simultaneously uttering a didactic death wish and a last battle cry—casts the worm as a forceful actor in these contested stories, as something deserving of being considered not just as a vector, but an ethnographic subject in its own right. For in the end, this account is not about anything so simple as two sides colliding. It is the much more intricate story of how these forces unpredictably mingled and slowly changed each other—the worms acting too, their unexpected persistence and very gradual disappearance conveying something that neither the health workers nor the local villagers could fully articulate to one another, as the mediating parasites themselves were all along exerting a force of their own (Serres 1982).

Many of the issues discussed here will outlive the guinea worm. These Dagomba communities will likely continue to fear other traces of witchcraft, divine new ancestral messages. Their families will continue farming peanuts and tubers, in poverty and in hope of better things ahead. Some lucky villagers will now have clean water systems (at least until locally irreplaceable grommets and gears begin to malfunction). Others have new roles as village health volunteers, a brittle network that will perhaps inflect claims to other futures. It will be interesting to see how long guinea worm filters continue hanging, talisman-like, in villagers' doorways and bedrooms.

With equally staunch hopes for things ahead, the majority of dedicated guinea worm campaign workers will go on with bolstered résumés to work for other tropical disease programs, perhaps trachoma control or malaria eradication, collating data and likely distributing new "magic bullet" pills and devices in other poor regions of West Africa. In this sense, neither side will likely reevaluate its ritual forms, or lose its faith. Still, this moment when guinea worm eradication allowed public health officials' and Dagomba villagers' respective technological and ancestral magics to cross paths can help us glimpse the risks, causalities, and potentials that these diverse groups of people see in each other, as refracted through "the other" living within us. For whether in reverence or disgust, nostalgia or triumphant defeat, the trajectory of humankind's largest bodily worm is a history worth remembering—inseparable as any parasite, it is our history too.

As for the guinea worm itself, it is not so clear where its story will definitively end. Although the parasite is not medically recognized as having any animal reservoirs (this niche historically being filled by the guinea worm's veterinary counterpart *Dracunculus insignis*), genetic sequencing recently showed that a guinea worm living in a dog in rural Ghana was, in fact, the human worm *Dracunculus medinensis*. Over time, several countries officially certified as free of guinea worm, from India to Uzbekistan, have also reported cases of human guinea worms found living as secret refugees inside the bodies of dogs and raccoons.[19] No one can say with certainty whether this is random accident, elegant adaptation, or if the last surviving guinea worms are patiently waiting to return home.[20]

Notes

1. I am extremely grateful to Ghana Health Services, the Ghana Guinea Worm Eradication Program, Ministry of Health personnel, and members of the Carter Center in both Tamale and Atlanta for their early support of this research. This ethnographic description of the campaign's social complexities and cultural ambiguities—anthropological interpretations that are mine alone, and for which I accept full responsibility—are offered here in the spirit of mutual care and critical inquiry, with respect for their dedication and difficult work. This research was approved by the Ghana Health Services Ethical Review Committee and the Princeton University Institutional Review Board. Fieldwork was funded in part by the West African Research Association, the Princeton Center for Health and Wellbeing, the Princeton Health Grand Challenges Initiative, and the Princeton Development Grand Challenges Initiative. An American University Dean's Research Grant also supported related archival work in its earliest stages. I thank João Biehl, Carolyn Rouse, Jim Boon, Carol Greenhouse, Joseph Amon, Ari Samsky, Erin Kane, Pat Moran-Thomas, and the participants in the "When People Come First" workshop for their thoughtful readings. Warm thanks to the Department of Anthropology at Princeton, and to Andrew Seidu Korkor, John Gyapong, Mr. Suly, Alfred O. K., and the many people in Tamale and the surrounding villages of Northern Ghana who shared their hospitality, reflections, and experiences with me.

2. See Kwasi Sarpong (2004:12).

3. This genus has technically been subdivided into three: *Mesocyclops*, *Metacyclops*, and *Thermocyclops*. The guinea worm larvae go from stage 1 to stage 3 within the bodies of these copepods, further complicating the guinea worm's intricate life cycle.

4. The male guinea worm's life cycle is significantly shorter than that of the females—although neither the male nor the female guinea worm survives beyond the birth of their first-stage larvae. Such short life cycles are of course hardly exceptional in the lower animal kingdom.

5. The guinea worm's Latin name, *Dracunculus* for "fiery dragon," comes from this trait.

6. The blister is caused by the release of a few larvae into the subdermis, so the bursting of the ulcer can occur even if the guinea worm never reaches water.

7. Stubbs and Bligh 1931:18.

8. This resemblance is also the reason guinea worm was historically once called not only the "medina worm" but also the "medina vein" (Grove 1994).

9. Some other interesting ethnomedical texts about perceptions of general worm diseases include Vecchiato (1997), Green (1997), Zondi and Kvalsig (1996), Reis (1994), Nichter (1989:164–65), and Hoeppli (1959).

10. For those interested in further reading about the social histories of Dagbon, see Bierlich (2007), Staniland (1975), Palmer (2010), and Tait (1963). J. Goody (1962), E. Goody (1973), and Hawkins (2002) examine the micropolitics of the supernatural elsewhere in Northern Ghana. The geography of these accusations also reflects profound north-south inequalities and regional imaginations that persist in Ghana (see Goldstone 2012; Parker 2006; Pellow 2011; World Bank 2011); for a comparative view of the occult from southern Ghana, see Meyer 1998; Gray 2005; Parish 2000. Of course, these realities in Ghana today are part of much larger permutations in occult politics emerging throughout neoliberal Africa. For a sampling of this vast ethnographic literature, see Apter 1993; Ashforth 2005; Austen 1993; Bayart 1993; Comaroff and Comaroff 2001; Ferguson 2006; Geschiere 1997; Masquelier 1999; Mbembe 2003; Schmoll 1993; West and Sanders 2003.

11. In Northern Ghana, some villagers spoke at length about President Carter's local visits, but many had not heard of Don Hopkins by name—yet another reminder of the divergent meanings, myths, and characters that global health campaigns hold for different people (*Global Health Chronicles* 2009; also see PBS 2006).

12. In 1997, a team from the World Bank and the Carter Center estimated that the economic rate of return for guinea worm eradication would be an impressive 29 percent (Kim et al. 1997). As Cairncross et al. detail (2002), attempts to estimate the economic impact of guinea worm disease have often relied on multiplying the number of days of labor lost by the mean production value per day, despite criticisms that such equations do not factor in what policymakers call "coping strategies" (see Paul 1998). But as Cairncross and colleagues also note, such economic arguments have been effective at galvanizing national policymakers in many African countries, whether or not these calculations were ultimately accurate.

13. See Carter Center 2004; Hopkins 1992:630; Huttly et al. 1990. In South Sudan, 444 of the 463 villages reporting guinea worm cases in 2011 did not have a single source of safe drinking water (World Health Organization 2012:184).

14. In 2002, the *Yaa-Naa* of Dagbon was killed, and the isolated pockets of political insecurity that followed the chief's death surely also impacted the Guinea Worm Eradication Program's success rates during that time, as in 1994–1995 (see MacGaffey 2006). Yet the repeated annual increases in guinea worm disease over more than a decade are not simply *reducible* to these chieftaincy disputes either, although American campaign workers frequently glossed setbacks in this way. The political instability in Northern Ghana was thus very different from that in the Sudan, where decades of violent military conflict have embroiled millions of people, dramatically affecting all areas of health care delivery. This tumultuous history is the primary reason why most of the remaining cases of guinea worm are found in South Sudan (see Hopkins and Withers 2002).

15. On a brief methodological note, I spent four months in Northern Ghana preparing for and conducting this ethnographic research on Dagomba community health issues between 2008 and 2009, including four weeks spent working closely

with the Guinea Worm Eradication Campaign itself. During this time I attended program staff meetings, visited the Tamale Case Containment Center during daily bandagings of emerging worms, interviewed the National Program head and various staff members, and visited numerous endemic villages with the program's field officers, sometimes observing their regular field activities and other times conducting my own interviews with guinea worm volunteers and local community members. Like much salvage ethnography, this period of anthropological engagement was much shorter than would have been ideal, a time frame with obvious shortcomings. I relied on whatever scraps of ethnographic information I was able to gather during these brief trips, as well as on the deep local knowledges and guidance of campaign workers themselves. By the time I was ready for a full year of intensive dissertation research, the guinea worm had already been eradicated from Ghana.

16. Other valuable snapshots from this phase include Centers for Disease Control 2011b; Greenway 2004; Hopkins et al. 2000; Hopkins et al. 2005; Iriemenan et al. 2008; Morenikeji and Asiatu 2010; Ruiz-Tiben and Hopkins 2006; and Seidu Korkor and Afele 2009.

17. In public health circles, debates about eradication rage on (especially see Cueto 2007; Henderson 2012; Rinaldi 2009; Stepan 2011). Those who support eradication point out the obvious long-term benefits of ridding the world of even a single disease once and for all. Having such a popular "targeted" aim also increases public and donor support, giving the campaign a more compelling storyline. Meanwhile, advocates of disease "control" rather than all-out eradication argue that building sustainable health systems should be the goal rather than campaigns, which cost a great deal of extra money in the final push of surveillance; in efforts to isolate a country's final cases, the guinea worm campaign has occasionally resorted to paying up to US$112 per "hanging worm" (World Health Organization 2012:185; see Rwakimari 2006:5). Yet on the ground in northern Ghana, eradication meant something different still (see Carter Center 2006).

18. I had to condense his original text at certain points and omit a few lines for reasons of space here, with much gratitude to Alfred for sharing his poem and for giving permission for its inclusion in this essay.

19. Cairncross et al. (2002) provide an insightful overview of this literature on the history of guinea worm infection within animal populations, and Muller (2005) reviews this apparent incident of a human species of guinea worm living in a dog in Ghana. Bimi et al. (2005) describe the breakthrough genetic sequencing tools of 18S-rRNA used to differentiate *D. medinensis* from *D. insignis*, including their finding from Ghana that suggested the guinea worm extracted from a dog was in fact the human worm *D. medinensis*. The authors additionally document reports of human guinea worm in dogs in Mauritania and a donkey in Mali. See also country-specific accounts of *D. medinensis* infection in animal populations of formerly endemic areas, including Pakistan (Muhammad et al. 2005), Uzbekistan (Litvinov and Litvinov 1981; Litvinov and Lysenko 1982), and India (Lalitha and Anandan 1980).

20. Obviously, guinea worms do not have the affective capacity to consciously wait with patience, and this expression is a figurative reference to the evolutionary accidents and persistent force of nature over time, which often thwart or outlast

human efforts to decisively predict and fully control disease. By playing here with the way that the guinea worm has already been anthropomorphized by various actors in this story, I mean to suggest that versions of the social complexities and conflicting priorities that unfolded during this eradication campaign will repeat themselves in other times and places; if not for guinea worm in Ghana, then for guinea worm in South Sudan—and one day in the future, when guinea worm is finally eradicated, this story will resurface again within the tales of numerous other diseases for which eradication has proven a more elusive goal than anyone expected, as polio and malaria take their place as the next frontrunners on the global eradication agenda. Even smallpox, the disease so often pointed to as proof that eradication is truly possible, has recently returned anew to intervention debates: there is now talk about resuming public smallpox vaccinations, owing to concerns that the eradicated disease could be intentionally reintroduced as a biological weapon (Carter Center 2002; see Hopkins 2002 [1982]; Henderson 2009). With epidemiologists already constructing contingency plans and control scenarios in case the only disease ever to have been successfully eradicated from the world someday returns, it is worth wondering whether a similarly unexpected plot twist may one day present itself in the wake of guinea worm eradication.

III

MARKETS

Overview

Various movements are afoot in the field of global health: from the collective control of epidemics to the personalization of disease; from trial and error to the standardization of evidence and policy; from health as a public good to the pharmaceuticalization of health care; from governmental detachment to the industrialization of the nongovernmental sector and a privatized politics of survival. Alongside them, critical questions abound: Has the biopolitical morphed into a multilevel turf war of private versus public stakeholders battling over the utility of government? Where does this leave the majority and the "surplus" poor and diseased subjects who are not targets of specific interventions? Is their biomedical rehabilitation "futile" in a world where health policies are increasingly oriented by market principles? How does this underside of global health speak to the decline of civil society as a viable "transactional locus" for the guarantee of social justice?

The chapters by Ecks and Harper, Han, Whitmarsh, and Biehl and Petryna provide valuable examples of the ways in which the movement of global health toward ever-greater scientization and private-sector involvement can be creatively studied by anthropologists. Strategically located at the sites where pharmaceutical industries, public health care providers, and patient-citizen-consumers intersect, these case studies provide a fertile ground from which to rethink the role of science, the state, and the market in global health and to evaluate alternative configurations, protagonists, dynamics, and possibilities.

How are the interpenetrating domains of ill health, therapeutic markets, and the law emerging as implicit and explicit sites for claiming political rights and confronting political failures? Are the subjects of rights and economic subjects—once understood as distinct entities—now included or excluded through shared mechanisms shaped by the market of global medicine? Is the market, then, what is ultimately produced by government and by the people?

Case studies in this section show how health policy debates about risk and compliance, as well as patient struggles for access to pharmaceuticals, are part of a changed health care landscape that the concept of the medicalization of social problems cannot fully address (Conrad 2007; Lock 2003; Scheper-Hughes 1992). While the culture of biomedicine is undeniably powerful, it is also speculative and improvised, and patients do not simply become the diagnostic categories and treatments that are applied to them. People may inhabit them to greater or lesser degrees, but they are also able to refuse them, or to redefine and deploy them to unanticipated ends. Understanding today's capacious pharmaceuticalization of health care requires analytical tools and methods that can account for the entanglement of multiple social forces and markets in defining the politics of health, the unregulated circulation of pharmaceuticals and their chemical effects, and the role of patients in creating demand.

In their contribution, Stefan Ecks and Ian Harper offer a way to see how the landscape of tuberculosis treatment in India emerges at the intersection of global business and political schemes and the local constraints of providing care. They follow the pharmaceutical industry's efforts to shape the diagnosis and treatment of TB, homing in on interactions between medical representatives (MRs) and doctors, and showing how the very materiality of global health interventions (drugs, protocols, policies, recordkeeping) provides the context for the expansion of a private therapeutic market.

India has the world's largest number of people suffering from TB, and most patients receive their care from private practitioners. The sphere of these private caregivers has been for the most part unregulated, producing "therapeutic anarchy," a situation in which the standards of care set by the WHO are altered or ignored, and where determining the extent of such informal practices has become nearly impossible. The WHO, working together with the Indian government, has sought to tackle the TB emergency in the country by involving an array of voluntary, corporate, and private providers and by extending collaborations via "Public-Private Mixes" (PPMs). The WHO now relies on directly observed treatment, short-course (DOTS) as the standard of care. This mixed partnership has also allowed the Indian state, and by extension the WHO, to gain some control over the therapeutic practices of the private side of the system.

As the majority of TB sufferers continue to receive help through private practitioners, however, DOTS wilts by the wayside. The reasons for this are manifold, but in general they reflect the ineffective organization of the Indian health care system, doctors' reluctance to take on additional administrative recordkeeping chores, and the widely held perception among practitioners and patients (reinforced by the pharmaceutical industry through its medical representatives) that DOTS provides subpar treatment and is ill-equipped to handle multidrug-resistant TB. Here, as in the Ugandan account, the move toward public-private mixes and the standardization of evaluations of care offer the state a prop on which to hang its own legitimacy. The supposed retreat of the state that these partnerships signal is in fact a strategic renegotiation of the state's responsibilities and a bid to grab a hold on an otherwise unruly industry.

Ecks and Harper show that flexibility in tailoring treatment is available to different health practitioners in various degrees, and they show how this flexibility positions practitioners within the commodity chains of pharmaceuticals. While general practitioners are more likely to prescribe the cheaper, predetermined combinations, so-called top doctors use the wider selection of drugs and information provided by Lupin Ltd., India's leading producer of anti-TB drugs. They provide highly personalized care and are directly remunerated for their brand loyalty. Lupin, on the other hand, benefits by having a larger share of the market, which not only means more direct profit, but also invites further outside investment because it demonstrates a solid grasp of local markets, which is especially convenient when applying for contracts from the WHO. Moreover, feedback from health practitioners and patients makes its way back to the pharmaceutical industry. What might at first sight seem to be an entirely top-down industry thus emerges in this ethnographic account as a somewhat surprisingly responsive and well-connected model of knowledge production and service provision.

From the thick description of these apparently out-of-the-way exchanges, we gain a more processual understanding of the entanglement of public and private health-related institutions and of the possibilities of action within and through them. By refusing outright condemnation of the market and its representatives, Ecks and Harper help us imagine different ways of negotiating the increasingly complex terrain of global health, of looking for possibilities where before we could only see limitations.

* * *

Clara Han's chapter brings into focus informal economies of care and the ways in which domestic relations transform health interventions, while at the same time drawing our attention to the ways in which neoliberal state reforms create an environment of uncertainty and scarcity that can redraw the boundaries of mental illness and health. Drawing from her long-term fieldwork in Santiago, Chile, Han dislodges the primacy of the institutional in global mental health discourse by positioning herself within poor neighborhoods and in homes, alongside extended networks that, over time and to varying degrees, convert neighbors into kin. This ethnographic move steers the study of global health away from biomedical understandings and policy framings toward a view of health that emanates from the duress of the social.

The ethnographer here confronts an economy of missed connections, frustrated exchanges, and uncertain outcomes. The violence inherited from the Pinochet regime continues to limit the health horizons of Chile's poorest citizens. And the regime's neoliberal policies, hailed as miraculous innovations in their time, continue to produce a context in which unemployment and underemployment are endemic, and credit, while it can give people a chance to buy some time, can also become a noose on which the future hangs. Meanwhile, a brittle idea of community, refracted through the technical languages of the state and conforming to the requirements of cost-effectiveness, has come to dominate mental health care planning for the poor in decentralized and mixed public-private health.

We get at different understandings of disease and different conceptions of health based on where we start our studies. By beginning in domestic networks in La Pincoya and not with a mental illness diagnosis or treatment program, Han's case study allows us to see the interactions between those who are diagnosed and those who are not. From this perspective, diagnosis and treatment are not the exclusive purview of the biomedical, but are, like almost anything else, wielded and exchanged for different things. The depressed, be they diagnosed or not, have to deal with labor insecurity while experiencing all kinds of nonspecific aches and pains.

Yet material scarcity also opens the possibility for other kinds of generosity in which medicines, particularly antidepressants made available by mental health programs, can be offered as a salve that keeps other kinds of sociability alive. Han redirects the notion of community that is prevalent in discourses of global health (as in epistemic communities of disease, or targets of intervention, or populations at risk) back to that of kith and kin, to the networks both ephemeral and durable that are vital to the survival of the urban poor and that depend on affective engagements and transactions.

By looking at the ways in which community mental health interventions actually affect the lives of their targets and the networks through which they materialize and acquire alternative meanings, this ethnographic study makes a compelling case for the need to rethink the standards of evaluation employed. If antidepressants can be exchanged among family and friends to help with their pain, if in this act of kindness a debt is paid and relationships are healed and fed, and if this in turn also alleviates some of the person's own pain, what kind of success can this intervention be said to have? What would a people-centered reorientation of the intervention in such a local economy of survival look like?

A reorientation of global mental health programs toward "the weave of life" demands a transformed understanding of health care, one in which health is enmeshed in networks of sociality, and care continuously subverts "the norms that life must overcome."

* * *

With rates of heart disease, diabetes, cancer, and asthma increasing worldwide, the treatment of chronic diseases has become a new frontier in global medicine and health policy. In his chapter, Ian Whitmarsh shows how this focus on chronic diseases is also transforming approaches in global health, marking a departure from the focus on urgent communicable conditions that have historically been the main objects of concern and intervention. He draws from multisited research conducted with medical scientists in the United States and health officials, doctors, and patients in Barbados and Trinidad and Tobago to problematize the constitution of population genetics as a powerful research and diagnostic tool and its deployment along the lines of race. A new figure of the patient is being fashioned in the twenty-first-century biomedical/market/policy focus on lifestyle diseases: "the locus of intervention shifts from attempts to remove structural barriers or expand access to medications, to getting individuals coming to see themselves as ill or potentially ill and acting accordingly."

In contrast to infectious diseases such as HIV/AIDS, there is no a priori agreed-upon knowledge that can inform interventions to curtail chronic diseases. Interventions targeting them are future-oriented and, in a sense, always partial, as the search for genetic predispositions for common diseases continues to unfold. While attending to genetic propensities, these interventions concentrate on producing information about who the afflicted will be and managing a condition that, ultimately, turns into the management of everyday life. The integration of genomics in population health, particularly in the management of chronic diseases, spurs new databases, institutes diagnostic tools and treatment guidelines for a distinctive patient figure, and locates potential markets for preventative pharmaceuticals. In this framework, poor countries play a much more complex role than that of recipients of aid or laboratories of experimentation.

If questions of delivery plagued previous efforts to combat infectious diseases, patient compliance becomes the new locus of intervention when disease states are anticipated. No longer limited to the timely taking of drugs, compliance comes to demand changes in cultural, social, and psychological proclivities along new lines defined by biomedical knowledge. Noncompliance thus becomes the disease itself. Through the interchangeability of research and intervention, a dual patient subjectivity comes into view: the patient is part of a biological population at risk, and thus not responsible for acquiring the disease, but at the same time requires individualized interventions at the level of choice and disposition.

Whitmarsh's ethnography and critique allows us to consider the ambivalences these subjects take on within a political, scientific, and cultural milieu populated by contradicting expectations and competing intentions. When global health efforts are increasingly framed in terms of experimentation, genomically racialized populations, and future diagnoses, the attentive eye of the ethnographer may help ferret out the technological and political-economic intermingling that ultimately shapes the possibilities of health care.

* * *

As public health actors and institutions around the globe contend with limiting public health paradigms and limited delivery systems, they must also struggle with how to guarantee the human right to health and how to fulfill promises for increased access to medical technologies. João Biehl and Adriana Petryna's chapter explores the emergence of novel arenas of contestation in which the role of the state and socioeconomic and medical rights are being reimagined and reshaped.

In 1996, Brazil became the first developing country to adopt an official policy granting free access to antiretroviral drugs through its broad-reaching but ailing public health care system (SUS). In the years since the launch of this therapeutic policy, Brazil has asserted itself as an innovator and leader in efforts to universalize access to AIDS therapies in poor contexts (through generic drug production, price negotiations, drug distribution schemes, and South-South technology exchange programs).

As the government opened the country to international financial capital and championed populist and much-needed social policies, it also strategically withdrew from strict market regulation. Today Brazil is the eighth largest pharmaceutical market in the world (total market value amounted to twenty-five billion dollars in 2011). It is estimated that more than half of the adult population (about sixty million) consumes pharmaceuticals daily. Multiple public and private actors are invested in making medical technology (and not for infectious diseases only) broadly accessible.

In the wake of the country's highly publicized antiretroviral drug rollout, public health and care have become increasingly pharmaceuticalized and privatized (Biehl 2007), and the rights-based demand for drug access has migrated from AIDS to other diseases and patient groups. A growing number of citizens are acting within the state to guarantee their right to health, understood as access to medicines of all kinds, whether or not they are available in official drug formularies. Widespread and often desperate patient demand, informed by physicians' prescriptions and mediated by public defenders and private lawyers, drives this phenomenon known as "the judicialization of the right to health."

The contribution by Biehl and Petryna examines the political subjects that emerge from this complex law-state-market ecology and shows how in this new chapter in the history of the right to health, the judiciary has become a crucial arbiter and purveyor of care and technology access. They draw on their efforts to empirically map right-to-health litigation in the state of Rio Grande do Sul (which has the highest number of such lawsuits in the country) and explore the impact that judicialization is having on health systems and on practices of citizenship and care. People's life chances and health outcomes are, in such a context, determined by what kind of subjects they are able to become through appeals to the judiciary, government, and research and health industries, amid drives for profit and the construction of new therapeutic market segments. Subjects here are not entirely atomized, nor are they seen as belonging to preexisting populations, but they are rather members of temporary collectives meant to aid in the navigation of the judiciary system.

As in other cases studied in this book, conjunctions of private and public interests in the new world of global health have produced in Brazil a complex arena in which the role and limits of the state and the benefits and obligations of pharmaceutical industries are constantly negotiated in ways that undermine the easy categorizations of neoliberalism or market fundamentalism. By charting the therapeutic trajectories of patient litigants and their families, Biehl and Petryna show that such negotiations are also available to those deemed targets of interventions or subjects of future medical policies and protocols, and not just to planners and implementers.

Economists have wrestled with the question of what variables determine improvements in health and survival. Some argue that the introduction of new knowledge, science, and technology always increases inequalities in health outcomes, both within and between countries—"at least for a time" (Cutler et al. 2006:117). Cutler and colleagues suggest not only that "knowledge, science, and technology are the keys to any coherent explanation" of declines in mortality (116), but also that health gradients between and within countries will continue to increase along with the accelerating pace of new medical inventions. Notwithstanding these initial inequalities of access, the authors argue that "help is on the way, not only for those who receive it first, but eventually for everyone" (117).

Biehl and Petryna question the assumptions that underpin economic trickle-down theories—namely, of the self-regulating capacities of free markets and the march of ever-expanding access to new, life-saving technologies. What they instead show ethnographically is that poor patients are in growing numbers not waiting for new medical technologies to reach them, but are demanding access now, even if one-by-one, one disease and one court case at a time.

Dropping in new medical technologies and treatments without attention to local public health infrastructures and without broader institutional reforms, however, leaves everything to the vicissitudes of the market. This, in turn, leads to a kind of "open-source anarchy" (Fidler 2007) in which, as Biehl and Petryna suggest, new strategies, rules, distributive schemes, and practical ethics of health care must be improvised and assembled piecemeal by a wide array of deeply unequal stakeholders on the ground. The plights of patient-litigants raise crucial questions over what appropriate political and legal mechanisms should exist to foster "the help that is supposedly on its way" and to offset the losses of life that may plague those who do not receive the new technology first.

In addressing the joint phenomena of the pharmaceuticalization and judicialization of health care in Brazil, Biehl and Petryna's case study captures the fluidity and fragility of biopolitical processes and their entanglement with the market. Both the milieus that these phenomena help to produce and the contestations that they allow are testing grounds for present-day techniques of governance. Different forms of social being emerge within and through these milieus and contestations, and they are always in potential flux.

—*João Biehl and Adriana Petryna*

9

Public-Private Mixes

The Market for Anti-Tuberculosis Drugs in India

STEFAN ECKS AND IAN HARPER

74 Percent

Ten years ago, Paul Farmer called tuberculosis the "forgotten plague" (Farmer 2000:185). While millions of people were dying every year of TB, the disease had become invisible for people living in rich countries. When the disease was rampant in the richer industrialized countries, it was at the forefront of public interest, but when, thanks to better nutrition, healthier living conditions, and more effective drugs, TB "ceased to bother the wealthy," it faded from sight (ibid.). Against this forgetfulness, Farmer urged anthropologists to listen to the voices of the poor and to record their stories of deprivation and discrimination. But he also said that ethnography was insufficient to grapple with the problem. A comprehensive perspective on tuberculosis "must link ethnography to political economy and ask how large-scale social forces become manifest in the morbidity of unequally positioned individuals in increasingly interconnected populations" (ibid.:197).

Since the WHO's declaration of TB as a global emergency in 1993, the fight against tuberculosis is receiving far more attention. Today even pessimists would find it difficult to call tuberculosis a "neglected" disease. Several global initiatives have emerged to bring effective anti-TB drugs to even the world's poorest regions. For example, the Global Fund to Fight AIDS, Tuberculosis and Malaria has distributed US\$19.3 billion to 572 programs in 144 countries (Global Fund 2010) since its founding in 2002. The WHO's push to spread directly observed treatment, short-course (DOTS) across all countries through their national TB control pro-grams has also been of great importance. DOTS aims to detect all smear-positive TB cases through sputum microscopy and to enroll all patients in a treatment regime lasting six to eight months. DOTS has had many successes, with the result that the global number of TB cases per capita has been falling by about one percent per year since 2004. However, the total number of cases is still growing due to overall population growth (WHO 2009c:1).

An increased awareness of the limitations of this approach has led to the expansion of DOTS since 2005. WHO's "Stop TB Strategy" (2010a) has six objectives: (1) to expand and enhance DOTS; (2) to focus on the poorest people, on HIV-comorbidity, and on multidrug-resistant TB (MDR-TB); (3) to strengthen primary health care; (4) to engage all care providers; (5) to empower people with TB; and (6) to promote research into new diagnostics, drugs, and vaccines. The strategy to "engage all care providers" entails plans to involve an array of voluntary, corporate, and private providers and to extend collaborations in "Public-Private Mixes (PPMs)" (WHO 2009c:34).

In this chapter, we will explore how public-private collaborations can be successful in India.[1] PPMs are an important part of the Stop TB cam-paign globally, but they are especially vital in India. One reason for this is the sheer number of TB patients. India has more people suffering from TB than any other country. Of the 9.27 million cases of TB worldwide in 2007, 2 million patients were in India (WHO 2009c:1). Another criti-cal reason is that an overwhelming number of these patients are being treated in the private sector and are often receiving a low quality of care. The WHO highlights that ensuring rational use of drugs *outside* the government-sponsored program is a particular concern in India. Previous research in the country has demonstrated poor compliance by private doctors with WHO treatment regimens, with mistakes in both drug dosaging and duration of treatment, and inflated charges for medicines (Arora et al. 2003; Uplekar and Shepard 1991; Singla et al. 1998; Prasad et al. 2002). In light of these findings, the WHO began a closer collaboration with the Indian Medical Association (IMA) to get a better grip on the situation (2009c:109). WHO claims that DOTS has been provided by 100 percent of the facilities under the Indian Ministry of Health since 2006, up from only 30 percent in 2000 (2009c:109) WHO also claims that PPMs are spreading rapidly, with nearly 21,000 Indian private practitioners now being involved in PPMs (ibid.:111). Yet these figures do not tell us what percentage of cases is actually being treated within DOTS or DOTS-allied PPMs. And they tell nothing about the scale of the problem: if there are *eight million* private prescribers in India (WHO 2010b:47), how can even a decent few of them be included?

Why private prescribers are such a headache for DOTS also emerges from research, commissioned by the Global TB Alliance, on how anti-TB medicines are distributed worldwide. Launched in 2000, the TB Alliance is itself a public-private collaboration between academics, donor organizations, and corporations that aims to speed up the development of faster-acting drugs against TB. Among its corporate stakeholders are Eli Lilly, Novartis India, and Lupin. In contrast to WHO research, the TB Alliance also draws on data from corporate sources, above all from IMS Health Inc., a world-leading market research firm. IMS data show the magnitude of private sector treatments of TB in India (TB Alliance 2007:8). Drugs procured through public tender for government-sponsored facilities make up only 12 percent of the entire Indian anti-TB market. A larger share of drugs supplied to DOTS centers comes from the Global Drug Facility (GDF), which was launched by the Stop TB Partnership in 2001. India is the world's number one destination for both GDF-supplied drugs and for GDF grant support (TB Alliance 2007:4). Yet GDF drugs only constitute another 14 percent of the Indian anti-TB market. The remaining 74 percent, the lion's share of the market, is entirely private and, therefore, entirely *outside* of DOTS. In light of these market data, the claim that DOTS covers "100 percent" of India's needs for treatment rings hollow.

The unusual position of India in the global anti-TB drugs market becomes clearer in a cross-country comparison (TB Alliance 2007:8). India not only consumes more TB drugs in the public sector than any other country (US$25 million in 2006), it also consumes more drugs in the private sector than any other country (nearly $70 million in 2006). According to the TB Alliance, there is no private market for first-line TB drugs in China, and high-income countries such as the United States, the United Kingdom, France, and Japan have no market whatsoever for private TB treatments. The language of public-private mixes suggests that the Indian Ministry of Health, with the support of the WHO, vertically controls TB treatments through its Revised National TB Control Programme (RNTCP). A number of recent studies suggest that Indian PPMs are successful at including private practitioners (e.g., Kelkar-Khambete et al. 2008). Official statements on PPMs never openly state that their ultimate aim is to gain control over private prescriptions, but in our interviews WHO-allied people routinely described this as one of their goals. For example, one of WHO's Delhi-based medical officers for TB told us in an interview in 2007 that Indian patients needed more protection from the private sector's "therapeutic anarchy," and that most private treatments were irrational and not compliant with WHO regulations. An officer for the German Leprosy and TB Relief Association, which promotes DOTS referrals among West Bengal's rural GPs, pharmacists, and unlicensed "quacks," said that PPMs were aimed at gradually smoking out treatments by private practitioners: "Only if we involve them, we can make them zero." But faced with a 74 percent market share of drugs prescribed outside of DOTS, the balance of power seems heavily skewed against public-sector control. PPMs in India are less about a strong vertical program generously inviting outside participants than a desperate effort to get a grip on a sprawling private market.

Farmer's call for more ethnographies of TB has certainly not been in vain, and many excellent studies have been written on how patients experience TB and how they navigate different paths to health. Such ethnographies can convey both detailed insights into people's everyday deprivation and also point to wider structural problems. For example, Veena Das and Ranendra K. Das's (2007) longitudinal study of health-seeking experiences in a Delhi slum shows that it is not always patients who fail DOTS, but that DOTS can also fail patients by "consistent institutional neglect and incoherence" (Das and Das 2007:85). For Nepal, Harper (2005) has shown how the very categories designed for entry into the public program also can be used to *deny* entry for those who do not fit the criteria.

To date, however, anthropologists have hardly looked beyond TB *patients*. Farmer's idea of linking ethnography to political economy suggests an essential difference between what can be studied through local ethnography and what can only be studied through political economy. This chapter—an ethnography of marketing practices by a private pharmaceutical corporation—offers a different yet complementary perspective. We look at pharmaceutical production, distribution, and retailing and present a snapshot of the upstream forces behind anti-TB drug prescriptions. Here we focus on sales representatives for Lupin Ltd., India's leading producer of anti-TB drugs. To our knowledge, no similar research has yet been published in relation to TB control. Farmer is right to say that ethnography alone cannot provide the full "structural" picture, but ethnography, we believe, can explore the point of view of the people whose daily work it is to actually build the political economy behind drug prescriptions.

The data we present are drawn from "Tracing Pharmaceuticals," a collaborative project on the production, distribution, regulation, and prescription of pharmaceuticals in India and Nepal. We took biomedicine's "magic bullet" paradigm of drug effects and turned it on its head: we selected molecules and followed them wherever they led. To start with treatments instead of symptoms is, to some extent, an inversion of Kleinman's (1980:104–118) classic formulation of explanatory models. Implicit in the idea of explanatory models is that they are ordered in a clear temporal sequence: first, people perceive illness symptoms; then they try to make sense of the symptoms; then they seek medical help; then a doctor gives a diagnosis; based on that diagnosis, treatment is prescribed. This order is so commonsensical that it appears counterintuitive to question it. Yet conceptual work done in the history of medicine and in science and technology studies has opened up other possibilities. For example, Ian Hacking's (1995) "looping effects" demonstrated that medical classifications interact with what they are classifying, and that it is often impossible to say which came first: the patients with the disease, or disease classification. Bruno Latour (1987, 1993, 2005) showed how relations between humans and nonhuman things can be traced. Taking these ideas and pushing them further, we wondered whether it might be possible to take a particular drug as a point of departure and to ask Kleinman's questions in reverse: What drugs are available? How does the availability of drugs influence the perceived causes of illness? How does the availability of drugs transform perceptions of illness? (Ecks 2008).

The three drugs that we selected for our collaborative project were rifampicin, oxytocin (Syntocinon), and fluoxetine (Prozac). Rifampicin was chosen from among the anti-TB drugs because it is an essential component of every short-course regimen, being the only first-line drug that combines early bactericidal activity, sterilizing effects, and the ability to prevent resistance. Indeed, the very rationale for the introduction of DOTS was to protect rifampicin against drug resistance. In the course of our research, we identified the leading brands of rifampicin in India and Nepal, traced them through various distribution channels, and explored the pathways by which they reached patients. Lupin Ltd. is the focus of this paper because of its dominant position both in the Indian private market and in the Indian and global anti-TB drugs procurement process.

"Champions of the Chest": The Rise of Lupin Ltd.

Lupin is one of India's largest pharmaceutical companies and has been among its top firms since the 1990s. Founded in 1968 with an initial capital of only Indian Rs. 5,000 (about US$700 at late 1960s exchange rates), Lupin established itself in the anti-TB product segment when it started bulk manufacturing of ethambutol in 1981. Calling itself "Champions of the Chest," the corporation is today especially well-known for its production of anti-tuberculosis medicines, controlling a globally dominant market share of the anti-TB drugs rifampicin, ethambutol, isoniazid, and pyrazinamide. Two of Lupin's bestselling brands, R-cinex and AKT, are tuberculostatic remedies (Lupin 2009:28). R-cinex is the brand name of a range of fixed-dose combinations (FDCs) of rifampicin, isoniazid, ethambutol, and pyrazinamide. AKT is a brand of "kits" that bundle separate tablets of these four molecules in different combinations and dosages; for example, AKT-4 contains separate tablets of rifampicin 450mg, isoniazid 300mg, ethambutol 800mg, and pyrazinamide 1500mg. Altogether, Lupin produces forty different antitubercular products, making it, in the words of one of its marketing directors, a "one-stop shop" for TB treatments. A recent addition to its product range is Ributin (rifabutin 150mg), which is marketed as an HIV-tuberculostatic. Lupin has market dominance not only in formulations, but also in active pharmaceutical ingredients (APIs): for rifampicin and ethambutol, Lupin is the world's leading bulk manufacturer (Chaudhuri 2005:51). Its API fermentation plant at Tarapur (Maharashtra), which was established in 1992, is the world's largest producer of rifampicin and one of only three global plants approved by the US Food and Drug Administration (FDA). Lupin is also one of only six global companies prequalified as a supplier for the Global Drug Facility, which distributes the company's products to fifty different national tuberculosis control programs worldwide. Since the Indian TB program is the world's number one recipient of GDF supplies (TB Alliance 2007:4), a good share of Lupin's products remains in India.

Lupin is trying to diversify its portfolio to produce a range of remedies for other ailments. It has become a world-leading bulk producer of cephalosporins, a class of antibiotics, and it is focusing also on cardiovascular, diabetic, asthma, and nonsteroidal anti-inflammatory drugs. In the course of these efforts, Lupin has become one of several Indian pharmaceutical firms that have managed to go global. In 2007–2008, for example, Lupin was the third fastest-growing company in the US prescription market, and acquired majority stakes in companies based in G8 countries, such as Germany's Hormosan and Japan's Kyowa.

Lupin's strong presence in the anti-TB drugs market, both in India and globally, went through several phases (Chaganti 2007). In the 1970s, Indian doctors treated TB with para-aminosalicylic acid (PAS), isoniazid, and thiacetazone. At that time, the Indian anti-TB market was held by Pfizer India and Biological E. Limited, then a medium-sized Indian company. But in the late 1970s, ethambutol, pyrazinamide, and rifampicin came onto the market. Internationally, rifampicin replaced injectable streptomycin, and ethambutol replaced PAS (Ryan 1992). Pfizer India and Biological E. had not anticipated such quick shifts in treatment regimes, and within a few years they lost their foothold in the anti-TB market. By the 1990s, the Indian market for the older generation of drugs had shrunk to 3 percent. Over the same period, Lupin, which "began flexing its muscles in the late seventies . . . was actively looking for opportunities to satiate its ravenous appetite for rapid growth" (Chaganti 2007:56). When Lupin introduced rifampicin, ethambutol, and pyrazinamide in 1981, it was only ranked number 62 in India. By 1988, it had captured nearly 30 percent of the anti-tubercular market and had risen to number 12. By 1992, Lupin's share had risen to 50 percent, and by 2006, it was ranked ninth among Indian pharmaceutical corporations overall with a 2.3 percent market share of pharmaceutical sales in India, and a 45.6 percent share of sales in the Indian anti-TB market. Lupin's annual report for 2008–2009 stated that it had become India's fifth-largest pharmaceutical company.

Combined data from three drug databases (CIMS, IDR, and MedCLIK) indicate that there are at least fifty-two Indian manufacturers of anti-TB drugs. Of the thirty-six companies listed in CIMS, thirty-four firms produce compounds of rifampicin and isoniazid; twelve produce compounds of isoniazid and ethambutol; nineteen produce compounds of isoniazid and pyrazinamide; and nineteen produce compounds of all four drugs. Despite this proliferation of brands, it is likely that the smaller companies are gradually being pushed out of the segment by the now-established leaders. For example, while the overall market for anti-tuberculars shrunk by 5.9 percent in 2009, Lupin's share grew by 5.6 percent (Lupin 2009:30). Bengal Chemicals, a government enterprise based in Kolkata, used to be one of the state's main suppliers of noncombined rifampicin, ethambutol, and pyrazinamide, but in an interview with us, its general manager of marketing explained that these were going to be abandoned because of shrinking profits. In Nepal, Lupin's increasing dominance of the market has resulted in local companies no longer being able to compete. Lupin's market share for rifampicin, ethambutol, isoniazid, and pyrazinamide is so solid that it no longer needs to fight off serious competitors. Instead, the company's challenge is to diversify its product range to shake off an overreliance on anti-TB drugs. If the TB Alliance actually succeeded in introducing faster-acting drugs in the next few years, Lupin's current market dominance would be up for grabs.

"The Most Vital Role": MRs' Views of the Anti-TB Drug Market

One of the main research methods used in the "Tracing Pharmaceuticals" project was the semistructured interview. We carried out a total of 475 interviews with people on all levels of the pharmaceutical business and in related regulatory and scientific bodies, most of them in Delhi, Kolkata, and Kathmandu, as well as in several smaller towns in Nepal and Northern India (Brhlikova et al. 2011). Among these were forty-two interviews with medical representatives (MRs), thirty in India and twelve in Nepal. This chapter highlights findings from interviews with eight MRs of Lupin Ltd., conducted in Delhi, Kolkata, Bijnor (Uttar Pradesh), and Kathmandu. Six of our interviewees were low-level reps charged with visiting private practitioners; one of them was an area manager; one a regional manager supervising several employees. Our questions ranged from the MRs' daily work experience to their views on the private anti-TB market. Depending on the respondent, the interview language was either English, Bengali, Hindi, or Nepali. All the interviews were recorded and transcribed into English.

All of the MRs said they were proud that Lupin was the leading company in the field, and one with an excellent reputation for quality. What distinguished Lupin from its competitors, they said, was that its drugs were readily available all over India, making it possible for patients to buy their prescribed doses from any shop as they traveled across regions. The quality of Lupin drugs was so high, they suggested, because the company produced its own active pharmaceutical ingredients: "No other company can provide that quality to the patients, only Lupin can do that, because almost all the companies are purchasing the raw materials from Lupin only." Their production plants were run in keeping with internationally established quality standards: "It is certified by WHO, it is approved by the US FDA, there are various certificates, it's really good." In short, the MRs felt that Lupin's commanding market presence was well deserved. It was a "good company" with a great sense of social responsibility. One MR pointed out that Lupin did not enter the anti-TB market during the 1980s for profit reasons, but out of a feeling of social commitment to the people of India. During this time, he said, multinational companies were withdrawing from the Indian market and were not meeting the Indian people's demand for these drugs, and this was when Lupin stepped in to help. Another MR said that after having worked in Lupin's anti-TB segment for several years, he felt more "like a social worker" than like a regular sales representative, and that his aspiration to fight tuberculosis transcended his day-to-day job. The MRs found that Lupin was also a good company in its relations with its workforce. While the job of a medical sales representative was tough and driven by tight sales targets, at least Lupin had a "humane culture compared to other companies." Even MRs who were active in the medical reps' trade union, the Federation of Medical Representatives Association of India (FMRAI), said that Lupin's work practices compared favorably to those of other companies. (By projecting the image that they work for the market leader, Lupin reps have acquired a reputation for arrogance among MRs working for other firms. This was especially evident in Nepal.)

Lupin's marketing sales force for anti-TB drugs is organized in the same way as other such divisions. There are area managers who monitor a group of medical representatives who go out and meet prescribers. Above the area managers, regional managers supervise larger geographic areas. For example, the regional manager for West Bengal and Sikkim oversees four area managers and nineteen medical reps. The overall supervision of all areas in India is the job of a product management team (PMT) at the Mumbai head office. The PMT develops overall strategies and tailors them to different regions: "Gross strategy has been formed at our headquarters where the product management team is there, the marketing team is there. They are seeing the total market scenario and the growth pattern and the prescription habits of the doctors and after observing everything, they are making the gross strategy. And then, according to the region, the strategy is formulated for West Bengal, Orissa, and all. It has been formulated according to the regions. The gross strategy is the same, a small plus-minus will be there."

Lupin MRs get regular updates on the company's overall performance. The MRs we interviewed portrayed the company in terms similar to those in its annual report, which says that Lupin is the world's leading manufacturer of rifampicin and ethambutol, but that the anti-TB segment shows a "de-growing" and that the product range therefore needs to be further diversified: the "TB segment is de-growing, that's why Lupin has ventured into vascular segment, now shortly we are going into gyne [gynecology] segment, into cardiac segment, and diabetic segment." Lupin's recent introduction of the anti-TB drug Ributin (rifabutin), which was approved by the US FDA as early as 1992, is seen as an exceptional event in an otherwise stagnant market. Rifampicin was developed in the 1950s by Sensi and colleagues (who named it after the 1955 heist movie *Rififi*). Given that rifampicin has been in use for over fifty years, one Lupin MR dryly noted: "The brand, as you know, is archaic." It seems that the Mumbai PMT team constantly changes marketing guidelines, not least because it feels the need to counter a sense of tedium that such a stagnant set of drugs induces in its sales force.

Since all the existing remedies against TB have been used for decades, and since no newer drugs have yet been developed, Lupin's dominant position in the market is based on producing high-quality drugs at the largest possible scale, in a wide variety of doses, and in a variety of combinations. In a market where all companies, even the largest, do not compete by holding exclusive product patents but rather by the quality, scale, dosages, and number of combinations they manufacture, marketing muscle greatly matters. In a market crowded by off-patent products that are all looking "similar" (see Hayden 2007), the lines between what counts as a "brand" and what counts as a "generic" are drawn in peculiar ways. In India, a "brand" is a recognized generic product from a "good" company. In turn, a "generic" drug is seen as a dubious product from a small or untrustworthy company. That is why Lupin's MRs speak condescendingly of the products of other companies as "generics." Even more than with other medicines, they point out, anti-TB drugs have to be of the highest possible quality. To accept anything less imperils not only the patient, but also the population at large through multidrug-resistant strains: "Tuberculosis is such a dangerous disease and bioavailability of each drug is very important. But it is important to have the quality for drugs. If there is a slight difference in the quality, then MDR-TB is spreading." For Lupin MRs, the biggest problem in their day-to-day business is the circulation of "generics." They perceived proliferation of companies and products as so pervasive that even Lupin has frequently been forced to introduce "me-too" combinations. About a new fixed-dose combination brought out by Macleods, a rival company, an MR at Lupin said that the company quickly introduced its own me-too version of the Macleods product. The lines between their own products and those of their competitors were so blurry that it was difficult to distinguish between a "generic" and an "unethical" or counterfeit drug: "These generics drugs, this is the number one problem. . . . Generics coming, plus unethical drugs also coming . . . it's a problem for patients, problem for medical representatives, problem for all the people." The MRs grumbled that the Indian government risked rising rates of MDR-TB by licensing companies that clearly had lower quality standards than Lupin.

Lupin MRs are also proud of knowing their customers better than their competitors. When asked what skills are needed in their line of work, they said that "identifying the customer" is of first importance, and "giving him what he wants" is second. This meant giving private physicians the products they want. It also meant providing services and gifts that convince them to prescribe Lupin products. MRs also have to liaise with retailers and distributors to ensure that Lupin products are widely available for sale: "In marketing, what is important is, first, we need to identify our customer, who is our customer, that's number one. And number two is, we need to give the customer our services. Like, we need to promote our brand continuously, we need to request for prescription, and we need to request the customer for our brand. . . . Plus ensuring availability. Our brand should be available everywhere."

Despite Lupin's dominant market share, even small fluctuations in demand have to be monitored carefully. A one percent drop in prescriptions is seen as a "big amount" that requires a quick response. The MRs rely on three sources to gauge market movements. First, Lupin's own sales data are fed back to the marketing team daily. Second, the MRs are briefed daily on data provided by the commercial research organization ORG-INS, which conducts sales audits with retailers and distributors on the market shares of different companies and products. Third, the MRs also monitor the career of their own products by keeping in touch with prescribers, retailers, and distributors. Through this mix of data sources, MRs are able to know precisely how many times individual doctors have prescribed their brands and how other companies are doing by comparison. Since there are different data sources, any mismatch can be picked up and further investigated. In other words, there is no hiding from an alert sales force: "ORG is giving some different data, that doctors are very fond of fixed-dose combination rather than kit, and I am getting the data that they are more fond of kit, then there is a mismatch. Then you have to intervene more in the market and we have to go more to the chemists and survey more doctors as to what goes wrong." Another MR described how he talks to retailers to know how much a doctor writes: "Normally, at a chemist near him, I go there and try to analyze—*Bhai, kitna likh rahe hain?* [Brother, how much is being written?]" The retailers usually provide this information without further ado. The MRs also ask from which distributor or wholesaler the retailers receive their products, and they can easily double-check to see if they have the true picture: "So, what I will do, I will nab those two distributors, see the records, if that chemist is telling the truth or not."

While the briefing of MRs is a "downward" feed of information top-down through the hierarchy, there is also an "upward" feed back from the field force to the area managers, regional managers, and ultimately the Mumbai PMT. The MRs in our survey did not see themselves as passive recipients of centralized information and sales targets, but as the best all-round source of information. A Kolkata-based regional manager proudly told us:

> Because [the MRs] keep better information on how is the market, how is the market reacting, how the patients are reacting, and how the prescription habits of the doctors are different. Suppose [the MR] meets two hundred doctors in a month. We have 19 representatives, so 19 times 200 doctors there are in total every month. So all these experiences first come to the area managers, then area managers again finalize on the important experiences that he will share with the regional manager, like me. Out of that, I will share with my sales manager and that will go to the GM [general manager] of the PMT department.

One MR summed up his position by saying that "medical representatives play the most vital role in the market," because they knew more about tuberculosis and its treatments than anyone else.

"Husbands and Wives": MRs' Perceptions of Private Prescribers

In India and Nepal, participant observation of MRs and doctors revealed that MRs were frequently treated like a nuisance by doctors. They often had to wait in a long queue and were given only one or two minutes to rush through their spiral-bound presentation charts and to leave a few product samples. In our interviews with them, MRs expressed annoyance that their job was held in low esteem, not only by doctors but also by society at large. It was a "mental blockage in society" that MRs were seen to be on a par with door-to-door salesmen. The MRs had to be *more* knowledgeable than doctors to convince them: "I should be able to have a better way of talking, a better knowledge."

Lupin MRs highlighted that they knew as much about correct prescription regimens as they knew about profits and markets. Being an MR meant more than mere selling: it was "concept selling." To convince the doctors to prescribe their drugs, they first had to be fully confident of what they were telling them: "Confidence is very necessary because, if confidence is not there, there won't be any confidence in the product." All the MRs said that this level of confidence was much easier to gain with a market leader than with a lesser company: "Doctors trust whatever Lupin speaks in TB. It is told to us that 'You are the leaders, whatever you speak, doctors understand that. So be positive and whatever you speak, it should be correct.'" In order to represent Lupin, one had to know everything about the right treatments, because "we are playing with the lives of people and doctor is trusting on us." The MRs' tremendous trust in Lupin was echoed by the doctors we interviewed. When asked what drugs they used, they frequently named Lupin's brands, such as "AKT," instead of the generic drug names.

The MRs said that they visited the widest possible array of doctors, both by specialty and by level of expertise: "*Every* doctor is treating TB. If he gets a single patient also in one year, he is treating them." Specialist pulmonologists received the most attention from Lupin's sales force, because they wrote up to four times more prescriptions than other types of doctors. After chest physicians came general practitioners, and thereafter other specialists such as pediatricians, orthopedic surgeons, and gynecologists. Specialists other than the pulmonologists had to be visited because tuberculosis does not exclusively affect the lungs but can also infect the bones, the intestines, or the eyes.

Different specializations made for different kinds of relations. The Lupin MRs whom we interviewed all felt that the doctors who valued their input most were those with the highest level of expertise: "They want to know of the latest developments and they are more interested because it's their subject." Knowledgeable doctors fully appreciated that they could learn much from the MRs: "They realize the importance of medical reps, because medical reps give them the information." Surprisingly, the specialist doctors were, in the opinion of the MRs, most eager for the MRs' input because they liked to *deviate* from treatment guidelines. They always experimented with their own regimens and preferred "individual choices" over an automatic implementation of WHO guidelines. Similarly, the fixed-dose combinations that had been brought to the market by Lupin and other companies were useful suggestions rather than a law that had to be followed always: "Few like to give fixed doses and then some other doctors like to administer individual drugs. So it entirely depends on their preference." One of the doctors' motivations for prescribing tailor-made doses, as opposed to fixed-dose combinations, was that toxic side effects could be better controlled: "Anywhere in India, leading chest specialists normally prefer individual therapy . . . maybe the patient is hepatotoxic to rifampicin . . . or maybe this drug is resistant and not giving him the proper results." Top prescribers used individualized regimens to minimize drug interactions and to maximize bioavailability: "Rifampicin: empty stomach. After breakfast: take ethambutol. And then after fifteen minutes, take pyrazinamide. Like that." Side effects of anti-TB drugs were inescapable and ranged from an alarming red discoloration of the patient's urine to irreversible liver damage. Getting the dosages right depended on a host of factors—for example, the patient's body weight and possible prior exposure to anti-TB drugs. Indeed, as we learned from interviews with chest physicians, one of the key complaints against DOTS was that it did not allow for enough dosage flexibility.

One MR even said that "there is no regulation, actually" for the range of doses and combinations in use. Adjusting treatment to the individual patient required taking into account a number of variables: "Suppose my weight is 40 kilograms today . . . I am prescribed as per my body weight. But after two months, after treatment, my body weight gets increased to 50 kilograms. So my doses will be increased." Pharmaceutical companies marketed an assortment of doses and combinations to allow private practitioners to fine-tune their treatment in any way they preferred: "Because of this, there are different varieties, different combinations available in the market." That individual drugs were more expensive than fixed-dose combinations was an added boon to the physicians, because more expensive regimens meant more rewards from the pharmaceutical industry.

While top doctors were receptive to Lupin's recommendations, general practitioners were less so, because they were busy with so many other diseases that they could not pay as much attention to what the MRs were telling them. The lack of interest shown by private doctors troubled the MRs since the MRs could, by their own account, save them from malpractice: "We are the only source for private practitioners. Even to the government doctors, because the government is not providing day-to-day updates . . . only pharmaceutical companies today, they are providing continuous medical education." The lower a doctor was in the hierarchy of specialization, the more likely he was to make decisions based on affordability rather than quality: "Price is a major factor in rural villages, and in areas where people are not that able to purchase . . . Low-end doctors, there, price matters." Lupin's prices are mostly pitched in the middle of the market: several companies have more expensive brands, but there are also many companies offering cheaper fare than Lupin.

Since the MRs always had to "know their customer," they would also visit prescribers at the lowest end: "quacks" without any medical qualifications. These so-called rural medical practitioners (RMPs), though unlicensed, are, in many areas of India, the only local source of medical care: "Basically they are quacks. So that is very dangerous." The MRs agreed that the RMPs' treatment of TB was appallingly bad. Although they did not know much about TB, RMPs treated it in their own way. For example, they would begin treatment and discontinue it after only one month. RMPs considered price far over quality, because their patients could not afford long-term treatments with quality brands. To convince RMPs to write Lupin products, the MRs had to resort to direct bribery: "For those kinds of doctors, you need money. Because in India, everybody is *paisa* [money]." In any case, RMPs could not choose quality "because they don't understand the quality."

According to the MRs, however, one should not blame the RMPs alone for the messy situation. Because, after all, anyone prescribing anti-TB drugs could make an error: "Even big, big doctors also make mistakes. Don't believe that only RMPs are committing mistakes." The basic health infrastructure was not in place: "The last thirty-seven years we [Lupin MRs] are telling, we are shouting. But tuberculosis, instead of finishing, it is flourishing. So there must be some basic problem at the root." The Indian government had failed to provide basic care to all its citizens, had failed to train health personnel. It fell to the Lupin MRs to pick up the pieces and inform providers of rational drug protocols where the government had left a void: "Because there is no other machinery to teach them, now pharmaceutical companies have also started village-level CMEs [continuing medical education]." That the easy availability of anti-TB drugs in the private market could be part of the problem rather than part of the solution was never mentioned by the MRs.

The many nuances involved in deciding upon dosages and drug combinations turned top doctors into opinion leaders. Lupin's overall marketing strategy used these leading physicians as spokespeople for the company. If marketing succeeded in getting *one* opinion leader to write a Lupin prescription, it would result in 100 prescriptions being written by other doctors: "One prescription gives 100 prescriptions . . . because if they are writing it, that means 'Oh yes, this doctor is writing,' that means, 'OK, this brand is good, this company is good.'"

The MRs knew precisely how much it cost Lupin to visit one doctor. Taking into account all the expenses—for salaries, training, transportation costs, gifts, and the samples handed out—each visit to an individual doctor cost between Rs. 250 (US$5.50) and Rs. 400 ($8.50). Given that an MR would only get a few minutes' face time with a doctor, or sometimes none at all, each visit was an investment that needed to bring a return: "Why [else] should I invest my money? I'm not a fool."

Such "investments" were not paid by Lupin alone. Two MRs active in the trade union said that newly recruited reps have to give up half their salaries to doctors and retailers to achieve their sales targets. Even area managers sometimes had to give "black money" to meet targets. This was a particular bone of contention with the Nepali MRs, who in 2007 were singled out for blame by that country's Department of Drug Administration (DDA) for unethical marketing practices (Harper, Rawal, and Subedi 2011).

Despite such questionable exchanges, the MRs said that they had "good relations" with doctors, especially if they worked with them over a long period of time. One MR even described the relationship as one between "husband" and "wife," with the MR as husband and the doctor as wife: the "wife" gives faithful service, and the "husband" gives gifts to express his gratitude: "My wife is daily making food for me and she is doing everything for me . . . so it's my duty to provide her love, maybe a sari, beautiful sari on her birthday, maybe on our anniversary." As with a married couple, the obligation to care for one another did not cease instantly when one side failed to live up to expectations. Hence even underperforming doctors continued to receive gifts from the MRs: "Commercially that doctor is not valuable, [but] . . . because of our relationship, we cannot leave that doctor." Nevertheless, the MRs still got most of their satisfaction when they were successful at attracting business: "I'm working hard and I get to see my brand's prescription written on a paper, on a prescription pad, and a patient is going to a chemist, and I'm standing there, it gives me real pleasure."

"Different Target Customers": MRs' Views on DOTS

In the anti-TB segment of the pharmaceutical industry, where all of the available drugs have been used for decades, companies compete in providing quality, availability, affordable prices, and perks for prescribers. What keeps the anti-TB market moving are not new active substances, but new combinations and new dosages. Treatment regimens recommended by the World Health Organization can give companies a welcome opportunity to reposition themselves in the private market. Lupin's own products always adhere to WHO guidelines, which favor fixed-dose combinations to minimize the risk of monotherapy and the effects of a patient's noncompliance. AKT and R-cinex, Lupin's two leading anti-TB brands, were formulated in response to WHO recommendations for a 4-dose fixed-dose combination (2002b). As an MR said, "WHO said, to increase the compliance, you should come up with fixed-dose combinations. So now companies have started manufacturing, and it is getting very very popular among doctors." Lupin's global reach was not the least of the factors that made it necessary for the company to focus on products endorsed by the WHO and the Global Drug Facility: "Internationally, you cannot market other than this." The MRs emphasized that the real challenge for marketing lay in exploiting differences without violating WHO guidelines. Lupin offered the same products in both private markets and public tenders, but the promotional pitch had to be adjusted according to the audience: "There is no separate strategy here. The company purely decides . . . how a product has to be promoted in front of a particular doctor, what kind of input to be given and what kinds of gifts are to be presented." The way that Lupin spins global regulatory guidelines to direct its products toward specific customers in local markets is a typical trait of "near-liberalism" (Ecks 2010).

While WHO guidelines directly informed Lupin's promotional strategies, DOTS was seen as a world of its own. An MR described patients' use of DOTS as follows: "You have a box mentioned in your name. You go there, you take one strip, eat that, put that empty strip there, go back. Next day, one day gap. Then once again." The Lupin MRs said that they promoted "market drugs" to private prescribers, and that such market drugs were different from the drugs given in DOTS centers. The MRs had no contact with DOTS because the drugs used there were supplied through a tendering process. There was no point in visiting the staff at DOTS centers because they were not in a position to select Lupin over other companies: "We have different target customers." There were contacts with doctors in government hospitals, because they could recommend that patients buy Lupin products from private shops instead of going to the DOTS—and because, usually, government doctors also have their own private offices, where they can prescribe as they wish.

What interested the MRs most about DOTS was whether or not the program decreased private sales. The MRs we interviewed were of two minds about this. Some said that Lupin's sales of anti-TB drugs were trending downward because of the expansion of DOTS. Others said that there was no change to sales, because the total number of TB patients was rising, and DOTS could not absorb them: "[DOTS] has not affected our strategies because we are working on one trend and they on another. The number of patients is growing very fast. That is the basic reason why there is no effect on the strategies of either." The Nepali MRs felt that sales were stagnant, because the relatively greater success of the Nepal DOTS program eliminated Lupin's gains in overall market share.

The MRs saw DOTS as neither the best answer to TB, nor as deserving of the support of the general population. Anyone who could afford private treatment should choose it instead, because it was more effective and more convenient. DOTS was for "poor people" only. In its current form, DOTS was, they believed, a near-complete failure: "If there are 100 DOTS program centers, only few, hardly five centers are functioning properly." The entire "system" around DOTS was faltering. First, the government did not do enough to advertise DOTS, so even the people who needed it most did not know about it: "The patient is very much uneducated and unaware also. Whether you give medicines free of cost or if you charge, they don't understand." Second, in their opinion, the staffs in DOTS centers were not diligent in carrying out their duties toward their patient.

For example, if a patient did not come into the clinic as scheduled, it was the duty of DOTS staff to visit him or her at home: "Sometimes patients are not getting the full course of medicines, right? If I am working in a DOTS center, then my job is to go to the patient's home and administer the medicine right in front of my eyes." This duty, they felt, was often neglected. Moreover, DOTS' target-driven audit culture incentivized center staff to manipulate the attendance records and cure rates. Finally, DOTS relied too much on sputum tests, in spite of the fact that there are many types of TB that cannot be diagnosed accurately through sputum only, for example, bone TB or abdominal TB. The emphasis on those forms of TB that can be identified through sputum tests created major blind spots: "DOTS therapy is . . . a partial therapy."

While DOTS was, for the MRs, a *near*-complete failure as a first-line treatment for TB, it was a *complete* failure in its approach to MDR-TB. This form of TB is caused by bacterial strains that do not respond to two or more of the first-line drugs, including rifampicin and isoniazid. MDR-TB is usually the result of a patient not taking the full course of medicines, or of doctors prescribing the wrong kinds of medicines. At the time of our interviews (2006–2008), the extension of DOTS to include the treatment of MDR-TB, an approach called DOTS-Plus, had only just begun.

For the MRs, MDR-TB was the Achilles's heel of DOTS. First, they alleged that DOTS success rates compared very unfavorably with the success rates of private treatments. In their view, in fact, the blame for rising numbers of MDR-TB patients lay with DOTS. DOTS was neither equipped to diagnose MDR-TB patients properly, nor to administer the right medicines. Even if an MDR-TB patient were to present herself to a DOTS center, she would never receive appropriate treatment. While the Revised National TB Control Programme was aware of this shortcoming, both the accreditation of laboratories to diagnose MDR-TB and the rollout of DOTS-Plus had been too slow.

The MRs' critique went on: DOTS was too inflexible to allow for treatment decisions that took into account the individual patient's needs. Such was its inflexibility that even those therapeutic choices that were entirely within the boundaries of international evidence-based best practice were disallowed. DOTS made it nearly impossible for patients to work in other areas or go traveling: "You cannot get DOTS treatment other than at your center. Suppose I am going for a marriage in some other city, I will not get the medicine [there], and you are not giving medicine for those periods to me."

Furthermore, the Indian DOTS program—as opposed to the programs introduced in several other countries, including Nepal—had opted for "intermittent" instead of daily doses. "Intermittent" meant that patients only had to come to the DOTS center every three days to receive their medicine, instead of making a daily visit. This has obvious advantages: for example, that patients would save the time and money spent on traveling.

In India, intermittent therapy was chosen because it was also cheaper for the program: fewer patients' visits to DOTS centers meant that fewer hours of staff time were needed. The downside of intermittent therapy was that it was much harder for patients to remember which days of the week they had to visit the DOTS center. Even worse, to miss a day's dose on the intermittent regimen effectively meant missing three days' doses. Therefore it was obvious to the MRs that daily therapy, as preferred by private practitioners, would have a higher success rate than intermittent therapy. In any case, it was ingrained in the habits of Indian patients to take their pills at the same time, every day: "It is the psychology of the patient, especially in India, to take the medicine daily. . . . But if you tell them that you will have to take this medicine intermittently . . . they may not follow that, because that is not tuned in their mind."

Finally, the MRs felt that DOTS was too obsessed with collecting statistical data, and that private practitioners would have no incentive to take on the paperwork requirements that they would have to meet if they were to participate in a DOTS public-private mix: "Many doctors are not ready to become DOTS in-charge because of so much administrative work which they have to do, so many records they have to maintain. So, because of that, they are reluctant." Our interviews with doctors made it clear that this was indeed the case.

Conclusions

In global health policy, tuberculosis is no longer a "forgotten plague" (Farmer 2000). Nor is TB a forgotten subject in medical anthropology. But more ethnographic engagement with perspectives beyond those of patients is needed. Specifically, while work has been done in the private sector, this has tended to focus on private doctors, with little attention paid to other players. This chapter highlighted the sheer magnitude of the private drug market in India and tried to capture ethnographically the perspective of one of its key actors: the medical representatives for Lupin Ltd., one of the world's leading producers of anti-TB drugs.

The RNTCP and the World Health Organization's move to involve the private sector in India has, so far, focused on promoting participation in public-private mixes to private prescribers. The problem they face is one of sheer scale: How can eight million private prescribers be convinced to support DOTS? The main point of contact, to date, has been the Indian Medical Association. Involving the IMA is a sensible tactic, but it is likely to have only limited success. The IMA has practically no influence over individual doctors' therapeutic choices. And as long as private doctors continue to depend on both the fees paid by patients and on kickbacks from pharmaceutical corporations, they will have little financial incentive to collaborate with the DOTS campaign. Moreover, we have learned from the Lupin MRs (as well as from interviews with doctors) that the opinion-makers among chest physicians prefer their own tailor-made treatments over those used in DOTS. Hence the doctors who would be most immediately in contact with the IMA are also the doctors least likely to believe in DOTS. That this is the case became evident on many levels. For example, we attended four DOTS awareness seminars presented to various groups of prescribers in West Bengal, and it was only at the IMA-sponsored event that the audience of doctors noisily challenged the presenters and generally disagreed with what they had to say about the benefits of DOTS. Audiences of municipal health workers and rural medical practitioners listened carefully and never openly questioned that the government-sponsored DOTS program should be the standard treatment.

Our ethnographic findings indicate that WHO treatment guidelines are becoming more accepted by private practitioners in India, but this does not appear to be the result of any educational efforts or of widened Public-Private Mixes. Instead, private doctors' prescribing habits have come closer to DOTS because of the increasing numbers of WHO-endorsed kits and fixed-dose combinations in the private market. The rise of kits and fixed-dose combinations in the market is corroborated by sales figures, such as

Lupin's report that R-cinex and AKT are their bestselling drugs (Lupin 2009:28). One crucial insight gained from the Lupin MR interviews is that WHO recommendations are becoming more common among doctors because of the availability and active promotion of these products, rather than because of any awareness-raising campaign by public health bodies. During an interview with a WHO TB officer in Delhi, we showed him a list of fifty-two Indian companies that produce rifampicin, either alone or in fixed-dose combinations. While he knew all the big brands, he was surprised by the huge range of companies and products, and said that this peculiar market needed to be better understood.

It is our contention that the Indian market for anti-TB drugs presents a unique opportunity for the WHO and other international organizations to extend public-private collaborations. Despite apparent therapeutic anarchy, there are only a handful of producers who have a major share both in the private market and in the procurement of drugs for DOTS. Leading corporations, above all Lupin, might be convinced that supporting DOTS would not decrease their overall product sales, but instead simply shift demand from the private to the public sphere. It could even be argued that such a shift toward the public domain would strengthen Lupin's competitive position, because the share of smaller companies would be further reduced. At the moment, however, Indian companies make more profits from promoting drugs to private practitioners than from supplying DOTS centers. If this balance of profits could be tilted in favor of the public system, companies such as Lupin would have a real incentive for promoting DOTS over private treatments.

Another potential inducement for companies to support DOTS lies in rights of access to *future* drugs. Just as Pfizer and Biological E. Ltd. lost their market shares when a new generation of anti-TB drugs came to the market, so are companies like Lupin threatened by more effective drugs. Once new drugs actually become available, Lupin must either get access to them or lose this market. Hence it makes perfect sense for Lupin to be one of the corporate stakeholders in the TB Alliance. From a public health point of view, it would be worth thinking about making access to future drugs dependent on providing active support for DOTS in the present.

Listening to the medical representatives provided several ideas about how corporate stakeholders might be able to build support for DOTS into their day-to-day work. Lupin MRs are proud of how much they know about WHO-endorsed treatments, and they crave more recognition from doctors. If the Revised National TB Control Programme and the WHO could tap into their desire for higher status, the MRs would be likely to gravitate to their side. That some of the MRs described themselves as "social workers" and as fighting against TB—in other words as having humanitarian concerns beyond narrow profit calculations—perhaps opens a door to drawing them into the public health field in new ways. The village-level awareness events that the MRs are already organizing could be better aligned with RNTCP/WHO campaigns. Also, if it is true that MRs have to give up parts of their own salaries to achieve their sales targets, might it be possible to allocate Global Fund resources to MRs who actively promote DOTS? Would it be worth discussing with Lupin's product management team in Mumbai whether persuading doctors to refer patients to DOTS centers might be built into the incentives of their sales force? At the same time, RNTCP and WHO must deal with the reality that MRs see DOTS as an all-out failure, and that they will need a lot of convincing before they agree that DOTS is workable. This will require RNTCP and WHO to reexamine their choice of the intermittent regimen and to allow greater flexibility in the direct observation regimens of patients.

The Lupin MRs take pride in seeing patients demand their company's brands at local medicine shops. If the incentives for MRs could be transformed so that they would take equal pride in seeing patients going to DOTS centers, then the strategy of involving the private sector through PPMs would have a much greater chance of success.

Notes

1. This chapter emerged from the collaborative research project *Tracing Pharmaceuticals in South Asia* (2006–2009) that was jointly funded by the Economic and Social Research Council and the Department for International Development (RES-167-25-0110). The project team comprised: Soumita Basu, Gitanjali Priti Bhatia, Samita Bhattarai, Petra Brhlikova, Erin Court, Abhijit Das, Stefan Ecks, Ian Harper, Patricia Jeffery, Roger Jeffery, Rachel Manners, Allyson Pollock, Nabin Rawal, Liz Richardson, Santhosh M. R., and Madhusudhan Subedi. Martin Chautari (Kathmandu) and the Centre for Health and Social Justice (New Delhi) provided resources drawn upon in writing this paper. Neither ESRC nor DFID is responsible for views advanced here. We would also like to thank Amy Davies and Reena Ricks for sharing their Edinburgh MSc dissertations on public-private mixes with us.

10

Labor Instability and Community Mental Health

The Work of Pharmaceuticals in Santiago, Chile

CLARA HAN

Take Away the Hunger

"If I give money, I exist," said Violeta. It was October 2004, and Violeta had hardly eaten for the past week. I came to visit her in her small shack situated behind her parents' house. Although it was a pleasantly cool night, she was wrapped in wool sweaters and had heaped blankets on top of herself. All I could see as she spoke to me was a pair of intense brown-black eyes, peering out from under the covers. Sparked by a violent argument with her parents over her need to contribute monetarily to the home, Violeta had attempted suicide by swallowing twenty tablets of fluoxetine. One decade earlier, she had been diagnosed with chronic depression after the death of her older sister from lupus. Violeta had "saved" the pills from years of prescriptions that she had received from the Psychiatric Institute, taking them only at moments of conflict with her parents. She could not finish the tablets, she told me, because she fainted. She woke up the next day to her daughter Marisol's persistent calls.

Violeta is thirty-seven years old, single, and has become the mother of her dead younger brother's daughter, Marisol. She shares a small shack with Marisol and her sister Jessica at the back of her parents' plot in La Pincoya, a *población* in the Northern Zone of Santiago, Chile, where I have worked since 1999. Formed by illegal land seizures, or *tomas*, between 1969 and 1970, La Pincoya consists of multigenerational homes, the majority of which are headed by women, many of whom arrived during or shortly after the *tomas* (Garcés 1997; Murphy 2007). In many of these homes, as in Violeta's case, both adult women and men are engaged in informal labor without a contract, as well as unstable labor on defined contracts or "indefinite contracts" which, as I discuss below, are often broken. Women primarily work at piecework sewing, domestic work, office cleaning, or in supermarkets, while men work primarily in construction, transport, and as security guards. Violeta told me that the situation in her family was getting worse. Her father Don Julio, seventy years old, had been out of work for six months. His last job was as a parking lot attendant, and he had worked without a contract and received 120,000 pesos (US$197) monthly.[1] He quit after his boss denied him three days off to visit his wife, Sra. Margarita. She had been hospitalized for complications arising from metastatic breast cancer and uncontrolled diabetes. Since then, the home depended on the contributions of two of his sons, who brought bread, tea, and vegetables, and at times on Violeta's unstable income from cleaning offices. Securing this work depended on contacts with local *contratistas*, subcontractors, who paid between 5000 and 7000 pesos (US$8–12) per week and hired according to the job. Violeta often spent several weeks at a time out of work.

One month earlier, Violeta had enrolled in the National Program for the Diagnosis and Treatment of Depression at La Pincoya's local primary care center. This program was, at the time, just beginning in La Pincoya. Consisting of six sessions of group "psychoeducation" and pharmacological treatment, with at least six months of follow-up, this community-based mental health program has served as a model for mental health programs within a primary care setting (Patel et al. 2009). Violeta quit the "group sessions" but continued saving her antidepressants. The group sessions, she told me, were "fantasy." "I liked being in the group, I never talked, but just listened to the psychologist talk and talk. I could even fall asleep for an hour there, in the group sessions. But, then, when the hour was up, it would be so *fome* [a downer] to return here [to the house] with the yelling and the insults. So I stopped going, because it was like being here (pointing to the sky) and then here (pointing around herself), and *me bajoneó* [it got me down]."

Of the pills, she told me, "I save them. It's a secret, Clarita. I keep them in a box under my bed, and when my parents yell at me, when they fight, I get hysterical, shaking. I start to take the pills. And they take away my hunger and make me high, high, like a *zombie*." She took out the box to show me. Packets of generic fluoxetine were interspersed with diazepam, boxes of brand-name antidepressants, and paracetamol. In the midst of this jumble of pills, she pointed to some antidepressants given to her by her friend Maria: "She gives them to me as gifts. She gave me two boxes. She told me, 'Take them, I don't need them, they make you sleep and make you feel better.' "

For Violeta, psychopharmaceuticals, domestic relations, and labor instability coalesced in producing both violence and care. The multiple ways in which her lived experience articulates the domestic, the state, and the market can help us critically assess the emergence of global mental health paradigms geared toward pharmacological treatment and to assess as well anthropological work on mental illness and pharmaceuticals geared toward the biosocial.

It would be possible to explore how Chile's national program for depression took shape from any number of perspectives, ranging from local politics to its interaction with labor insecurity issues to its impact on domestic relations. In this essay, I will instead explore how this program's local destiny was forged through pharmaceuticals.[2] How and when women use antidepressants reflect both their practical knowledge of everyday afflictions and the shifting affective configurations of their domestic lives. In La Pincoya, psychopharmaceuticals distributed by the local primary care center in the framework of community mental health are absorbed into domestic relations. As material substrates, they can manifest care among neighbors and kin when shared in a variety of ways. They have entered a local formulary of medications informed by practical knowledges of the bodily symptoms and afflictions that are often reactions to labor instability, kinship relations, and economic indebtedness. I will examine how these knowledges work in relation to "health," experienced locally, and how these knowledges—in tandem with institutional failures—can obscure rare disease processes.

Thus, rather than following the trajectory of this program and the associational identifications through a single disease category—assessing biosocial identifications through patient groups, for example—my work is instead positioned within the neighborhood and in homes, alongside extended and durable kinship networks that, to varying degrees and over time, convert neighbors into kin (Fullwiley 2007; Rabinow 1992). Such a positioning within the weave of life allows us to see how domestic relations transfigure state programs in their materiality. That is, we might appreciate the actual materiality of state programs by tracing how pharmaceuticals are taken up in daily life; how diagnoses are generated and received by physicians, patients, and their families; and how and when public-sector and private-sector health care is sought out in the face of disease and distress. Such a positioning, however, also asks that we analyze how these state programs emerge from and articulate other political and economic processes, such as health system reform and labor deregulation.

In Chile, reforms have emerged from specific historical conditions: the Pinochet regime's dismantling of a welfare state that left in its wake a subsidiary state, and, since the beginning of the democratic transition, the state's attempts to pay a social and historical debt to the poor (French-Davis 2004; Han 2012; Petras and Ignacio Leiva 1994; Schild 2000). Creating an account of the national program for depression within the register of the local may help us tether global health initiatives back into specific lifeworlds, lifeworlds that offer other modalities of care and notions of well-being. Before moving back to the lifeworld of La Pincoya, let me chart briefly how this community mental health initiative arose from particular political and moral stakes and became a model for Global Mental Health.

"Packages of Care"

In October 2008, the *Lancet* published a piece, "The *Lancet*'s Series on Global Mental Health: 1 Year On," succinctly assessing the "commitment of stakeholders" and support from leaders in global health for a call to integrate mental health fully into global public health policy. This series of five articles on global mental health, published in 2007, documented and evaluated evidence-based "packages of services" for mental health programs in low- and middle-income countries. Continuing this call for action and for the implementation of global mental health initiatives in such countries, the *Lancet* launched a "Movement for Global Mental Health," a global advocacy campaign of "support for the specific goals of scaling up services for and protecting the human rights of people living with mental disorders" (Patel et al. 2008:1356).

By privileging this "global" call to action and assessing its results over one year, however, the *Lancet* obscured the temporality of national initiatives as well as the political and moral struggles they entail. Dr. Ricardo Araya, a psychiatrist at the University of Bristol, Alberto Minoletti, the head of the Department of Mental Health of the Ministry of Health, and Rubén Alvarado, an epidemiologist at the University of Chile's School of Public Health—all architects of Chile's National Treatment Program for Depression—responded in a letter to the *Lancet* in August 2009, remarking that, "Introducing changes in mental health care can take a long time. A movement to improve the mental health of the population has been evolving for longer than a decade in Chile. What has been achieved amounts to a silent revolution, but a long chain of events prepared the ground for these transformations" (Araya, Alvarado, and Minoletti 2009:597). Araya and his colleagues drew upon key policy milestones of the past decade in charting this "silent revolution" and put their work into a historical perspective that makes clear how community mental health interventions were both morally and politically imagined in the context of the recuperation of democracy, and how they were constrained through health-sector reforms and the privileging of technical languages in state policy.

On the one hand, the Pinochet regime restructured the health care system, transforming a universal national health care service into a mixed public-private system (Araya et al. 2006; Barrientos 2000; Homedes and Ugalde 2004). Through municipalization, primary care was decentralized to the municipalities, making them responsible for the maintenance of primary health care facilities and the implementation of services (Gideon 2001). On the other hand, the regime dismantled an emerging community mental health movement that had gained a foothold at the University of Chile in the late 1960s. Founded by Dr. Juan Marconi, this movement, Intracommunity Psychiatry, was politically aligned with the left and drew from Chilean health professionals' deep roots in Social Medicine (Mendive 2004; see also Waitzkin et al. 2001). Between 1967 and 1990, no large-scale epidemiological studies had been conducted on mental illness in the population. With the democratic transition, psychiatrists and epidemiologists committed to community mental health returned to the state and university and faced the enormous task of reinvigorating a thoroughly debilitated mental health system. Researchers documented a 57.3 percent prevalence of mood disorders in primary care consults and a 25.1 percent prevalence of psychiatric morbidity in Santiago and concluded that these disorders were "intimately linked to situations of marginality, unemployment, low income levels, and education" (Araya 1995:10; see also Araya et al. 2001; Araya et al. 2006). These figures gave visible shape to what the 2000 National Plan for Psychiatry and Mental Health called the "historical debt to the mental health of the population" (MINSAL 2000).[3] But their calls for community mental health now were refracted and supported through the technical languages of the state.

In 2000, Chilean psychiatrists at the University of Chile and the University of Bristol led a study on a low-cost, primary care–centered treatment program for depression among low-income women in Santiago. The researchers chose three primary care clinics in poor areas of Santiago and divided a sample of 240 female patients diagnosed with major depressive disorder according to DSM-IV categories into two treatment regimens. The study was designed as a randomized controlled trial, and the experimental regime was a "stepped-care improvement program."

Those women in this regime who were diagnosed with severe or persistent depression, as measured on the Hamilton Rating Scale for Depression (a scale commonly used in psychiatric research to assess the severity of depressive symptoms), were given a combination of antidepressant medications (fluoxetine, amitriptyline, and imipramine) along with seven consecutive weeks of "psychoeducational group intervention" and two "booster sessions" at weeks nine and twelve. Social workers or nurses, who had been trained and observed by the researchers, covered a range of topics on depression, including "the symptoms and causes of depression, available treatment options, scheduling positive activities, problem-solving techniques, and basic cognitive and relapse-prevention techniques." The patients were each given a manual on depression that covered the content of each session and listed examples and exercises (Araya et al. 2003b:996).

Primary care physicians were also given training by the researchers on administering a pharmacotherapy protocol that included structured assessments at initial and follow-up visits for the patients with severe and persistent depression. In addition, the leaders of the group sessions monitored adherence to medication regimens for the patients receiving pharmacotherapy. The female patients in the control arm were given the usual care provided at the primary health care center, which included antidepressant medication and/or referral to specialty services. The patients were evaluated at three and six months.

The results were published in the *Lancet* in 2003 in an article entitled "Treating Depression in Primary Care in Low-Income Women in Santiago, Chile: A Randomised Controlled Trial." Comparing the two groups after six months, the researchers showed that those in the stepped-care program had significantly lower points on the Hamilton Rating Scale for Depression. After six months, 78 percent in the experimental group had 50 percent or less of their initial HDRS score. By comparison, only 34 percent of the control group had a 50 percent decrease in their depressive symptoms. Echoing a long history of Intracommunity Psychiatry in Chile, Araya and colleagues underscore that the "main innovative element was the role enhancement of the non-medical group leaders, most of whom were available in the clinics and were often closely connected to local neighborhoods" (Araya et al. 2003b:999). Yet, far from the "cultural revolution" proposed by Intracommunity Psychiatry, these researchers focused on "modest interventions" within the scope of existing limited structures of care:

> The combination of high rates of depressive illness, poverty, and scarce resources can easily induce nihilism in physicians and policymakers. Our findings should offer hope that modest interventions can have a substantial effect on depressive symptoms and functional impairment. (Araya et al. 2003b:999)

These "modest interventions," however, rested on an affective and ethical ethos of patient care, as well as on local political conditions. This ethos had been built into the community intervention study through careful attention to patient care and through the training of primary care physicians and nonmedical staff by the investigators themselves. These were their ethics of experiment as well as the conditions of "community" set forth by the study.

By 2004, this program had moved from the pilot stages to implementation across the country within primary care contexts. An assessment of the program's effectiveness in 2005 hinted at a disjuncture between psychosocial interventions geared toward creating identifications among the afflicted—by setting up self-help groups based on disease identity, for example—and the taking up of antidepressants in everyday life. In a sample of 229 patients, Alvarado et al. demonstrated that after three months, 73.3 percent of the women had achieved "complete adherence" to their medication regime, while, by contrast, 37.8 percent adhered to group intervention. Overall, 77.2 percent of the women showed a statistically significant improvement in depressive symptoms, according to the Beck Depression Index. The researchers stated that, "This data puts into relief the necessity of developing specific strategies to improve the adherence to treatment, in particular those strategies of the psychosocial type; the psychosocial intervention was unattended by close to 15 percent and had an irregular attendance of 40 percent" (Alvarado et al. 2005).

In 2006, depression, along with other ailments, was added to the list of fifty-six diseases covered by the state's health reform, Plan AUGE (Acceso Universal con Garantías Explícitas [Universal Access with Explicit Guarantees]). This plan, now fully implemented, prescribes clinical protocols for these specific diseases, detailing how they are to be diagnosed and treated, the maximum waiting time for treatment, the necessary qualifications of providers, and the amount of the co-pay. It extends to both public and private systems, and has opened the door to the enforcement of medical care through the judiciary, which so far has not been widely used.

For depression, six sessions of group cognitive behavioral therapy as well as six months of pharmacological treatment are fully covered for the indigent. For low-income patients (those earning less than 144,000 pesos per month), there is a 10 percent co-pay. As for other diseases, some specific treatments are covered, while others are not. And it is in this parsing out of what can be covered and when, and what cannot, that we begin to see how this system fails to comprehend the lives of the poor. As physicians Román and Muñoz remark in their assessment of Plan AUGE, "'A system of health' is much more than a simple 'system of disease'" (Román and Muñoz 2008).

By 2008, the Depression Treatment Program was treating and managing 84 percent of Chilean patients with depression in primary care, a total of over 200,000 patients across the country. This program for the treatment of common mental disorders in low-income countries advances "packages of care" consisting of screening, psychoeducation, and the prescription of generic antidepressants, and it has been the model for other national initiatives. As we shall see, however, the effectiveness of the package hinges upon community conditions that allow psychosocial interventions to gain traction and to work their way into everyday lifeworlds.

A Local Formulary for Adaptation

From 2004, I observed this program's implementation in the Municipality of Huechuraba, where La Pincoya is located. I arrived nine months before municipal elections, when there was significant tension between the center-left Concertación government's administration and oversight of programs through the Northern Metropolitan Health Service (Servicio de Salud Metropolitano Norte) and the municipal administration. The right-wing mayor had appointed a Director of Health trained as a commercial engineer. According to one psychologist, the director instilled a "culture of terror" in the health workers, who feared losing their jobs and not receiving their pay if they did not reach the number-of-patients-treated goals set by the National Program. High rates of burnout among the young psychologists hindered any sense of continuity between patients and their providers, as well as among the staff.[4]

As I followed a group of women enrolled in the program in October 2004, it became increasingly clear that the group psychoeducation sessions were not generating a potential patient self-help group or identification through disease or patienthood.[5] Because they were in search of work opportunities or had to care for sick children and other relatives, women often could not make the group sessions, and when they did, they often used the time to sleep. In this context, the "package of care" unraveled, and the antidepressants entered into a local formulary that was used to treat the aches and pains associated with unstable labor and economic indebtedness. Given to kin or friends in moments of crisis, antidepressants became one more material substrate for care, specifically, one that gave the body the vital energy or *ánimo* to look for work.

Consider Gladys. "We share them," Gladys told me. I met with her and her husband Jorge in the two-bedroom house that they shared with Gladys's daughter and granddaughter. Gladys and her husband were both in their fifties and had been married for the past thirty years. We sat in a sparsely furnished living room with freshly painted white walls. Only the overstuffed blue couches and an old green sewing machine gave the room some color. When I entered their house, Gladys apologized. "It's not very welcoming," she said, explaining that they had just finished constructing a second bedroom, off from the main house. Before, she told me, they were using the living room as a second bedroom, where her daughter slept.

Her daughter had been addicted, episodically, to *pasta base* (cocaine base paste) over several years. Attempting to break the addiction, she had smoked cigarette after cigarette in her room. "The walls were full of smoke," Gladys said. The smoke sunk into the walls, staining them yellow and giving the entire house an acrid smell. Once the second bedroom was constructed, they worked on cleaning the walls, coating them with white paint. They removed the furniture and bought new sofas on credit. The whiteness of the walls and the sparse, clean furniture gave the house and the family a chance at another narrative. But Gladys and Jorge would now have to contend with the demands of debt payments in the face of unemployment.

Seated next to Gladys, holding her hand, Jorge remarked, "All you see here, it was bought on credit." "*Credit*," he emphasized, "so it is not as if these sofas we are sitting on are really ours, they still belong to the department store. And we are paying the quotas, or we try to pay, but are behind." Gladys explained, "You see, we paid for everything on credit, and that is why I got ill. Jorge lost his job in construction. They said he was too old, that he could not carry as much as the others. And we could not keep up with the payments." She pulled her hand out of Jorge's and began to rub her wrists. "I could not get out of bed," she went on. "The debts, they were tying me to the bed. I woke up in the morning, and the first thing I thought of were the debts. My body was tied to the bed. So Jorge took me to the primary care center and they told me I had depression, and so I started taking the pills and going to the meetings with the psychologist."

A month had passed since the group sessions, and I asked her if the group meetings had helped her. "No, no, poor thing. The psychologist is such a good person, and pretty. I wanted to help her." She continued, "But the pills they gave me, they help my body get up. They told me to take one pill a day. But I only take them when my body cannot get up from bed. The pills raise the spirit/energy [*te levanta el ánimo*]. So last month Jorge started to look for work, but he wasn't finding anything. He rode his bicycle so far from here. He was riding his bicycle, because we cannot pay bus fare. And I thought, my poor *viejo*, going around on bicycle all around the city. And he comes home for tea, and a half of a round of bread. We had not even a peso for bread! I tried to start again in piecework sewing, but my body would not get up. I took the pills to get my body up from bed. I got a few *pololitos* [temporary jobs] and we had a little money to get through to the end of the month." But at that point, Gladys remarked, Jorge also became ill: "He got sick, it [unemployment] was eating his nerves. . . . So, we shared the pills. I told him, take them, they help."

Jorge took up the story: "I have worked my whole life in construction. And my wife, I never wanted to see her have to work again. For many years, she worked in sewing, but her wrists started to hurt. Sometimes she could not even pick up her cup of tea. It was too painful. When I got a contracted job in construction, I was earning well. And I told myself, I will never let that happen again. My wife, she can relax, she can be a grandmother to her grandchild. But then I lost my job. They told me I was too old to work. They fired me. It was like in one moment, we were doing well, moving up, renovating the house, and the next moment we did not even have a *peso* for bread. It was hard to look for work. At my age. . . . They ask for young men thirty-five years old or younger. I am fifty-seven years old. Where will I find work? I rode all over the city looking for work and found one *pololito*, very hard labor. Yes, I took the pills that Gladys gave me. They helped me with *ánimo*. I took them for a few days, but then I stopped when I found work. It was like, whoosh [he made a sweeping movement over his head and smiled]. It does not last for a long time, three months, but we can pay the debts in the meantime."

Gladys continued: "Yes, it was a relief. I felt like we could breathe again. We could buy bread. We could pay our debts. But I still worry. Workers die in construction. It's dangerous. He works in the most dangerous part. They tie a rope around him, and he has to work on the outside of the buildings. He could fall, the rope could fail." I asked Gladys if, with all these ongoing worries, she was still taking the pills. "No," she said. "Now I save them for critical times, and it will be hard when Jorge has to look for work again. Why take them when we are better?"

The word *ánimo* in colloquial usage carries multiple significations: "the soul or the spirit that is the principle of human activity; value, force, energy; intention, will; attention and thought" (Real Academia 2010). For Gladys and Jorge, the pill was a dynamic and vital force felt immediately within the body. It was saved for "critical moments" that demanded will and activity, perhaps as an "adjuvant" for a "will to live" (Biehl 2007). The sharing of this pharmaceutical also revealed a vital force—a kind of care—generated by relationships themselves.

But in saving their pills for "critical moments," Jorge and Gladys also evidence the occasional and unpredictable moments of scarcity that result when employment is unstable. The precarious labor market is an outcome of the Pinochet regime's reform of the Labor Code, which fragmented organized labor while giving the employer the power to unilaterally terminate work contracts with thirty days notice. While notable modifications were achieved during the democratic transition, such as legally demanding that employers justify in writing a worker's dismissal, Article 161 of the current Labor Code continues to allow employers to dismiss workers on the basis of "business interests."[6]

As sociologist Volker Frank has pointed out, this regulatory environment has produced "an ever increasing tendency to substitute permanent contract workers with temporary and subcontracted labor, a lowering of income for the total labor force, a decrease in fixed individual incomes for Chile's workers, and an increase in incomes tied to productivity gains, bonuses, and other 'incentives'" (2004:74). For historian Gabriel Salazar Vergara, this "logic of employment," in which "no work contract should be permanent and every worker, according to business interests, is dispensable," has become "the third vertex of the 'social pact' of neoliberalism" (2005:88). Indeed, by 2005 the Decree Laws' legacy and the current Labor Code produced an extremely precarious labor situation in which over 93 percent of new work contracts remained in effect for less than one year, and 50 percent for less than four months (Riesco 2005:59). This situation places specific demands on women who work in the informal sector of the economy. For home-based work such as piecework sewing, they are paid per unit, and thus work long and intensive hours while at the same time trying to cover domestic activities such as child care, cleaning, and food preparation (Díaz 2009; Díaz and Mauro 2010).

In the face of this unpredictability, the consumer credit system has become a resource that low-income people use to tide themselves over, though at the cost of monthly debt payments.[7] Department stores such as Almacenes París and Falabella not only offer credit cards but have also opened their own banks. Supermarkets, such as Supermercados Líder, offer cash advances. Pharmacy chains have partnered with department stores to allow the purchase of pharmaceuticals on department store credit. By 2006, the national census showed that low-income populations earning between US$110 and $300 per month were paying 36 percent of their monthly income to consumer debts (MIDEPLAN 2006).

In Gladys's case, the unpredictability of her husband's work contract paired with the constant pressures of debts were experienced as an external force pressing down on her and impeding her body from "getting up." For others, it is the pain of "adaptation" that calls for medication. As friends in La Pincoya say, "*Hay que adaptarse*" [One has to adapt]. What constitutes "adaptation"?

Héctor and Ruby, a couple in their midforties, allowed me to closely follow their work activities. They lived with their three children, ages eighteen, fifteen, and three, in La Pincoya. Table 10.1 outlines their employment trajectory from 1999 to 2005.

The trajectory, however, does not allow us to appreciate the depths of the daily instability in Héctor and Ruby's life. Let me turn, therefore, to the layers of activity that made and unmade their everyday routines. In June 2005, Ruby began piecework sewing in *la rueda* [the wheel]. *La rueda* is a form of labor common in piecework sewing, in which one person is responsible for one task only—for example, attaching the collar to a fine silk blouse. Contracted by a clothing company, the leader of *la rueda*, who most often lives outside the *población*, finds the workers through neighborhood connections. Workers are often not given contracts. The leader drives from one house to the next, picking up a ready batch to send to the next woman in *la rueda*. The tempo of *la rueda* depends on the pressure of the leader, but also on the women themselves. The women are paid according to the units of pieces finished. If one woman finishes several units, the pressure is on the next woman to finish those units within the

Table 10.1

Ruby	Héctor
July 1999: office cleaning	August 1999–March 2003: hospital parking lot attendant
August 1999–February 2000: piecework sewing	April 2003–September 2003: unemployed
February 2000–April 2002: nanny in La Dehaesa	October 2003–June 2005: DVD/CD warehouse inventory
May 2002–July 2002: Hush Puppy factory worker	
August 2002–June 2003: piecework sewing	
July 2003–May 2005: nanny in Nuñoa	
June 2005: piecework sewing	

same time period to avoid having her units divided between herself and another woman.[8]

Ruby's first assignment was to put zippers into fuzzy pink baby jumpers, for which she was paid 100 pesos (17 cents) for every 50 jumpers. Between sewing sessions, she also took care of her three-year-old son, cleaned, cooked, supervised her older children's homework, checked on her mother, and ran errands. She made 6,000 pesos (US$10) in three weeks. She was then switched to sewing very fine frills into the chest darts of silk blouses. For this work she received 200 pesos (33 cents) for 13 blouses. But the work was painstaking, and it was new to her: the fabric, the type of stitching, and the placement of the stitches all required practice. It took Ruby three hours to make 13 blouses. The leader of *la rueda*, Sra. Teresa, returned the sample unit Ruby made. The frills were not done correctly. Ruby would have to remove the extremely fine stitching without ruining the material, or pay the cost of the fabric. As I sat with her taking out the stitches, we found that the task was nearly impossible. Sra. Teresa switched Ruby from sewing the frills to collars and cuffs. Ruby aimed to make 20,000 pesos ($33) for the month, but she ended up only making 8,000 pesos ($13) in her four weeks of work on the blouses.

Economic pressures started to build. Héctor's income of 160,000 pesos would not cover the household expenses and also leave enough money for food, the 40,000-peso mortgage payment on their house, Héctor's daily bus fare, their department store debts, the quotas on the sewing machine, their utility bills, and the cost of private medical visits for her three-year-old son's persistent loss of weight. Exacerbating the situation, the leader of *la rueda* was late in her bimonthly payments. Héctor and Ruby skipped the June mortgage payment. Ruby drank black coffee and sewed. The hum of the machine pervaded the house, underneath the sound track of the *Toy Story* video that she played repeatedly for her three-year-old. The child, however, often preferred to sit in Ruby's lap and cried when he could not. Sitting in the same position for long periods, hunched over to look so closely at tiny seams, is extremely fatiguing, particularly for the eyes. "I can't get a rhythm," Ruby lamented, rubbing her eyes.

After one month, Ruby decided to look for work *afuera* [outside the house]. She hoped to find a job close to home, but she dreaded work as a nanny. She could not imagine caring for other children while her own son continued to have little appetite and was underweight for his age. It was "a daily agony," she said. I accompanied her to the Municipal Office for Labor Information (Oficina Muncipal de Información Laboral, OMIL). She received the *tarjeta de cesantía* [unemployment card] that gave her access to an unemployment subsidy and to the "database" of job opportunities: a bulletin board and Rolodex. Companies also called into the OMIL to ask for names of people looking for low-paid, subcontracted, and temporary labor. As we walked down the street, I asked Ruby what OMIL stood for. "OMIL, OMIL. I don't know for sure. Something to do with emergency. Because not having work is an emergency, so they must deal with crisis situations."

The office was small and run down with dim yellow lighting and a few chairs. The chairs were empty, but several men and women were standing around a glass-covered bulletin board with notices of potential employment. "Looking for domestic employee [*empleada doméstica*]. Live in [*Puertas adentro*]. 160,000 monthly (US$268)." "Office looks for employee for cleaning, Monday, Tuesday, Wednesday, at night. 90,000 monthly ($151)." Ruby wrote down several telephone numbers, the amount paid, and the schedule. She made phone calls, a month passed, but there was no answer.

In the meantime, Héctor too was facing daily instability of another kind. Héctor worked shifts. In June, he was working nights, waking up at 2:00 pm, preparing lunch for himself and the children while Ruby continued working, then getting to work by 7:00 pm. He did warehouse inventory until 7:00 am, arrived back home by 9:00 am, and promptly went to sleep. The last weekend in June, he had no time off. The warehouse needed people working "extra hours," but the "extra hours" began in the morning. Héctor came home for two hours, then returned to the warehouse until 7:00 pm. The following week, he was assigned mornings again. But that assignment was interrupted when his boss suddenly moved him to nights in the middle of the week. "*Me descompagina*" [It unsettles me], said Ruby.

With Héctor's schedule in flux, routines that would otherwise provide a temporal grounding for the everyday cannot be maintained. Héctor looks tired and is unshaven. He has a perpetual spasm in his neck. Compounding the physical toll, Héctor has been told to do manual labor, unloading immense wooden shipping crates of primary materials used to make compact discs. This work was not part of his contract. Three years earlier, he had been diagnosed with osteoporosis, rare for a man of his age, and he suffered from a chronic lower back injury. He now begins to have severe back pain.

By the end of July, Banco del Estado had mailed the next mortgage bill. Héctor and Ruby owe 40,000, plus another 13,000 for interest and late fees, as well as the next 40,000, for a total of 93,000. Other bills arrive. Department stores Johnson's and Hites, the Lider supermarket, and Bansolución add up to 65,000 in monthly debt payments. Ruby tells me, "If I pay these bills, there will neither be money for the bus, nor money for food, nothing. So, I need to look for *pitutitos* [contracts for little jobs] selling music [pirated CDs]." She decides to pay one dividend and half the monthly debt. Her sister Lorena lends her 10,000 for the month.

One week later, Ruby has a terrible headache. I meet her at her house. "I have a stabbing in my eye," she tells me. "I have a headache. But, all in the eye. I think I will vomit. The stress has me *embarrada* [covered in mud/ dragged in the dirt] from the nerves. All the time, you're with this pressure. I go to bed thinking, I get up thinking. The organism is angry with me because my mind *no me deja tranquila* [doesn't allow me to be tranquil]. The pressure is so much. There are so many people in the same situation as me, and so it's so difficult that one fixes one's situation because all of us are in the same situation. *Este sistema maldito nos tiene cagado a todo los pobres* [This evil system has all of us poor people screwed]."

Ruby and Héctor's experiences show how daily routines are not a given of everyday life, but rather an achievement that must be secured against the odds.[9] Confronting moments of economic scarcity, they must find ways to adapt, living "unsettled" routines that they try to bring into a new form of regularity. This process of adapting has a temporality. It is one of the body catching up with conditions that outstrip it. Unable to predict, to anticipate, to count on a future, the body constantly struggles to adapt, manifesting in bodily aches and pains, sore arms and legs, headaches, insomnia, a lack of appetite, and painful eyes. Ruby provides her own diagnosis: these symptoms arise from specific life conditions produced by "the system."

In the wake of such commonly experienced symptoms, women and men have developed a practical knowledge base—a local formulary of go-to medications—for their alleviation: paracetamol for headaches and neck and back cramps, vitamins to boost the *ánimo*, benzodiazepines to quell *los nervios*. In this constellation of "adaptation symptoms" and "adaptation medications," the specific role of the antidepressant is to provide the necessary vital energy so that the body can get up and look for work. Passed between neighbors and shared between kin, the pill renders immediate benefits—as a materiality that manifests how the self is enmeshed in relationships.

Dr. Chanta and Systemic Failures

These somatic complaints and recourses to "vital energy," folded into the everyday as recognizable symptoms of unstable employment, could provide a counterpoint to Global Mental Health's emphasis on "common mental disorders." Changing scales and registers from the population—as it is epidemiologically accounted for—to the textures of relationships and materialities of the local helps us critically question the temporality of the common disorder. We might ask, how is "common" understood across these scales and registers? That is, epidemiological studies account for "common mental disorders"—such as depression or generalized anxiety disorder—by charting the prevalence of symptoms that count toward such disease categories within a given population, symptoms that themselves must manifest with a certain temporality to be counted *as* depression. Ethnography, on the other hand, helps us attend to the unpredictable, singular, and discontinuous experience of unstable and changing work regimes and their relationship to the manifestation of depressive symptoms. In other words, ethnography helps us attend to those small events of precariousness in the household and how those events distribute across the kinship network. From the perspective of *the event*, there are variations and intensifications of symptoms, depending on the particular pressures of debt payments and conditions of employment.

In the dynamics between patients, families, and physicians, symptoms of "adaptation" express, in a sense, a locally experienced "health"—the very capacity to respond to shifting life environments. What I mean by "health" follows from Georges Canguilhem's delineation of "'pathology' as the vital contrary of 'health' and not the logical contradictory of 'normal.'" That is, "health is precisely a certain latitude, a certain play in the norms of life and behavior. What characterizes health is a capacity to tolerate variations in norms on which only the stability of situations and milieus—seemingly guaranteed yet in fact always necessarily precarious—confers a deceptive value of definitive normalcy" (Canguilhem 2008:131–32). The pains of adapting illustrate the cost of health today in a milieu of work regimes that make staying afloat a daily achievement.

For many in La Pincoya, treating these symptoms with the local formulary is what it takes to make it to the next day, to have a functioning body that allows one to search for work and "adapt." However, these implicit practical knowledges and locally experienced adaptabilities and latitudes may themselves facilitate the reception of such pains as "common mental disorders" of the poor not only by physicians, but also by those afflicted—in other words, as the normal aches and pains of living. And sometimes they can also obscure rare disease processes. Exploring how such local knowledges fail in concert with the failure of medical institutions, and how these joint failures shape a patient's chances in the health reform's framework of universal access and explicit guarantees is the subject to which I now turn.

This is the story of Soledad, Ruby's sister. Soledad and I sit in the shady patio of her sister's house. It is September 2005. In her one-room shack just up the street, her partner Johnny has passed out from a night of consuming *pasta base*. She stayed up all night waiting for him to come home, but he never did. He only arrived in the morning, with bloodshot eyes and reeking of alcohol. Soledad lives on her mother's property, as do the families of her three other siblings. She is forty-five years old and has a twelve-year-old son and a one-year-old baby, Pepito. Johnny first became addicted to *pasta base* fifteen years earlier. After seven years of episodic use, he entered an evangelical therapeutic community, where, in Soledad's words, he was "touched by God" and returned "different, transformed." But eight years later, shortly after the birth of their second son in 2004, Johnny relapsed. As a result, he lost his stable job as a security guard and could only sustain temporary work.

Soledad had also recently lost her job and was searching for temporary work in office cleaning and piecework sewing. After eight years of work as a nanny, her *patrones* fired her after she gave birth to Pepito. Before Johnny's relapse and the loss of both their jobs, however, they had bought a house, three houses down the street from Soledad's mother. A one-bedroom house with yellow-painted, cracked brick walls and an outside patio of weeds and mud, it was in need of significant repairs. The monthly mortgage for the house was 50,000 pesos (US$83). In addition, they had taken out a bank loan of 300,000 pesos ($500) from Banco del Estado for household repairs, for which they paid 20,000 pesos ($33) a month. Because of the instability of their income, Soledad had rented out the house, but the renters left without notice, leaving two months of rent unpaid.

Soledad and Johnny had no income for the month of September, so Soledad was counting on the money from the renters, a family from the south of Chile, to at least cover the mortgage and monthly loan payments. To complicate matters, Johnny had sold the stereo, TV, and DVD player to pay for drugs. He knocked on doors asking for money, and Soledad estimated from what her neighbors told her that he owed them at least 75,000 pesos (US$125). She sold family heirlooms—her grandmother's three-panel antique mirror and her deceased father's collection of vinyl records—to cover the debts to department stores and the supermarket.

Soledad had been diagnosed with depression at the primary care center. She had a constant headache, and her body, she said, was rigid from anxiety. As we spoke, she rubbed her neck and shoulders. The week before, a legal demand had arrived from Banco del Estado for two months of unpaid mortgage. She had asked her brother José for the 50,000 pesos (US$83) that he owed her. But he was also out of work. "It frustrates me," she said. "José buys and buys, and I gave him the money to pay his debts when I was doing well. And when I need the money, it is not there." José later told me that he felt *bajoneado* [down] because he could not pay

Soledad back. But he was also frustrated that Soledad continued to allow Johnny to stay with her. Johnny, José said, was the problem. "Why can't she just throw him out? He sells our things to buy *pasta base*."

A few days after our conversation, Soledad got a loan from her niece Vali, her sister Lorena's daughter. Vali gave Soledad all of her savings to pay for the two overdue monthly payments on her bank loan. Soledad felt ashamed. Vali had been saving the money to buy her own house. "I need to pay her back urgently. Vali gave me the money, but I know that she now walks around *angustiada* [anguished] and *bajoneada* [down], and this makes me feel worse." As the aunt, Soledad was now in the shameful position of owing money to a niece, who, according to kinship norms, she should protect as a mother would her child. She said, "I practically raised Vali. She's as much my daughter as Lorena's. How could I take her savings?" We were standing in the doorway of her shack. She was angry with Johnny. But she was even angrier at herself for staying with Johnny. "After all these years of struggle, we have nothing. I thought I could save Johnny, but he is weak. I love him, but he is weak. I spent my life trying to save a lost case."

"Did you ever consider separating from him?" I asked.

She responded, "I think if I could go back in time, I would never have gotten back together with him. But it's not so easy to throw him out. He has nowhere else to go, and I think of my son. His father is his idol. If I threw him out and something happened to him, if he were stabbed or killed, my son would never forgive me." Soledad's patience was wearing thin, but her impatience was directed mostly at herself. "I recognize that I am very intolerant. It makes me angry, gives me rage, and makes me down. But this is because of what is happening in my surroundings. It's so much at times that I want to take an eraser and erase myself." With "erase myself" Soledad voices the multiple contradictory relational demands that she embodies and that overwhelm her. As a mother, Soledad seeks to protect her relationship to her son. As the eldest daughter, she has sold the heirlooms that connect her to past generations in order to pay off debts to secure a possible future. By owing a debt to her niece, Soledad has to absorb the shame of a reversal of kinship obligations, even as the debt revives the possibility that one day Soledad, her sons, and even Johnny might once again inhabit their own home.

Over the next four years, Soledad continued to be torn between these pressing relational demands as she sought work. In 2006, she worked in an office cleaning, a job acquired through a local *contratista* in the Business City of Huechuraba, which houses international advertising firms. Afterward, she worked in outsourced food prep for private Catholic schools. In 2007, she did piecework sewing from home. But then her wrists and hands, injured by repetitive strain, became so painful that she could no longer continue to sew. She used a home remedy, warmed paraffin compresses, for symptomatic relief, and found work as a nanny. But throughout 2007 Soledad developed fatigue and body aches and pains. She went to the primary care center, where she was diagnosed again with depression and prescribed antidepressants.

Soledad continued to have body aches and pains until early 2009, and her wrists were not improving. She had now stopped treatment for depression, and she, as well as her family, had, in her sister's words, concluded "that these were the pains of the everyday." In mid-2009, Soledad began to have problems with her vision. She was given a referral to an ophthalmologist and waited a month for the appointment. Upon examination, she was referred to a neurologist for a "possible brain tumor." At this point, Soledad's sister Ruby was accompanying her to her appointments. Ruby and her husband Héctor and their three children had managed to buy a house in 2004 and lived one street over. Soledad had such severe bodily aches and pains that her sister Ruby was convinced of the brain tumor. (Their mother had required surgical resection of a benign brain tumor years earlier.) But after a cursory exam, the neurologist, Dr. R, told her, "Don't worry, it's depression."

Remaining unconvinced, Ruby took her sister for a private consultation (*consulta particular*), paying for lab tests and scans out of her own pocket, which in Ruby's case meant taking out a personal loan of 1 million pesos from her employer, Marta, who ran an NGO for community development in La Pincoya. Marta's husband was a wealthy businessman, and Marta herself had been quite successful in securing state funds for local development projects. The lending of money between employers and workers to finance private consultations among the poor and the use of private consultations for second opinions in the face of medical uncertainty are areas that warrant further research. By the end of

November 2009, Soledad finally received the diagnosis of a massive growth hormone–secreting pituitary adenoma. The tumor had to be surgically resected. Unable to afford the surgery and hospitalization out of pocket, Soledad and Ruby returned to the neurologist in the public system with the private clinic's diagnosis in hand. Dr. R told them that Soledad would have to wait five months for neurosurgical resection, although, according to Plan AUGE, treatment should begin within thirty days.

At Ruby's insistence, Soledad was scheduled for surgery in early February 2010. By this time, however, the tumor had become so massive that the neurosurgeon had to perform two separate surgeries, and still only 10 percent was resected. I spoke to Ruby on the phone shortly after the second surgery. Soledad was convalescing in her home. She told me that after the surgery the neurosurgeon, "a young man, he pulled me aside, and said he would have never waited to do the surgery. He did not understand why the doctor waited so long for the surgery." Dr. R came later and apprised Ruby of the neurosurgeon's findings. She said that she "exploded" at him: "Does one have to pay millions of pesos to be considered a human being?! The only name I can give him is Dr. Chanta, Dr. Chanta [Dr. Charlatan]." Dr. Chanta, she said, told her that Soledad would eventually grow blind from the tumor impinging on her optic nerves and could suffer a heart attack. Soledad's only option now was to begin medication that could possibly shrink the tumor and alleviate the deleterious effects of excessive growth hormone.

In the face of the "complication" created by the collusion of the practical knowledge of the people of La Pincoya, physicians' preconceptions about the "common mental disorders" of the poor, and medical negligence, Ruby and Soledad were confronting medical uncertainties that departed from the protocols of Plan AUGE. At this point, Soledad had moved into Ruby's house because she needed constant care. Ruby was left trying to untangle the complicated vocabularies of medicine that tied into the complexity of health care coverage, while also caring for her sister, her sister's children, and her own family, and holding down a job.[10]

As a result of the excess growth hormone secreted by her adenoma, Soledad is now suffering from acromegaly. Her hands and feet are growing larger, and her face is becoming more coarse. But Plan AUGE only covers surgical resection, post-op medications, and in some cases radiation therapy—that is, treatments for the predictable after-effects of Soledad's surgery. It does not cover the costs of her real and unpredicted need for medications that she will have to take daily to prevent blindness and eventually death. As Dannreuther and Gideon have pointed out, "One limitation of the Plan AUGE is that users requiring a different course of treatment to that specified in the protocols for a particular health condition . . . will not be covered by the AUGE. They must continue to use the preexisting system and decide between FONASA [the public financing system] and ISAPRES [the private insurers]" (Dannreuther and Gideon 2008:858).

Ruby alternated between sadness and rage. *Me cambió*, she said, "It changed me. *Trato de ponerme dura* [I try to put on a thick skin]. I have had neighbors die, but this changed me. This is my sister. We have endured this life together. I should take her to that doctor so that he sees what state she is in now!" She began to cry, "How is she going to be able to live in her home? The home that she has rented out and never been able to live in? She will not be able to work again. Can you imagine it, paying dividends on a pension? The situation is not for this, economically."

Uncertainty also surrounds possible medical treatments for Soledad. She was to begin taking medications to shrink the tumor and mitigate the effects of excessive growth hormone, but Ruby told me that a month's supply would cost about 1 million pesos. She was going to organize a neighborhood bingo game to raise funds for the medication, but while that was in its planning stages, surgical resection was again advanced as a potential treatment.

As of this writing, Soledad is once again preparing for surgical resection. She has married her partner Johnny. Johnny had been separated from his first wife for several years, and upon Soledad's illness, he filed for divorce. Ruby told me that Johnny had relapsed into using *pasta base*. Dark feelings of resentment and fears of betrayal color the marriage, feelings that are lived in silence by Soledad's sisters. The sisters fear that Johnny's divorce and remarriage to Soledad is motivated by an interest in securing the inheritance of her house upon her death. Thus, Soledad's family now faces a delicate task. They hope to encourage Soledad to file for a "separation of assets," so that Johnny cannot have access to her house, which the family together might manage to maintain for her children's future, although not without financial struggle.

Health and Care

In the midst of unstable work and the monthly demands of debt payments, women and men in La Pincoya are struggling to adapt and keep up with labor conditions that constantly outrun them in their unpredictability. Within this context, securing daily routines is a daily achievement, a locally experienced "health"—a feat that requires both responding to the variability of environment and responding to the needs of their kin. Such precarious achievement comes with significant costs and involves, as we have seen, a whole range of dangers and threats, not the least of which is the possibility that disease processes might be obscured. These pains of adaptation take shape in affective configurations of the domestic that implicate corporeally different experiences for men and women. As Soledad and Ruby's struggles have shown, it is the women who are most often caught between the multiple and often counterposed tensions of kinship relations, relations that can entail both care and violence.

Antidepressants have gained a life in a local formulary of medications that treat these aches and pains. Through their effects of conferring the "vital energy" one needs to look for work, antidepressants function as adjuvants to the vitality of domestic relations that already make up ordinary life. I realize that such a perspective sits in awkward tension with Global Mental Health's calls for the treatment of "common mental disorders" through packages of care. While care for mental illness is certainly desirable and necessary, attention to how "health" is locally experienced and how the costs of health are mitigated in everyday life can allow us to approach "care" differently. Ethnographic work within the weave of life permits an exploration of the norms that life must overcome and helps us critically consider the desirability of such norms as they work in tandem with the care provided by Global Mental Health.

Notes

1. Based on the October 2004 exchange rate: 609.27CLP/1USD. Source: Banco Central Base de Datos. http://si2.bcentral.cl/Basededatoseconomicos/951_417. asp?LlamadaPortada=SI [last accessed July 2, 2010].

2. I would like to thank the families in La Pincoya for inviting me into their lives. Thanks very much to João Biehl and Adriana Petryna for organizing and leading the "When People Come First" seminar at Princeton University and for

their encouragement. Thanks also to the seminar participants whose comments were very helpful. The research for this work was funded by the National Science Foundation Graduate Fellowship, the National Institutes of Mental Health Ruth L. Kirschstein National Research Service Award Individual MD/PhD Fellowship Grant No. 5 F30 MH064979-06, and the Social Science Research Council-IDRF.

3. The social, political, and moral commitments of mental health professionals in Chile's public health system blur the differentiation made by Andrew Lakoff between the "biological" disease category of depression and the social and political basis of pharmaceutical marketing in Argentina. As Lakoff points out, in his interviews with sales representatives, a social science critique of medicalization of suffering was redundant: "the very salience of social accounts of suffering served not as a critique of the role of pharmaceutical marketing, but as its *basis*" (Lakoff 2004:251). But Chilean mental health researchers have consistently posed their studies in terms of the complex linkages between biological processes and social inequalities, advancing the diagnostic category of depression not solely as a "biomedicalized psychiatry," but rather by means of efforts to promote community mental health with depression understood as a complex biopsychosocial process (see Araya et al. 2003a; Rojas et al. 2005). Indeed, given their nuanced understandings of mental health, neither a simplistic critique of medicalization nor one that advances a solely political or economic etiology would suffice. A mistaken focus on which etiology the psychiatrists are privileging or not—since indeed their etiological bases are multiple—evades the question of *how* the antidepressant is being used by ordinary people. For this anthropologist, what is at stake is how pharmaceuticals come to be used in everyday lifeworlds to treat actual everyday aches and pains, elucidating bodily-affective experience tied into general life conditions. The point here is not to argue that Chilean mental health researchers are medicalizing a complex reality, but rather to show and reflect on a different view of health, through symptoms, a view that close attention to both the use of pharmaceuticals and daily activities affords.

4. Indeed, in the midst of this municipal election year, it took nine months for me to receive permission from the municipality to observe group sessions in the local primary health care clinic, difficulties that may have been inspired by the institutional letters of support I received from the Ministry of Health's Mental Health Unit and from the Northern Metropolitan Health Service.

5. This trajectory contrasted sharply with the pilot program's results in the *población* La Bandera located in the Southern Zone of Santiago, where I visited at the suggestion of Dr. Rojas. There, the group sessions became a new "test site" for the formation of affective community through the marker of depression—not as a strict disease category, but rather as a set of conditions that women struggled with in their everyday lives. The group sessions expanded into a "self-help group" with legal status and over fifty members. The difference again illustrates how local political conditions and an affective ethos of experiment can determine to a large extent the success of decentralized programs. It is not just the provision of a technical infrastructure that matters, but the qualities of commitments and care evident in the health workers and administration. At the same time, it confirms the findings of medical anthropologists and physicians who have shown how affects

and ethics "hold together" local institutions of care, generating belonging and enhancing treatment adherence (Behforouz et al. 2004; Biehl 2007).

6. Art. 161. Sin perjuicio de lo señalado en los artículos precedentes, el empleador podrá poner término al contrato de trabajo invocando como causal las necesidades de la empresa, establecimiento o servicio, tales como las derivadas de la racionalización o modernización de los mismos, bajas en la productividad, cambios en las condiciones del mercado o de la economía, que hagan (and per "hagan" [make] above) necesaria la separación de uno o más trabajadores (Ministerio de Trabajo y Previsión Social, Gobierno de Chile, 2003). [The employer can terminate the work contract invoking as a cause the needs of the company, establishment, or service, such as those derived from the rationalization or modernization of those same entities, lowering of productivity, or changes in market conditions or the economy, which make the separation of one or more workers necessary.]

7. However, for families the consequences of the contraction of credit with the global economic crisis must be further examined.

8. Most of the costs of production are absorbed by the women themselves: electricity to run sewing machines and ambient lighting are part of household bills. The sewing machines and overlocks are usually bought on credit by the women with subsidies from the state.

9. As a counterpoint, much of the philosophical and anthropological literature on embodiment and practice has asked the question how improvisation—or the new—is possible against the background of habit. For example, Pierre Bourdieu struggles with the question of how new patterns of thought and practice are forged in relation to the *habitus* (Bourdieu 2000). Merleau-Ponty asks how perception leaves open an indeterminate horizon in relation to the sedimentation of history and habit within the body (Merleau-Ponty 1962). However, we might also ask ourselves how habit itself is achieved in contexts in which the minute activities that make up everyday life are constantly shifting.

10. How Plan AUGE could be changing patterns and intensities of care for the ill within the home is suggested by sociologist Irma Arriagada: "Even when the improvement in basic health care coverage allows for the access by all to hospitalization and medical care (including the most poor and migrant persons), the medical and technological advances along with a new conception of efficiency in hospital management have provoked a reduction of hospitalization time and a steering of care towards the home, which establishes a series of difficulties for some poor and migrant families to provide this care. Thus, it is sustained that the model of attention defined in the health reform that articulates the institutional systems of health and the domestic/community continues to rest on the mediating role of women" (Arriagada 2010:16–17). This insight points to an area of much needed research.

11

The Ascetic Subject of Compliance

The Turn to Chronic Diseases in Global Health

IAN WHITMARSH

In 2002 the World Health Organization issued a World Health Report that focused on noninfectious chronic diseases (2002c). The report noted that diseases such as heart disease, diabetes, cancer, and asthma were increasing globally. This attention to chronic conditions marks a departure from a focus on the urgent communicable diseases that have historically been the objects of global public health initiatives. In this new arena, there are no infections to prevent, no contagion to stanch, no immunizations or treatments to make mandatory. I explore here the medical subject that emerges out of this twenty-first-century global health focus on diseases of "lifestyle."

These chronic conditions are considered to be spread by modernization. A new meaning of "communicable" is being proffered to describe conditions carried by industrialization, by increased exposure or access to pollutants, fast foods, sedentary employment, and leisure. Obesity is a paragon of such conditions, tied by researchers to diabetes, cancer, and heart disease. The WHO noted in its report that for the first time in history there are more obese people in the world than malnourished people.

What might it mean to juxtapose the malnourished with the obese as objects of public health? "Malnourishment" marks deprivation, a call to redress a lack in possibilities; "obesity" marks excess, an overabundance of possibility that demands control. With chronic diseases, the locus of intervention shifts from attempting to remove structural barriers or expand access to medications to convincing individuals to see themselves as ill or potentially ill and to act accordingly—eating and drinking differently, taking their medications, becoming more physically fit.[1] Compliance is thereby becoming a principal public health issue of the twenty-first century,[2] and compliance posits a figure with a responsibility to continually work to discipline the self into a biomedical subject. In what follows, I draw on fieldwork in the Caribbean and the United States on the science and medicine of the chronic diseases of asthma, diabetes, and obesity to explore this subject.[3] Moving from scientists in the United States to health officials, doctors, and patients in Barbados and Trinidad and Tobago, I explore the ways in which biomedical science and global health become intertwined, creating particular forms of health intervention.

I argue here that the figure that inhabits biomedical compliance is not the familiar (neo)liberal individual found by recent social science analyses to be at the center of global science, markets, and governing (Rose 2007). Current American biomedical research and policy around obesity, asthma, and other chronic conditions is a turn away from any individualized liberal subject that might inhere in medicine: the science of biological predispositions to illness and structural causes of noncompliance rejects the perceived moralizing discourse that sees the sick individual as responsible for his or her condition. Instead, this expertise focuses on factors causing sickness outside the individual's control, including cultural traditions, psychological issues, and socioeconomic context. Global health expertise and governance of chronic diseases organizes not around a volitional individual, but instead around a cultural and psychological concept of the community. Compliance techniques attempt to affect community behaviors and cultural attitudes toward food, beauty, children, and medicine. This expertise approaches the community as a source of biological, psychological, and cultural predispositions that affect health. I argue here that this expertise on predispositions intersects with the current emphasis on access to "information" to fashion a new subject of compliance.

Medical Dystopias

In the countries of Barbados and Trinidad and Tobago, American biomedicine is critical to government health interventions. Despite its population of only 269,000, Barbados attracts biomedical research from all over the world. American and British academic teams explore genetic propensities for heart disease, diabetes, cancers, asthma, even acute lung injury. Multinational pharmaceutical companies conduct clinical trials on medications for asthma, heart disease, blood pressure, and cancer. Barbados has a national drug formulary that is taken as a model by the World Health Organization, which believes that the pharmaceutical industry should have a central role to play in medical education and government policy making around public health (Whitmarsh 2008a). Trinidad also attempts to partake in the future of biomedicine by attracting British and American geneticists and other medical researchers exploring cancer, diabetes, and heart disease. Both countries have made chronic disease central to their public health interventions. In Trinidad, the Ministry of Health has implemented a "Chronic Disease Assistance Programme," which "provides citizens with free prescription drugs and other pharmaceutical items [including free blood glucose testing technologies] to combat many chronic health conditions." These include diabetes, asthma, and heart disease. In Barbados, the government similarly offers free pharmaceuticals to citizens for five chronic conditions: epilepsy, asthma, hypertension, diabetes, and cancer. This integration of the bioscience and biomedicine of chronic conditions into the public health interventions of poorer (but not among the poorest) countries turns compliance into a central issue in public health.

The chronic diseases of obesity, diabetes, asthma, and heart disease have followed other public health crises in being called "epidemics." Asthma diagnoses are increasing worldwide, particularly in urban areas and in countries undergoing rapid development. Obesity is similarly increasing in what American biomedical researchers routinely refer to as "the fattening of the world," and this condition is now a transnational focus of medical, governmental, private, and nongovernmental institutions. National governments from western Europe to East Asia, in both postcolonial and postsocialist countries, have adopted policies to intervene on obesity among their citizens. One result is that cultural domains that anthropologists have traditionally examined, from the aesthetics of physical beauty and desirability to childrearing and food choices, now fall under the purview of "health."

At biomedical conferences and lectures in the United States, researchers communicate this crisis through statistics mapping the future thirty years ahead. At a 2009 conference on obesity that I attended in California, a researcher brought up a slide showing the expected number of obese people in 2040: "I know you have probably seen these slides many times. It's always shocking." An audience member nodded, "Every time." The speaker went on, "It's really scary." These maps are dystopias, spatial representations of the suffering to come and, like all dystopias, they give coordinates to both a judgment and an intervention. Part of what must be done about the crisis of noncommunicable chronic diseases is to get patients (and potential patients) to believe that there is a crisis. As the researcher giving the lecture on obesity continued, "Thankfully, the public is coming to realize that there is an epidemic of type 2 diabetes."

With lifestyle diseases, a primary intervention on the pandemic is "behavior." Compliance as a problem area calls for an extension of the biomedical perspective (recognizing there is a problem, knowing the risks, getting a diagnosis, understanding the significance of taking medication and eating and drinking appropriately, valuing health, acting in healthy ways). This solution distinguishes the crisis from the cause of disease: medical researchers, practitioners, and officials consider chronic diseases of modernization to be caused by political, economic, social, cultural, and sometimes psychological and genetic factors. But compliance makes the *crisis* not these structures that cause disease, but the lack of a medical perspective. Consider asthma. Medical researchers, from immunologists to epidemiologists to geneticists, all take asthma to be a multifactorial disease, caused by a complex of environmental and hereditary factors. But asthma can be managed with an inhaled steroid—and uncontrolled asthma is then the result either of a lack of access to that medication or of not taking it correctly. Access to the medication is a field of its own, but increasingly science and states turn to what happens to those medications that are available. In biomedical literature, low compliance rates for asthma medication are a primary site requiring intervention (Apter et al. 1998; Bender 2002; Glauber and Fuhlbrigge 2002; Weinstein et al. n.d.). Medical research on compliance explores patient beliefs and views about available medications, their dosage, efficacy, purpose, side effects, and mechanisms. In Barbados, the government frames the extremely high levels of asthma as a problem of noncompliance with brand inhalers.[4] A widespread underuse of "preventer inhalers" (those that include an inhaled steroid) is the critical public health issue related to asthma according to medical practitioners, government health officials, and nongovernmental organizations alike.

This logic creates the possibility of intervening in the health crisis by making the pharmaceutical more desirable. In asthma medications, pharmaceutical companies GlaxoSmithKline and AstraZeneca have patented inhalers that combine long-acting beta2-agonists with inhaled steroids (both "preventer inhalers"). These are reformulations of available medications, allowing extension of the company's right to exclusivity. GlaxoSmithKline's combination inhaler, sold as Advair in the United States and Seretide elsewhere, was the fourth bestselling drug in the world in 2004, according to the *New York Times* (Grady 2005). In the absence of evidence showing that these new combination inhalers have better efficacy or safety than what was previously available, GlaxoSmithKline and AstraZeneca position them as improving compliance. In Barbados, the multinational drug companies hold lavish conferences for influential medical practitioners around new pharmaceuticals like the combination inhaler. These conferences are designed to introduce the medication and suggest the significance of getting the drug onto the National Formulary. I attended one such event that was held for a combination inhaler. The speaker, an asthma researcher flown in for the event, talked about "how to make asthma treatment simple." During his lecture, he explained the successive stages of complexity in asthma intervention: "First we administer the correct medication. Then we make sure they are taking the medication. Then we go into the home to do environmental changes. Because this is complicated. The first is simpler, the second is expensive." The speaker explicitly suggested the relevance of this metric to Barbados as a poor country: in his view, given the economics of medical care, going into the patient's home was not viable. He went on, "We are trying to be simple: talk to the patient about what is achievable, what is acceptable. You cannot say, 'You must move.' It's easier for patients to use one device." The pharmaceutical was presented here as a kind of social medicine, responsive to structural causes and cheaper than moving families, implementing antipollution policies, or entering the patient's home. The combination inhaler is thus made into a vaguely economical-through-simplicity response for poorer countries. AstraZeneca's combination inhaler Symbicort made it onto the Barbadian National Drug Formulary in 2003, as did Glaxo-SmithKline's Seretide in a more provisional way. Symbicort in particular was very quickly picked up by urban-area private and public medical practitioners. As one public-system pediatrician told me about treating asthma a few months after Symbicort was added to the Formulary, "All the children over ten I put on a combination inhaler." Compliance as a public health issue creates new ways for pharmaceuticals to act as social medicine.

But stories like this about pharmaceuticals are perhaps familiar by now. Overemphasizing the pharmaceutical risks making it exceptional, according some power to its "thereness" as commodity or chemical, as tactile or potent or fetishized. In the biomedicine of compliance, the pharmaceutical is simply one among many rituals invoked to improve global health. In the case of the obesity epidemic, weight-loss drugs are in the background of public health campaigns; compliance is about food and drink and daily activity. American research and public health outreach around obesity reveals several different routes to compliance. In the United States, public health programs use outreach campaigns; parent groups pressure schools to change available foods; officials back food legislation (such as the controversial sugar tax now proposed in several states); and extensive media coverage is given to researchers and practitioners who describe the economic and health toll of being overweight. Again, these interventions are not reducible to an individualized approach to medicine. The question of "community" versus "individual" approaches to public health is a robust area of contestation within public health these days. Such discordance came across at a California conference on diabetes in 2008 that brought together state public health officials, medical researchers, and community nurses and medical practitioners. At one point, a researcher and a public health official were discussing ways to intervene in the high rates of diabetes in California. The researcher argued for tele-medicine, in which phone calls with informative electronic voice messages are strategically made to patients: "Tele-medicine promotes more effective targeted communication and management for patients. We think it might help prevent diabetes for patients who may be at high risk. It's an interactive health technology that can be tailored (reaching people who have less literacy and medical skills). Now we're doing a project on pharmacy data to target those with low adherence to try to get their use of medications to be better." Like the combination inhalers, tele-medicine was considered particularly relevant to poorer communities. In later discussions at the conference, medical staff talked about using tele-medicine as a substitute in facilities that lack funding: two representatives from state clinics mentioned that they would be exploring using tele-medicine since they had lost funding and staff. Tele-medicine could become a kind of proxy for medical interactions in the low-income communities of California. The public health official talking with the tele-medicine researcher took exception to his emphasis on compliance with medication protocols. She emphasized instead reducing the consumption of unhealthy foods and drink. The means to this form of compliance was the soda tax measure recently introduced in California cities, which would increase the tax on sweetened beverages, and thereby presumably reduce their consumption. Again, this intervention was considered to be focused on poor communities—for obvious reasons—and was lauded as potentially generating new revenue for state public health outreach.

All three of these interventions—the new easy-to-use pharmaceutical, the electronic phone health message, and the tax on unhealthy choices—are considered particularly suited to poorer communities. These interventions diverge in the traditional metric of "individualized" versus "community" approaches. The public health official told the researcher that it was time to shift from "self-advocacy," such as information for patients, to "community advocacy," such as taxing unhealthy foods. But this community/individual distinction can remain contentious because both alternatives leave intact the shared logic that increasing compliance is the object of public health intervention. The conversation continued:

PUBLIC HEALTH OFFICIAL: When I was in the medical field, we asked how can we improve self-management skills. Then I switched over to public health, and started doing *community* based work. So what do you, as a guru of self-advocacy, think about moving from self-advocacy to group-advocacy.
RESEARCHER: I totally agree. It's the process of acculturation that is leading to diabetes. It's the environment.

In both of these approaches to chronic disease, the citizens are seen as undermining themselves, and the public health intervention is the process of bringing them closer to a biomedical way of understanding and living. The intervention here reveals precisely what is out of control in the dystopia of lifestyle pandemics: the community's behaviors, attitudes, or affect—a noncompliant subjectivity.

Biomedical Asceticism

This public health approach to compliance organizes market, state, and public institutions internationally, including in the English-speaking Caribbean. In Trinidad, the Ministry of Health gives free blood glucose meters to all diabetics and works with some large local companies to educate their employees about the health risks of being overweight, while the Ministry of Culture and Gender Affairs conducts lectures about healthy foods and healthy weight at community centers, which become social events. A nongovernmental organization (NGO) made up of diabetics goes to schools, workplace events, and health fairs to offer free blood sugar testing and to give talks on the importance of early testing for diabetes. In Barbados, asthma inhalers are similarly a focal point across private, public, and state organizations. In addition to Ministry of Health lectures and literature distribution, the NGO Mothers of Asthmatics focuses on getting mothers to give their children controller inhalers, holding lectures and distributing pharmaceutical company materials about controlling asthma in schools. These techniques and institutions around compliance are supplemented by the common informal mechanisms—the commercial diet industry, private gyms, purveyors of health foods, and radio programs and newspaper editorials about the dangers of overeating or not taking medications appropriately. Compliance is not restricted to techniques of the clinic but rather extends to a logic for a more biomedical populace. This logic carries an asceticism. Compliance is about minimizing unhealthy attitudes, desires, and behaviors. In Barbados, noncompliance with standard pharmaceutical prescriptions is considered the cause of the asthma crisis. Practitioners' accounts tell of asthmatics stockpiling oral steroids, refusing to take the newer and safer inhaled steroids, and overusing "reliever inhalers" (short-acting beta2-agonists). Most medical practitioners and pharmaceutical company representatives argue that undue fear and strange beliefs cause this inappropriate use of medicines. In this logic, asthmatics and the families of asthmatics must work to overcome these irrational impulses in order to properly take their medications. A similar logic of an inability to control oneself is found for obesity. In the American biomedical context, this subject position is most often depicted as a kind of unintentional excess caused by psychological issues, social forces, or biological disposition. At times, the peculiarly American shame around fat is used to generate sympathy for the sufferer at conferences and in outreach contexts: a recent public health program put out by the state of California included posters displayed in urban areas that simply depicted a midriff of a heavy black or Hispanic person with text warning of the dangerous effects of such weight. New York City's public health department had their own version of such posters, showing a coffee mug overflowing with congealed fat. Efforts like these play on the American disgust with fat, discussed by many (Schwartz 1986; Stearns 2002). In Trinidad, obesity is less likely to be figured as being about shame than it is about hedonism—a lack of wanting to control. As one Ministry of Health official put it, "Locals overindulge in saturated fats, cholesterol and refined carbohydrates." This overindulgence is tied to a sense of luxury. A general practitioner at a public clinic explained, "There is an idea that Trinidad lives with a lavish lifestyle. People are not satisfied with the necessities, they always want a little extra. The patient knows what to eat." The more authoritarian medical culture of Trinidad makes for a disciplinary tone to such remarks. These desires run amok are associated with America. A public health official in Trinidad told me, "Since the oil boom people have more affluence, people stop working, and the Kentucky [Fried Chicken], the fast foods, are always full. One in eight people is overweight in Trinidad because . . . they have money so they acquire American tastes, the hamburgers, the hot dogs." And a newspaper editorial read, "Four million Americans are reported to be morbidly obese. In light of the popular culture of 'supersized meals' and 'dollar menus' in the US, this may not be surprising." At a seminar on the metabolic syndrome, a doctor simply told the audience: "Trinis eat too much! [to which nurses and pharmacists attending answered "Yes"]. We are becoming more Americanized."

But whether the obese person is a hedonist or a collection of unwanted but compulsive appetites, the answer is more biomedical asceticism, a work on the self through the discipline of taking in expertise. Biomedicine is often seen as having removed the interiorized subject. The patient of biomedicine is considered a biological object, a body, a set of neurological chemicals, or an otherwise unknowing individual. Accordingly, the discourse of "compliance" attempts to replace discernment of a patient's wants and needs with a pragmatics of getting the patient to act in healthy ways. But this pragmatism masks that in the biomedicine of compliance, an interiorized subject is read into the acts and motives of the patient. Asceticism runs throughout the notion of compliance in biomedicine: the daily betterment of the self is each individual's calling, a coming together of *I must* and *I desire*; the patient must not only continually learn, he must *want to* learn. Knowing oneself biomedically—the health risks, the treatments, the proper course of action—is posited as available to anyone, and so becomes a labor expected of everyone. This new science of compliance contains critique: social and institutional forms are analyzed for their harmful effects, but this critique must be registered in terms of health and so remains an intimate expertise. The objects of social critique from the 1960s and 1970s are here turned into medical maladies: plastics in bottles, pollution, smoking, alcohol, fat, processed foods, video games, television—today are all pathologized as sickening as they retard mental and physical growth. In the 1970s' social critique, television was the "idiot box," purveyor of propaganda, helping the machinery to operate; today, TV reduces attention spans, causes obesity, makes children apathetic. With germs, vaccines, violent entertainment, fast foods, plastics, noise, and stress, we have an array of "environmental toxins" that the subject must learn to identify and avoid. This is accomplished by coming to recognize their medical import. And the results will be emancipatory as noncompliance becomes a public health issue and intervention is oriented around changing patients' behaviors in an emphasis increasingly called "patient empowerment." This focus on patient autonomy draws on the social movement to give patients more agency that came out of the 1960s and 1970s. Today this notion of agency is used to fashion a patient as self-advocate.[5] Failure to do so, to *be* so, is a failure of discipline. The noncompliant subject, which includes almost everyone in the case of "lifestyle" diseases such as obesity, is thereby made into a kind of complicit sufferer.

This ascetic subject of compliance is a different figure from that in other, competing approaches to public health. During the summer of 2008,

Trinidad newspapers reported on a debate occurring in their parliament about the role of Cubans in Trinidad's medical system. Several Cuban doctors and nurses worked in the country's hospitals, clinics, dispensaries, and other public medical facilities, as part of the Cuban government's policy of sending medical practitioners as trainees/aides to poor countries in the Americas, parts of Africa, and elsewhere. The political debate was about whether these doctors and nurses were helping Trinidadians or taking jobs away from them. During this much-publicized discussion, I talked with a Cuban nurse who was living in Trinidad for two years as part of her training, working in a government-run hospital. She contrasted medical care in Trinidad with the well-known Cuban public health approach, in particular with the Cuban policy of having a designated doctor for each neighborhood. Like many others, she extolled the Cuban system's success in dramatically reducing or eradicating sexually transmitted diseases and other common conditions through the minute attentions of the state's neighborhood doctor. The doctor in her account was an intimate state presence, coming around to each household periodically, recording health information about each family member, knowing who the daughter was dating and what illnesses ran in the family. This public health model reveals by contrast the peculiar features of the biomedical public health figure. Like biomedical science and practice, the Cuban health care system in the nurse's account—with its doctor who amasses information about every facet of health in the home in his or her jurisdiction—might be called a biopolitics: a system of measuring social, psychological, and personal practices around something called life (that is, an amalgam of health, reproduction, longevity, and labor as physical productivity). But the Cuban doctor's knowing each citizen in his neighborhood is a recording of this information to be passed along to the state, which modifies itself in response to the cultural, the social, and the psychological habits of its citizenry/patients. In American and Caribbean biomedicine, by contrast, the site of modification is the citizenry—biomedicine only provides an expertise that enables the citizen as potential patient to become biomedical by taking in this expertise, to modify his or her cultural, social, and psychological proclivities.

This, then, is a call for the power of biomedical discipline. One public health coordinator in Trinidad told me, "We try to teach discipline to people who are very delinquent. We have too many new people with diabetes."

The obese and the asthmatic must learn to improve the self by internalizing another's expertise. As Foucault writes, "'Know thyself'" has obscured 'Take care of yourself' because our morality, a morality of asceticism, insists that the self is that which one can reject" (Foucault 1994a:228). Here the desires, cultural attitudes, and familial traditions create a self that can be denied through the rigorous internalizing of knowledge. This biomedicine of compliance is intimate without familiarity—the patient must conform his innermost desires and convictions to the knowledge furnished by medical expertise. In biomedicine the injunction is not to surrender to some authority, but to come to see the value *to the self* of being compliant. This injunction takes the form of knowing yourself biomedically. And today, another name for knowledge is "information."

Measuring Compliance

Compliance as a public health issue is intimately tied to the valorization of information, which is a crucial means to overcoming deleterious cultural traditions, family habits, or beliefs. This information is an eclectic collection—diagnoses, data about health risks, and precise prognoses of a given disease (and not, for instance, the historical excesses of biomedicine or the painful results of attempts at rational social control, or whatever we call what is learned from personal experience). The act of attaining health information, of being open to and wanting more of it, is the making of a subjectivity of compliance. Medical researchers routinely argue that patients are not objective about their health risks, and, as Stanley Cavell notes, "objectivity is a spiritual achievement" (Cavell 1979:98). In Barbados, as in the United States, poorer communities use the emergency room for primary care. Medical caregivers in Barbados contrast this posited excess use by patients of state facilities such as the public hospital against the responsible consumption of medical resources, in which a disciplined practice toward medicine is achieved. The figure of the asthmatic takes on an economic meaning as the toll of noncompliance is discussed in economic terms. In Ministry of Health policy reports experts estimate the cost of asthma to the Barbadian economy. In interviews, government officials talked with me about the loss of workdays caused by asthmatic patients' improper use of their medication. And government medical practitioners talked about the state burden created by parents not adequately controlling their children's asthma with preventer inhalers. In these state rhetorics, the patient is an individual deemed politically and morally responsible for consuming medications appropriately so as to alleviate the financial burdens of the state. Diabetes is similarly talked about as taking a toll on the state through medical costs. Excessive eating and drinking, oversized food portions, and not taking care of one's health are considered to be a drain on the state's (and therefore citizens') resources in the Caribbean. Public clinic practitioners spoke often with frustration about patients returning to the chronic disease clinics in Trinidad each week while continuing to eat poorly, drink alcohol, and not take their insulin. The cost to Trinidad's public healthcare system was considered unsustainable. Compliance here becomes a moral duty: not eating to excess, not drinking to excess, and faithfully taking one's medications is a responsibility to oneself, to one's children, and to the nation.

This knowing and caring for the self by taking in expertise relies on precise diagnostics. The ministries of health in Barbados and in Trinidad and Tobago (like American public health programs) push for more extensive testing, for weighing people and taking blood glucose readings in schools and in work environments. As one official in Trinidad told me, simply, "We do a lot of blood testing here in Trinidad. *A lot* of blood testing." Such measurements reveal the patient's concordance with biomedical norms underneath their words. A diabetes expert, in an interview with a local newspaper, explained, "Too many people believe that they have the natural ability to manage their weight without resorting to expert assistance." She made the case that obesity was *caused* by "resisting helpful information," with life-threatening consequences. Diagnostics are medical information that will help patients know themselves, and so know how to act: the patient must learn to listen to the expert, but also to the blood and lung measurements that can stand in as proxies for this authority. As a Trinidadian official told me, "We are asking them to do their own blood sugar levels. We talk about patient empowerment. They need to know their medication, their A1Cs, their bp [blood pressure]." Glucose and blood pressure levels allow the patient to know himself anew with regard to his self-destructive tendencies. A Trinidadian researcher of diabetes and heart disease explained to a group of nurses and pharmacists, "Go to the mall and watch. You will see a family eating together, mother, dad, sister, brother—all overweight. You lose the perception of what a normal portion is. We think we should have our children fat and plump. A lot of people are not doing tests at home. . . . Lots of patients have the strips, have the meters, they're not doing it."

Expanding Diagnostics

This increasing emphasis on diagnostic techniques for noncommunicable diseases allows the designation of the "predisposition" of those who are "potentially ill." In the case of diabetes, there is the "prediabetic," an individual with high blood sugar levels (but not high enough to be diagnosed with diabetes [Greene 2008]). In the United States—as in Trinidad and Barbados—the diagnosis "prediabetic" is increasingly used to indicate individuals who are expected to become diabetic, whether because of diet, family history, or predisposition. The diagnosis of asthma has undergone a similar expansion. In Barbados, a diathesis has been created of a "potential asthmatic": a child diagnosed with asthma without ever having had an attack (Whitmarsh 2008b). In both potential asthma and prediabetes, the diagnostics are considered crucial to public health because they reveal that the sickness resides as potential in so many, that even the healthy are in some sense ill. As in American biomedicine around obesity, there is a sense in Trinidad that the obese fail to see themselves medically. To quote a local news column: "A substantial number of people in Trinidad are obese, but don't perceive themselves in that manner. They use words like—thick, well-rounded, meaty and full-figured when describing their own physiques." Diagnosing overweight and prediabetes allows their vision to be corrected. They are not the "well"; they are the not-yet-ill.

This extension of diagnostic categories is linked to what Biehl calls pharmaceuticalization (Biehl 2004; see also Whyte, van der Geest, and Hardon 2002; Dumit and Greenslit 2006; Petryna, Lakoff, and Kleinman 2006; Nguyen 2010). The potential asthmatic in Barbados emerges out of a confluence of attention given to the American genetic research occurring there with the integration of the pharmaceutical industry into public healthcare, as I have argued elsewhere (Whitmarsh 2008a). In public and private practice, multiple diagnostic criteria are used, with each deemed independently sufficient to diagnose and warrant treatment for asthma.

As a result, in addition to the many potential asthmatics I met, I came across several asthmatics who were being prescribed multiple preventive inhalers and several oral medications for their condition. This has led to widely voiced criticism among families of asthmatics of the government's focus on patent pharmaceuticals as the solution to the public health crisis of asthma. In the case of Trinidad, where patent pharmaceuticals are not the center of the national formulary, pharmaceuticalization is less centralized. But a similar orientation exists around the need to medicate those who are potentially ill. As one doctor who is involved in government interventions on diabetes explained:

> We no longer say six months of lifestyle, then medication. There has been a paradigm shift. The longer you keep blood sugars high, and cholesterol high, it not only damages the eyes, the kidney. . . . So the quicker we bring down blood glucose, the better. That is why we are going to dual or combination therapy. . . . Personally I think the ADA's level [American Diabetes Association's cut-off levels for diagnosing diabetes] is too high. We are trying here to simplify for patients. If a patient has to take the medication four times a day, it's much less likely, especially here in Trinidad. I don't know what it's like in the US, but here, it's much less likely they will take it.

Like combination inhalers, combination diabetic medications are made part of public health care as an intervention on compliance. This focus on medication carries the public health necessity of diagnosing the pre-ill.

Public Health Predisposition

The concept of the pre-ill today connotes a predisposition toward a particular condition. This predisposition is increasingly cast as biological. And here the emphasis on extending compliance intersects with the notion of genetics.

The shift toward biomedical science within the field of public health includes a call to integrate genetics, the cutting edge of biomedical research. In the United States, there is an increasing discourse calling for the inclusion of medical genetics into public health interventions. Muin Khoury of the Centers for Disease Control and Prevention has been a particularly strong herald. He writes:

With the increasing discovery of genes for [single gene disorders] the number of genetic tests (molecular, biochemical, physiological, and other) will rise, thereby challenging the delivery of quality genetic testing and counseling services. These challenges have called for public health action to develop partnerships with the provider and laboratory communities. They also have motivated academic and government groups to develop guidelines for integrating genetic services into routine healthcare and public health programs. (Khoury 2003:263)

Francis Collins, director of the National Institutes of Health, also stresses the forthcoming importance of genomics to the population's health: "The implications [of genomic research] for diagnostics, preventive medicine, and therapeutics will be profound" (Collins and McKusick 2001:540). Others echo this optimism: "Public health approaches will need to adapt to meet new challenges so that applications of genomics to a broad range of human diseases can become a reality" (Rasmussen and Moore 2004). This public health genetics relies on the promise of a future of genomics: Collins, Khoury, and others refer to the pending availability of genetic tests for common disease susceptibility and the rapidly lowering costs of conducting such tests (Collins and McKusick 2001). Such advocacy for genetics in public health depends on the historically twofold meaning of public health in the United States as both intervention and information gathering. Until particular genetic techniques that affect disease processes materialize, surveillance and monitoring are touted as genetic technologies that are likely to have an impact on public health. Rasmussen and Moore build on early public health approaches to birth defects to produce a "model infrastructure" for monitoring diseases by creating "genetic disease-specific clinical databases" (2004). Surveillance in the form of an increased awareness of genetic propensities and allele frequencies becomes a "public health service" in such accounts (Grosse et al. 2006). The search for genetic predispositions for common diseases is part of the quest for personalized medicine. As one American obesity researcher explained, "We want to relate these [diabetes] changes to SNPs identified as risk alleles in the genome-wide association studies of diseases. And then use this information to create personalized dietary recommendations and drugs and so forth." In the absence of any current application of genomics research to the treatment of diabetes or asthma, what the science promises to contribute to the lifestyle diseases is a better understanding of who the patient is. Research aims to determine the biological predisposition or the neurochemical imbalance that causes the patient to be asthmatic, or to overeat, or to be addicted. The science becomes another tool to help the sufferer of a lifestyle disease to know himself or herself.

The emphasis on genomics as the medicine of tomorrow has given rise to a kind of research as global health intervention. Increasingly, national governments try to join in on cutting-edge biomedicine as a way to intervene in the health of their populations (e.g., Canada's health genome project [Hinterberger 2010], and Estonia and Iceland's national genomic databases [Fortun 2008; Pálsson and Rabinow 1999]). These governments place their citizenry at the center of large-scale genomics ventures. In Barbados, the government poses the population as biologically black in the interests of attracting international genetics research, reflecting on the nation's vulnerable position in the global economy and its desire to access cutting-edge biomedicine. As the minister of health put it, "The possibilities are limitless. . . . We must not be left behind." As genetic analysis makes use of national databases of biomedical records and biological samples, governments position their participation in genome projects as a public health program, improving the lives of their populations. Such a search for genetic predispositions as a health act changes public medicine in ways often hidden by a bioethics focus on informed consent and privacy. In the Caribbean, these shifts include a biologization of more than the etiology of disease.

Chronic Racial Dispositions

Race is the reason for the extensive international genetics research that takes place in the Caribbean. Populations in the area are targeted as either Afro-Caribbean or Indo-Caribbean (depending on the region) in genetics projects that search for race-specific causes of disease (Whitmarsh 2009a). This research fits with the broader and growing body of research that attempts to link racial disparities in the prevalence and severity of common diseases (e.g., cancer, heart disease, asthma) with genetic propensities.[6]

These projects posit racially specific genetic predispositions that come to fruition in particular environments. In American genetic studies on asthma conducted in Barbados, genetic predispositions are considered to interact with an environment that includes the dust from roadwork, pollution, housing demographics, and living arrangements, which are translated by the research into IgE levels or the presence of gram-negative bacteria. In the case of obesity and diabetes, this emphasis on environment is replaced by excess behaviors, which interact with genetic predispositions considered specific to particular racial and ethnic communities. Diabetes is considered to be caused by a kind of "ethnic pathology"—an amalgam of the cultural, psychological, and biological. As with all chronic diseases, particular ethnic groups are considered susceptible (particularly Hispanic women, women of African descent, and South Asians).

Again, biomedical science here rejects the individual figure as the basis for ethics and governance. The genetics of race and disease is intended by researchers to remove moral stigma, recognizing that obesity or diabetes or asthma or heart disease are not the fault of the communities that suffer from them. The turn to biological predisposition is a banishment of the moralizing language that blames the individual for his or her excesses. What takes the place of this liberal subject is an internally flawed group. The attempt to explain racial disparities in health with genetics is a biological predisposition posited retroactively.

In the Caribbean, this constitutes a new approach to global health. As I have argued elsewhere, the wealth of international research projects on the genetics of race and disease in Barbados is changing medical care (Whitmarsh 2009a). Genetics is associated with the forefront of biomedicine and considered centrally involved in asthma, giving shape to environmental and other explanations without providing a precise etiology for Barbadian medical practitioners. The extraordinary precision that genotyping technologies promise in describing race and disease are valued for increasing "objectivity," even as their authority is undermined for being arcane and inconsequential to the realities of Bajan health. The future of public health genetics is denigrated while at the same time new medical interpretations of illness etiologies are created around the hyperspecificity of technologies of race and disease. Such an integration of genetics with medical care and public health occurs around the new category of the "metabolic syndrome."

The designation "syndrome" in biomedicine denotes a kind of intentional categorical ambiguity. Syndrome is another way of saying symptom ambiguity, a moment where medicine appears to return to its preclinical gaze, to the disease as a collection of symptoms, not having a fixed origin (Foucault 1994a). But what makes this current use so radically different from the preclinical period is the felt lack. The fixed point of origin of the disease isn't just absent—it's missing. This is what the term "syndrome" draws attention to, in contrast to "disease": syndrome points to a lack in biomedicine, which then allows for multiplicity. The metabolic syndrome is one such moniker, a collection of medical characteristics that are thought to be risk factors for diabetes and heart disease: high body fat, high blood pressure, insulin resistance, high triglycerides, and too much bad cholesterol in proportion to good cholesterol. A diagnosis of metabolic syndrome relies on cutoff measurements of these characteristics. The cutoff points for the syndrome are lower than those needed to make a diagnosis of each condition separately, the idea being that if one has a given blood pressure, or cholesterol level, or blood glucose level alone, there is little cause for concern, but taken together they comprise a syndrome, a predisposition for heart disease. There is controversy around each component of this diagnosis: how to take these measurements, what numbers to use as cutoff points, and which ones together comprise the syndrome. This contestation makes the metabolic syndrome a controversial category, even within the biomedical world: critics, including the highly influential American Diabetes Association, have questioned the definition and utility of the condition, and have called for further research before the diagnosis enters clinical use, a position that placed them in opposition to the American Heart Association and the National Heart, Lung, and Blood Institute. In the meantime, the metabolic syndrome is increasingly used internationally in medical research, diagnostics, and care.

Over the last fifteen years, the metabolic syndrome has taken shape as an object of clinical, pharmaceutical, and research practice. The condition is considered to have reached epidemic levels, and funding, research, and clinical use have increased dramatically. Dietary and exercise regimens are recommended, alongside the use of pharmaceuticals, including antihypertensives, ACE inhibitors, and therapeutics for diabetes. Differentiation by ethnicity is increasingly used in research and is already common in medical practice: Hispanic women and African-American women are particularly targeted as at-risk populations. In Trinidad the metabolic syndrome is being taken up in public medical clinics to intervene on heart disease. As a doctor at a government clinic explained to me, "Metabolic syndrome, if we see one of diabetes, hypertension, cholesterol, we diagnose one, we diagnose it." This allows for an expansive diagnostic, as is the case with potential asthma in Barbados. Particular ethnic groups are considered especially susceptible to the predisposition. Public and private doctors talk about the biological and cultural proclivities toward hypertension and obesity among Afro-Trinidadians, or diabetes among Indo-Trinidadians. The metabolic syndrome category itself becomes a way to diagnose a tendency toward the condition without requiring precise measurements. As one Trinidad doctor in a public clinic explained to me, "Doctors will actually refer patients, and on the record it will say metabolic syndrome. We will get referrals for *family members*." This diagnosis of a familial tendency turns ethnic histories and traditions into biological predispositions. As genomics is increasingly used to understand common diseases, the biological, the psychological, the social, and the cultural become intertwined with little reason to disentangle them. Chronic and common diseases—diabetes, heart disease, asthma—become vaguely associated with a diathesis that blurs cultural, biological, and personal habits.

Such a predisposition is like a fate found after it comes true, only legible in the unlikely events that brought it to fruition, yet somehow always there already. In Barbados, this constitutes an intervention on that disease of modernity, asthma, that reconfigures the illness as a biological racial predisposition brought about in the tropical home that can only be grasped through genotyping technologies. In Trinidad and Tobago, a conceived diathesis toward diabetes biologizes cultural, psychological, and personal histories. The result is that medical care and public health interventions are transformed. The public health imperative of increasing compliance turns these racial "fates" into arenas of intervention. A biomedical orientation becomes a necessity for everyone, but some are considered particularly disoriented.

Like pharmaceuticals, genetics has been a focal point of social critique in the last twenty years, in a way that has perhaps reified some characteristics as supposedly intrinsic. In the biomedical logic of compliance, racial health disparities are critical, but distinguishing between the genetic predispositions and socioeconomic structures that account for them isn't.

Genetic, socioeconomic, and cultural factors can seamlessly intertwine in a predisposition to chronic diseases that requires racially specific interventions to increase compliance. An extensive amount of research and governing techniques are organized around compliance among particular races in the United States. Public health departments provide pamphlets in Spanish about unhealthy culinary traditions for Hispanic immigrants; both pharmaceutical companies and nongovernmental asthma organizations offer literatures designed to persuade African-American mothers to get their children to regularly take their preventer inhaler; and an extensive field of scientific research investigates how to encourage disadvantaged minorities to eat and drink in healthier ways. These interventions make the contemporary biomedical emphasis on the pre-ill carry race. As compliance figures a culturally, biologically, and socially particular object, governance targets particular communities.

Patient Futures

The growing emphasis on chronic diseases in global health is a focus on the future. Discussions of the various noncommunicable disease epidemics extrapolate decades ahead, where modernization is leading countries. Poorer countries are cast as tardy versions of the G8 countries, where chronic disease rates exceed those of infectious disease. And just as diseases are projected forward, so is intervention: the increasing speed and scale of genomic science, the expansion of disease identification, and research on gene-environment interactions is expected to shift our approaches to common diseases. As a result, taking part in global biomedical research becomes a form of public health intervention. Amid this talk about the future, changes are occurring in the meaning of public health. As genetic diagnostics are configured as a social good, health "information" is valorized, and compliance to biomedical norms becomes paramount. An ethical imperative is created: individuals must fashion themselves into people who collect information, conduct proper risk analysis, follow prescriptions, and adequately test and measure themselves.

Medical cultures in Trinidad, Barbados, and the United States differ by traditional bioethical measures: practitioners in Trinidad in particular traditionally tend toward an authoritarian paternalism toward patients, and consequently toward more explicit judgments of patients' health and medical choices. In the United States, by contrast, social movements have given rise to "patient advocacy," a turning away from blaming the ill for their conditions and toward a more sympathetic medicine. The search for genetic predispositions and for the causes of noncompliance is a search for a more personal medicine, one that will account for the mix of genetics and social factors that make this particular subject ill. As is common in American ideals, this pragmatism is paradoxically populist: biomedical personalization is a route to a more just medicine. On the way to a future of personalized medicine, genomics increasingly uses race. This constitutes a rejection of the individualized liberal subject of free choice held accountable for his or her illness. But as in other structuralist relations, renunciation can bring the object of renunciation ever closer. The attempt to banish moral judgment by finding biological predispositions for lifestyle conditions can create a fixed, distancing fate that precludes the radically relational uses of "race."

Similarly, an emphasis on "patient empowerment" can produce a subject with the ethical obligation to know and so to care for himself or herself through biomedical logics. Public health programs and discourses about chronic diseases increasingly rely on this ethical injunction to fashion the self through biomedical knowledge and information. As global health takes up chronic diseases, this figure becomes international, while simultaneously biological predispositions and expanding diagnostics extend the communities considered already ill. These predispositions and proclivities bring race, ethnicity, and culture into the crisis of "compliance." An expertise of cultural and social mores and traditions thereby becomes necessary to any techniques of making a public healthier. In the United States, this makes for pamphlets and educational outreach that target the dietary, aesthetic, and medical attitudes of particular communities—African Americans, Puerto Ricans and Mexicans. In the English-speaking Caribbean, this gives rise to education programs for Hindus and Afro-Caribbeans. These governing techniques target whole communities, cancelling the distinction between the ill and the healthy. The object of global health intervention on chronic diseases is everyone, each with his or her peculiar (racial, cultural, biological) subjectivity, a peculiarity to be overcome in favor of becoming a modern subject of compliance.

Notes

1. For anthropological analyses of access to pharmaceuticals as a peculiar form of governance, see Biehl 2004; Ecks 2005.

2. For interpretations of the contemporary emphasis on biomedical compliance, see Kaljee and Beardsley 1992; Ferzacca 2000; and Maskovsky 2005. For anthropological troubling of a notion of irrational compliance, see Veena Das and Ranendra Das 2006; Trostle 1996; Kamat and Nichter 1998; Nancy Scheper-Hughes 1992.

3. "Addiction" is another chronic disease that is fraught with unexpected and contradictory meanings, a subject that several anthropologists have been exploring. For excellent examples, see Garcia 2008; Raikhel 2010; Schull 2006.

4. These pharmaceuticals carry a sense of biomedical expertise, along with other things, all multivalently interpreted as the medicines travel (Whyte, van der Geest, and Hardon 2002).

5. For example, in the conference in Barbados to launch one of the combination inhalers, the literature given to us at each table referred to the new easier-to-use formulation as "empowering the patient."

6. For anthropological and sociological critiques of this field, see Braun et al. 2007; Duster 2005; Fullwiley 2007; Jones and Perlis 2006; Kahn 2004; Kaufman and Hall 2003; Koenig, Lee, and Richardson 2008; Montoya 2007 and 2011; Shields et al. 2005.

12

Legal Remedies

Therapeutic Markets and the Judicialization of the Right to Health

JOÃO BIEHL AND ADRIANA PETRYNA

> Justice does not exist! Human Rights do not exist. What
> matters is jurisprudence. This is the invention of Law. . . .
> The challenge is to create and not to make Human Rights
> applicable. It is a matter of inventing jurisprudences so that,
> for each case, such and such thing could not have been
> possible. . . . Many times, life can be seen case by case. . . .
> It is not a matter of right of this or of that, but of situations that
> evolve . . . to struggle for jurisprudence . . . to create the right.
>
> —*Gilles Deleuze*[1]

Entering Justice, One by One

Seven children lie in a hospital room, each hooked up to an intravenous drip.[2] Their parents stand near them, bantering with each other and with the doctors who circulate in and out. Every week these parents bring their young children, who suffer from a disorder called mucopolysaccharidosis (MPS) here, to the Research Unit of Hospital Universitário, a public teaching hospital in Porto Alegre, the capital of the southern state of Rio

Grande do Sul, Brazil.[3] The children are receiving enzyme replacement therapy (ERT), which can cost up to US$200,000 dollars per year per patient.[4]

MPS encompasses a group of inherited metabolic disorders in which mucopolysaccharide, a complex carbohydrate, builds up in body tissues in a dangerously nonmetabolized form due to the lack of activity of a specific enzyme (Beck 2007). MPS disorders affect approximately 1 in 25,000 individuals (Clarke 2008) and usually manifest in early childhood. They are characterized by skeletal and joint deformities, stunted growth, and facial changes caused by accumulation of mucopolysaccharide in the underlying facial bone. MPS leads to neurological, cardiovascular, and respiratory impairments, as well as liver and spleen enlargement and hearing loss. Severe cases are fatal in the first decade of life and milder cases may entail a normal lifespan but have significant disease morbidity (Clarke 2007). MPS disorders are not curable, but ERTs have proven useful in reducing some of their symptoms, improving quality of life, and, in certain cases, increasing lifespan.

All the children with MPS in this room are patient-litigants. Their parents are suing the government so that they can receive treatment for life. Between 2008 and 2011, we spoke to multiple actors involved in this new and increasingly ubiquitous practice of litigation against the state for treatment access, a phenomenon known as the "judicialization of the right to health." Though patients are suing all levels of government for everything from baby formula to complex surgeries, a large portion of lawsuits are for medicines.

Brazil is among the approximately one hundred countries that recognize a constitutional right to health (Gauri and Brinks 2008:1). An important part of this right is access to medicines. Although Brazil has one of the world's most advanced HIV/AIDS treatment programs, many of its citizens still go to local pharmacies only to find that essential medicines are not available. With a population of almost 200 million and an economy on the rise, Brazil is one of the fastest growing pharmaceutical markets in the world today. Doctors increasingly prescribe and patients demand new medical technologies.

The US Food and Drug Administration (FDA) and the Brazilian National Health Surveillance Agency (ANVISA) have approved some MPS treatments; others are still in clinical trials.[5] Biotechnology companies are entering the field of orphan disease treatments, breaking new ground beyond the blockbuster model of drug development (Petryna 2009).[6]

Doctors at Hospital Universitário were excited about the possibility of finally offering patients something more than just an accurate diagnosis of their genetic ailment. But they were also cautious about hyped claims of efficacy. "It is a new world," said Dr. Maria, who monitors these children. "I think we are bringing new things from genetics to SUS [Brazil's Unified Health System]. Some here were in clinical trials, but all are SUS patients now. To guarantee treatment access and to follow up on the effectiveness is very problematic." The interests of clinical research, public health, and biomedical markets fold into the injured bodies of these young patient-citizen-litigants.

The children here come from low- and middle-income families that would never have been able to afford these genetic therapies on their own. They obtain them as a result of lawsuits their parents have filed against the state of Rio Grande do Sul in the name of the right to health. Article 196 of the 1988 democratic constitution affirms health as a right of the people and a duty of the state, "guaranteed by social and economic policies that reduce the risk of disease and other adversities and by universal and equal access to actions and services" (Constituição Federal do Brasil). The parents told us that, in order to make the claim, they must have a diagnosis and medical documents proving the benefits of the costly treatment. In most cases, district judges immediately issue injunctions that force the state to provide the treatment for a month or two. A final ruling by the higher courts might take several years as state prosecutors file multiple appeals, expert-committees review medical evidence, and the case might find its circuitous way to the country's Supreme Court in Brasília, the country's capital.

Only one of the seven children has some of her infusions paid for by the drug manufacturer. Rita, who is twelve years old and "in a near-vegetative state" (according to her mother Ilse), took part in the first clinical trial that led to drug approval in Brazil. In 2004, after the trial ended and the trial sponsor stopped providing the enzyme on a compassionate-use basis, Rita became one of the first MPS patient-litigants in the state. She won an initial court injunction that had to be periodically renewed, since state prosecutors were appealing the ruling. A physician told us that, in the meantime, the manufacturer had agreed to share the cost of Rita's treatment with the state, most likely to avoid becoming a defendant in the higher court. For all of these children, the uncertain and potentially fatal natural history of their disease now meshes with hope-inspiring, cutting-edge genetic therapies and a time-consuming juridical quest. The critical question of who will pay for the therapy—the family, the government, or the manufacturer—is bound to the emerging field of jurisprudence over the right to treatment.

The three-hour infusion time is over and the children are awake, talking and playing—all except Rita. Ilse caresses her daughter's face. Like all the MPS children in the room, Rita's stature is short and her head is enlarged. Her facial features are coarse and her skeleton slightly deformed. Her mental development "was delayed," Ilse states. A red folder containing the latest medical records and court rulings lies at Rita's feet. "After the study ended, we contacted a private lawyer, Mr. Moura, and we filed a lawsuit against the state to get the enzyme. Other parents followed suit," Ilse states. "Rita is a citizen. Here in Brazil, she has the right to health." Ilse, like the other parents in the infusion room, uses the expression *entrar na justiça* "to enter the judiciary" (or literally, "to enter justice") to refer to their lawsuits.

All over Brazil, patients are turning to courts to access prescribed medicines (Azevedo 2007; Colluci 2009). Although lawsuits secure access for thousands of people, at least temporarily, this judicialization of the right to health generates intensely complex sociomedical realities (as embodied by the MPS families) and significant administrative and fiscal challenges which, officials argue, have the potential to widen inequalities in health care delivery (Ferraz 2009). In this chapter, we explore how right-to-health litigation became (in the wake of a successful universal AIDS treatment policy) an alternative route for Brazilians to access health care, now understood as access to medicines that are either on governmental formularies or are only available through the market. Is the judicial system an effective venue in which to implement socioeconomic rights? Which practices of citizenship and governance are crystallized in these struggles over drug access and administrative accountability?

Government-purchased medicines make up a formidable market in Brazil and, as we will show, treatment litigation takes place in the context of a dysfunctional decentralized public health system. The role of market forces in judicialization—a mix of pharmaceutical marketing strategies targeting physicians' prescriptions and fueling patient demand, as well as limited regulatory oversight—must not be overlooked, either. But a key point here is that low-income patients are not just waiting for new and high-cost medical technologies to "trickle down": they are using public legal assistance and the levers of a responsive judiciary to gain full access now.

The twin phenomena of the *pharmaceuticalization* of health care and the *judicialization* of socioeconomic rights raise crucial issues that are at the heart of global health debates today: technology access and care delivery, the financing and sustainability of treatment programs, the strengthening of health systems, and the improvement of outcomes. We need a deeper understanding of the political economy of pharmaceuticals that informs large-scale treatment initiatives, and we need to know how information, science, and technology impact health systems and life projects on the ground.

Pharmaceuticalization and Judicialization

Brazil's adoption of a constitutional right to health in 1988 was accompanied by the creation of the Sistema Único de Saúde (SUS), extending health coverage to all citizens. To improve the management of the public health care system, the Ministry of Health divided responsibilities for pharmaceutical distribution among three levels of government as part of a broader process of decentralization. While the federal government retained some of its central role in financing public health (administering some high-priority disease programs that required high-cost treatments), state and municipal health secretariats had to develop new structures to assess health needs and to administer federal and local funds for drug provision. Through this infrastructure, citizens are guaranteed access to medicines specified on formularies drafted by government administrators.[7] These actions delegated responsibility, but they did not ensure sustainable funding and technical capacity at local levels. Medications are frequently out of stock and lists of newer, high-cost medicines are infrequently updated (Campos 2007; Homedes and Ugalde 2005). A private health care system exists as well but does not cover medicines, and many health providers participate in both systems.

AIDS activists were among the first to successfully equate the constitutional right to health with access to pharmaceuticals (Scheffer, Salazar, and Grou 2005). And in 1996, at a time when global responses to HIV/ AIDS were largely prevention-based, Brazil became the first developing country to sign into law and enact a policy of free and universal distribution of antiretroviral drugs (ARVs). In the years that followed, Brazil has seen unprecedented alliances among activists, government reformers, multilateral agencies, and the pharmaceutical industry, and it asserted itself as a leader in the global push to universalize access to AIDS treatment. An incremental change in the concept of public health materialized through the AIDS policy (Berkman et al. 2005; Galvão 2002; Okie 2006; Parker 2009; Scheffer, Salazar, and Grou 2005). In terms of both delivery and demand, public health is now understood less as prevention and primary care and more as access to medicines and community-outsourced care—that is, public health has become increasingly pharmaceuticalized and privatized (Biehl 2007).

Treatment access is a central tenet of global health activism and interventions today (Adams, Novotny, and Leslie 2008; Brown, Cueto, and Fee 2006). Public-private health initiatives are booming and drug companies are rebranding themselves as global health companies, making older treatments more widely available and expediting access to newer ones. Some critics contend that public-private treatment partnerships can be used by corporations as a good public relations move, offsetting public scrutiny of the pharmaceutical industry's political influence and the opaqueness of its drug-pricing practices (Applbaum 2010; Samsky 2011). Companies can, of course, also use such partnerships to gain footholds in developing country markets, to influence national drug policies, and to improve drug distribution networks.

Such is the case of Brazil. From a market perspective, it is once again the country of the future. The federal government has successfully juggled demands for market openness *and* poverty reduction: it has strategically withdrawn from strict market regulation, and while championing much-needed social policies, it has consolidated itself as a strong state, way beyond a minimally involved neoliberal one. In 2009, Brazil's GDP was US$1.796 trillion, and its GDP per capita was, US$10,427, ranking 103rd in the world (World Bank 2009). In 2004, about 20 percent of the population lived below the poverty line, a number that had fallen to 7 percent by 2009. Brazil's income inequality (as measured by the Gini coefficient) is one of the highest in the world, but according to the World Bank, it has been falling due to "low inflation, consistent economic growth, well-focused social programs, and a policy of real increases for the minimum wage" (World Bank 2009).

Today, a variety of actors—patient associations, industry advocates, and public health physicians—have vested interests in making high-technology medicine accessible to all. In the process, the country is becoming a profitable platform for global medicine. About half of the adult population takes medicines on a daily basis (Carvalho 2005). And this is where the state comes into the picture: pharmaceutical access.

In a conversation about unequal drug pricing worldwide, a pharmaceutical executive suggested that his company was adapting to the human rights and social justice frameworks that had successfully politicized access to treatments and health care in the recent past. Referring, for example, to the ongoing struggle over continued access to state-of-the-art antiretroviral therapies in Brazil, he said rather bluntly that his company had co-opted the activist role. To make government act properly, he suggested, "You don't need the activists, just buy our drugs and you will save money." Yet, we know that drug prices in Brazil are 1.9 times higher than in Sweden and 13.1 times higher than the world index (Nóbrega et al. 2007).

Brazil is now experiencing the types of problems and conflicts that other middle- and low-income countries treating AIDS are beginning to face. It has an inexpensive first line of ARVs, but a growing number of patients are starting new, more expensive drug regimens, either because of drug resistance or because newer patented drugs have fewer side effects. Between 2004 and 2005, the cost of treating a single AIDS patient rose from US$1,220 to $2,577, and the total cost of providing AIDS therapies more than doubled from 193 million to 414 million dollars (Nunn et al. 2009). In 2009, thirty-two different drugs were available in the Brazilian HIV/AIDS program: 59 percent of them (19 drugs) were imported, and their cost comprised 72 percent of the total amount spent.

State-purchased high-cost medicines now make up a formidable market in Brazil—one that has grown from US$208 million in 2004 to $377 million in 2005. In 2002, the Health Ministry spent more than US$1 billion on essential and high-cost drugs. In 2007, it spent about US$5 billion.[8] Drug expenditures grew 252 percent between 2002 and 2007 (Vieira 2009).

The rights-based model for demanding AIDS treatment access has been taken up by other patients' groups that are now also claiming the right to pharmaceuticals in courts. People of all social and economic backgrounds are mobilizing for increased and sustained access to drugs that either are covered by government programs and are not available to them, or are for specialized treatments not yet included in official formularies. (These include treatments for prevalent as well as uncommon and rare disorders, among them diabetes, bipolar disorder, asthma, hepatitis C, and such rare genetic disorders as MPS.)

Ana Márcia Messeder and her colleagues (2005) profiled this medical-judicial phenomenon in the state of Rio de Janeiro. The authors identified a total of 2,733 medicinal lawsuits filed between January 1991 and December 2002 and analyzed a representative sample of 389 of them. The majority of cases were initiated by public defenders or pro bono lawyers from nongovernmental organizations (NGOs) or universities, and only 16 percent of the lawsuits came from patients being treated outside of SUS. Until 1998, plaintiffs almost exclusively demanded medications for HIV/AIDS.

Beginning in 1999, two years into the universal AIDS treatment policy, there was significant diversification in the kinds of treatments and pathologies that were the subjects of right-to-health litigation. The diseases now included diabetes, cancer, and other conditions besides HIV/AIDS. As more and more patients adopted the rights discourse and legal practices pioneered by AIDS activists, the number of lawsuits dramatically increased. In 1995, only four such lawsuits were filed against the state of Rio de Janeiro. In 1997, this number had increased to 314, and in 2002 it was 1,144. In their study, Messeder and colleagues show that patients were "exerting greater organizational and lobbying skills to secure their rights" (2005:532), but public defenders and judges lacked clarity about the division of pharmaceutical responsibility among various administrative levels. Indeed, they were found to show "disregard for the rational use of medicines and for possible harms that come with misprescription and misuse" (2005:533).

These Brazilian patient-litigants were exhibiting knowledge and skill that their class position typically did not confer and were working within the state, challenging public health administrations to fulfill their mandates. Though the public debate over judicialization has tended to focus on demands for experimental and high-cost drugs, two important studies of right-to-health litigation (from the state of Rio de Janeiro, Pepe et al. 2010; and from the municipality of São Paulo, Vieira and Zucchi 2007) show that in the majority of cases, the drugs requested were already part of drug formularies and that about three-quarters of the off-list drugs requested had publicly available generic equivalents. This newer phenomenon—demanding access to drugs already on official formularies—could be an indicator of the failures of municipal administrations (the alleged providers) and state health secretariats (the supposed cofinancers) to fulfill their public health duties.

While claims for pharmaceutical access have migrated well beyond HIV/AIDS and right-to-health litigation has become an alternative pathway for accessing healthcare in Brazil, a ruling by the Supreme Court in 2000 concerning a patient's access to a newer antiretroviral drug still constitutes the precedent for judicial intervention in both state and federal courts. In his ruling, Justice Celso de Mello understands the AIDS pharmaceutical assistance program as the actualization of the government's constitutional duty to implement policies that secure the population's health. As the concrete embodiment of the need for "programmatic norms," the AIDS program acquires an inherent judicial value in Mello's ruling. As soon as citizens in need have medicines, the government's legal responsibility for implementing programmatic norms that secure health is fulfilled and ceases to be "an inconsequential constitutional promise." In this rendering, the immediate assurance of the right to health through pharmaceuticals circumvents questions about the limitations of policy and resources, as well as the evidentiary basis of new drugs' efficacy.

Public health actors and institutions around the globe are currently struggling with how to guarantee the human right to health and fulfill promises for increased access to treatments while contending with the perennial debates over prevention versus treatment and the limitations of delivery systems. As the judicialization of the right to health grows in volume and importance in Brazil, it signals the beginning of a new chapter in the construction and management of the country's universal health care system, as well as of the evolving pharmaceutical sector of its economy—the eighth-largest pharmaceutical market in the world (with an estimated total market value of US$30 billion in 2012 according to the Sindicato das Indústrias Farmacêuticas do Estado de São Paulo).

Brazil's response to the judicialization of the right to health is an important litmus test for other low- and middle-income countries where increased pharmaceutical access is underway.

Right-to-Health Litigation

Young Rita's legal process, like that of the other patients receiving enzyme replacement therapy at Hospital Universitário, remained unresolved. The paperwork had grown "to half a meter high," in the words of Mr. Moura, the lawyer who represented several of these families. Mr. Moura sees litigation as the only way forward, because "the state does not fulfill its role. Health is the duty of the state and the right of the patient." He insists that in almost all cases initial rulings are in favor of the patients. Genetic therapies are a new threshold in the judicialization of the right to health, he adds. Why? "Because these are medicines with a *slightly* elevated cost."

Brazilian states are seeing the number of successful lawsuits brought in their courts reaching into the tens of thousands, a process that is redefining the roles and responsibilities of the state, altering administrative practices, and encroaching upon health budgets. With a population of 11 million, the state of Rio Grande do Sul faces one of the highest numbers of health-related lawsuits in the country (Hoffmann and Bentes 2008). In 2009 alone, there were over 12,000 lawsuits in the state seeking access to medicines, a staggering increase from 1,126 in 2002. In 2008, the state spent US$30.2 million on court-mandated drugs, an expense that represented 22 percent of the state's expenditure on medicines for that year (Biehl et al. 2009).

Consider Lizete, who is suing the state for medication to treat her pulmonary hypertension. She is fifty years old and lives with her husband, a taxi-driver, in one of the shanty towns of Porto Alegre. Lizete found out she was HIV-positive in 2002. Unlike her AIDS therapies, which she receives for free at the local health post, the drug that she most urgently needs is not offered through the public system and would cost her about US$1,300 a month. On her doctor's advice, Lizete went to the public defender's office, where she qualified for free legal representation, and sued the state. She initially lost her lawsuit, but later won on appeal. Though a district judge ordered the state to begin immediate provision of the medication, when she was interviewed in August of 2009, several months had passed and Lizete had yet to receive the drug. She had hoped to get better so that she could return to work and better care for her eleven-year-old adopted son.

Past research has suggested that right-to-treatment litigation is for the most part a practice of the financially better off (Chieffi and Barata 2009; Da Silva and Terrazas 2011; Vieira and Zucchi 2007) and that low-income patients tend to sue for low-cost medicines, while higher-income patients tend to sue for very expensive medicines (Da Silva and Terrazas 2011:12). By contrast, an analysis of information we collected from 1,080 medicinal lawsuits against the state of Rio Grande do Sul[9] suggests that patients who procure treatments through the courts are mostly poor individuals who are not working and who depend on the public system for both health care and legal representation (Biehl et al. 2012). Among the plaintiffs who reported their employment status, more than half were retired and about a fifth were unemployed. Among those who reported income, over half earned less than the monthly national minimum wage (about US$300) and relied on the free legal services of public defenders.

Roughly two-thirds of the medicines requested in our database were already on drug formularies. About a quarter of lawsuits were exclusively for access to on-list, high-cost drugs, though low-cost essential medicines were frequently requested alongside other medicines. Off-list drugs requested by plaintiffs were also often low-cost and many had been available in the market for a long time. This suggests that government pharmaceutical distribution programs are failing to fulfill their role of expanding access and rationalizing use (DECIT 2006; Guimarães 2004).

Moreover, judges at district and higher court levels almost universally grant access to all medicines requested, recognizing that their provision is consistent with Brazil's constitutional right to health. For example, in almost all of the 1,080 lawsuits examined, district judges granted plaintiffs an immediate injunction for access to medicines; in cases where the initial ruling was in favor of the provision of medicines, the state's higher court upheld the decision most of the time.

According to legal scholar David Fidler, developments in health jurisprudence "have produced open-source anarchy and a more elastic relationship between power and ideas in global politics." In such an elastic relationship, "changes in material capabilities of state and non-state actors, and changes in the world of ideas, have more impact on each other than in the closed, state-centric system that prevailed during the Cold War" (Fidler 2008:410). Fidler recognizes a "deeper importance for law in public health endeavors within and between countries" (Fidler 2008:394; see also Fidler 2007).

Anthropologists John and Jean Comaroff have been attending to such a "judicialization of politics" in post-apartheid South Africa and how it has affected social mobilization, particularly in the field of HIV/AIDS. Class struggles, they argue, "seem to have metamorphosed into class actions. Citizens, subjects, governments, and corporations litigate against one another, often at the intersection of tort law, human rights law, and the criminal law, in an ever mutating kaleidoscope of coalitions and cleavages" (Comaroff and Comaroff 2006:26; see also Vianna and Burgos 2005; Yamin and Parra-Vera 2010).

Right-to-health litigation speaks to a productive "open-source anarchy" (Fidler 2008) at both macro and micro levels in Brazil as well. Interviews we conducted with judges, attorneys, and public health officials revealed divergent and conflicting views on the litigation pathway that, as we have been suggesting, has become an alternative route to health care. Many judges working on right-to-health cases feel they are responding to state failures to provide needed drugs and that these waves of lawsuits are a milestone in the democratization of a culture of rights. Whether this goal can be attained through individual claims, however, is contested. The fact is that judges employ idiosyncratic rationales and create their own standards in adjudicating right-to-health cases. They cite the "risk of death" and the "right to life" and base their rulings for the most part on jurisprudence (such as Justice Mello's, referred to earlier) and personal experiences—they cite specific tragic stories in which they think treatment provision would have made a difference.

Administrators, on the other hand, contend that the judiciary is overstepping its role and that judicialization skews budgets and increases inequalities in health care access. Some acknowledge, however, that legal pressure has improved the distribution of some drugs. In the meantime, private law offices specializing in right-to-health lawsuits, such as Mr. Moura's, have multiplied, and local public officials are capitalizing politically on such court cases, using them to gain media attention and popular support. Many patients are indeed poor and are represented in court by attorneys from the state's independent public defense office. The public defenders we interviewed see their work as a mode of guaranteeing accountability; they also seek greater visibility and political significance within state institutions for themselves. Patient associations play a highly contested role. Officials claim that at least some of them are funded by pharmaceutical companies eager to sell the government high-cost drugs whose efficacy might be questionable and widespread prescription unwarranted.

Judicialization has indeed become a parallel infrastructure in which various public and private health actors and sectors come into contact, face off, and enact one-by-one rescue missions. In April 2009, the Brazilian Supreme Court held a rare public hearing to examine the pressing challenges posed by right-to-health litigation.[10] Public health officials, lawyers, physicians, activists, and academics testified before the Court, providing varied viewpoints and recommendations on how to respond to the enormous judicial demand for medical goods. An immediate outcome was a long-overdue updating of formularies for specialized high-cost drugs. The Brazilian National Council of Justice also issued a set of recommendations for local judges, asking them to attend more carefully to scientific evidence and to strive for "more efficiency" when ruling over health-related cases.[11]

If access to AIDS therapies was the litmus test of the right to health in the 1990s, now it is access to genetic therapies. The latest right-to-health landmark ruling involved a request for a medicine to treat a genetic disease. This treatment was not recommended by the Ministry of Health's therapeutic guidelines and was not publicly available. In March 2010, the court rejected the argument that the state was not responsible and decided in favor of the provision of the high-cost therapy. In his ruling, Justice Gilmar Mendes stated that once the disease was medically confirmed and treatment was indicated, the "Ministry of Health's therapeutic guidelines can be questioned." Moreover, "the state has to provide resources, not only to support and fund the provision of universal care for its citizens, but also has to provide variable resources to attend to the needs of each individual citizen."

There is a heated debate in Brazilian courts on the positive duty the constitutional right to health imposes on the state and the extent to which the courts must enforce this right. But the country is yet to have a substantial public debate about the meaning of the right to health in light of new medical advancements. Although a "right to pharmaceuticals" is being consolidated in Brazil, the various branches of government have yet to develop robust health technology assessments. Moreover, bolder regulatory steps in drug pricing are needed, along with a reconsideration of the responsibilities of private health insurance plans in covering drug costs (which they currently do not). Attention must also be paid to broader aspects of the right to health, including structural-rights interventions and social determinants of health, such as education, water, sanitation, vector control, air pollution, and violence prevention. Meanwhile, hard-to-pin-down patient-citizen-consumers draw from human rights language and jurisprudence and make governments work for them as they negotiate the vagaries of the market and survival.

To look at the ways and means of right-to-health litigation is to enter an intensely contentious political-economic-experiential field. Here the penetration of market principles in health care delivery is unexpectedly aligned with the juridical subject of rights. The rational choice-making economic subject (necessarily a consumer of technology) is also the subject of legal rights. This dual subject position complicates Michel Foucault's concept of biopower—the way in which natural life has become an object of modern politics (1980; 2007). In judicialization we do not see a top-down biopolitical model of governance in which population well-being is the object of knowledge and control, but rather a contestation over the utility of government by multiple private and public stakeholders. There is an economic reason within governmental reason.[12] At stake here are the ways in which government (qua drug regulator, purchaser, and distributor) facilitates a more *direct* relationship of atomized subjects of rights/interests to the biomedical market in the form of technology access alongside the continual creation of commercial horizons.

Patient-Citizen-Consumer

Rita has a "severe case" of MPS, Dr. Maria tells us. "She walked until she was four," her mother Ilse adds. "She even went to nursery school, but now her whole body is damaged. The organs, liver, and spleen have enlarged, and she also has respiratory problems." Ilse insists that Rita improved while in the clinical trial, but that she also knew that the enzyme does not "stop the neurological damage." Later Dr. Maria told us that she believed that in Rita's case, the neurological damage was so far along that the enzyme would not be effective. Yet all of the parents we spoke to suggested that not obtaining this treatment (whose access they had to renew periodically in the courts) would be unconscionable or tantamount to killing their children.

Dr. Daniel Muller, who coordinates MPS trials at Hospital Universitário, does not see high-tech treatments for MPS as magic bullets. "They can stabilize the disease," he told us, "or maybe lead to small improvements." He also emphasized the need for a community genetics approach: "We have tools to go to the community and to work preventatively at the level of prenatal screening and early care of the child." But while new genetic diagnostics are now beginning to circulate in the public health care system, "doctors cannot offer termination of pregnancy as an option," he added, "given this predominantly Catholic country's anti-abortion laws."

The therapeutic imperative voiced by the families we spoke to—"we would do anything and go anywhere to get the treatment"—is embedded in a complex medical-legal-religious context, a "conservative continental problem" in Dr. Muller's words. To complicate matters further, the family's affective tissue has become a catalyst for a grassroots and somewhat troubling uptake of high-tech treatments. According to Dr. Muller, many families make "emotional rather than rational" decisions: "Even though we have clinical scales to differentiate between severe, intermediate, or mild forms of the disease that can help us to decide which cases should or should not be treated . . . today, with judicialization, treatment depends on the family and on the judge's understanding. If we don't give the family a prescription, they can go to another doctor."

The initial MPS clinical trials in which Rita participated tested the efficacy of the enzyme on older children and young adults. Now that it is approved and in the market, new trials are testing its safe use in younger children. The study that Dr. Muller coordinates at Hospital Universitário has attracted twelve new families from all over Brazil and also from Chile and Bolivia, he told us.

Whether such trials are a public good or an exploitative mechanism is a complicated matter (Petryna 2009). Pharmaceutical companies are increasingly enlisting specialized public treatment centers in middle-income countries, such as the genetics service at Hospital Universitário, to run trials. These centers have highly qualified staff and the capability of re-cruiting specific patient pools. For example, there are some six hundred patients diagnosed with MPS 6 (one of the subtypes of the mucopolysac-charidoses) globally, and a quarter of them live in Brazil. As clinical trials unfold and evidence is produced, they morph into powerful marketing tools as multiple players struggle to make the treatment standard via a protocol and reimbursable by insurance companies (in the United States) or by the government (in countries like judicialized Brazil).

Ilse stated that taking care of Rita is "my work, full time." Her second husband, Rita's father, is the breadwinner. After discovering the girl's condition and wishing to avoid "the 75 percent chance of having another MPS child," the couple adopted a son. He brings "joy to the house," Ilse said. The parents want the courts to grant the treatment for Rita's "whole life" (*vida inteira*). The mother continued, "She will not be cured of her MPS. There is no cure. But she needs the enzyme." For Ilse, the therapeutic imperative is not a push for cure but an effort to keep Rita alive. Arguably, here the biopolitics of the state is tied to technology access and "making live and letting die" has become a familial affair. "The state should give it to her. It's stressful to have a sick child and to have to fight for her to get the medicine which she has a right to. It is Rita's right as a Brazilian citizen. But we must always fight with judges, prosecutors . . . it is so ex-hausting. This is my work, day and night."

Mirta and her two children with MPS come from the rural town of Fronteira. Her first child "had it too, but she died at the age of three. She would be twenty-two years old now. There was no treatment at the time." When asked their age, Jessica mumbled a number to which the mother said *mais alto*, louder. "Ten." Pedro was eight. Their infusions had just ended and both were watching cartoons on TV.

"It is a struggle," Mirta said, conveying how her family had to learn to operate as dual subject of rights and interests in this therapeutic state-market complex. "Every week we leave Fronteira at 1:30 am. The city hall transports us by van. We get here at 6:30 am and when the infusion ends we return home." Mirta's husband manages garbage collection for the town. "Jessica walks, but Pedro walks very little. They go to school in the afternoon." When asked what she does for a living, Mirta plainly states, "I take care of them." We had heard that these children are having difficulties accessing enzyme replacement therapy. "Yes," Mirta says, "We have to sue all the time."

For years, Jessica and Pedro had been coming to the genetic service for clinical observation and palliative care. When a study was launched to test the enzyme, "They did not meet the age criteria of six and above," Mirta lamented. She interpreted this exclusion in constitutional terms: "They did not have *the right to be researched.*" Excluded, the family kept a close eye on the MPS study. Once it was published and the therapy was approved by ANVISA and available in Brazil, "the doctors called us and asked if we wanted *entrar na justiça* [to file a lawsuit] to see whether we could get it. Of course, we said yes. The doctors and the MPS association are in constant contact with us."

There is no pre-given biopolitical population to which these atomized subjects of rights belong. And so, in their private efforts to become such subjects, these children and guardians have to rely on temporary collectivities such as the patients' associations that crop up at the intersection of patient/family demand, pharmaceutical marketing, and legal activism. Mirta is thankful for the lawyer whom the "MPS association hired for us," but she cannot recall his name or the terms in which Jessica and Pedro's cases were argued before judges who were ruling on their claims. Nor did she have a clear sense of how to act in her scripted legal subject position, and she suffered from the constant uncertainties and court fights that renewing access to the ERT entailed. "Jessica got the treatment for ninety days and Pedro for forty days. Their cases never fall into the hands of the same judge."

Technology Access and Privatized Health

The issue of treatment continuity weighs heavily on doctors who place their patients in clinical trials or who prescribe these genetic therapies. Several of the doctors we interviewed mentioned that when studies end, trial sponsors sometimes do continue to provide the drug for a while, either as part of an extended-access or compassionate-use program. "But all this is at the company's discretion." Dr. Maria emphasized that these children's biologies are wrecked by treatment discontinuity: "Sometimes they get it, sometimes they don't." Pedro and Jessica suffer from a "complete lack of consistency" of access to the therapy.

Not only are these children's biologies precariously tethered to new medical commodities, but the timing of rulings and court injunctions unleash their own kinds of hazards. "Patients go for some time without the treatment until a court injunction comes," Dr. Maria told us. Doctors provide crucial means of veridiction for patients' legal claims for treatment, but then the courts become battlefields of veridiction-falsification as the state's general attorney's office has created a taskforce of rotating medical experts who support or disqualify claims for treatment access and efficacy.

Conflicts over evidence in courts create yet another set of medical problems. According to Dr. Maria, "It is worse to have the treatment and stop it than to not have it. When treatment is interrupted and then restarted when a new ruling or injunction comes, patients almost always have an adverse reaction to the therapy. The protein in the therapy is foreign to their bodies. In the medical reports we file as part of the lawsuit, we try to make the case that treatment should not be interrupted, but we know that this argument does not necessarily work."

How does the celebrated economic equation "more technology equals better health outcomes" (Cutler and McClellan 2001; Cutler, Deaton, and Lleras-Muney 2006) square with the judicialization of health care? A major challenge facing clinicians such as Dr. Maria and her colleagues is how to assess whether the enzyme is actually improving the patient's condition. Even in the therapy's postmarketing stage, patients remain in a kind of experimental state. "What does the treatment actually improve in the patient? They have had the disease for a very long time, eight or nine years, and have had very little treatment over those years. We know that the enzyme improves lung function. But when it comes to other markers, we need more time to really assess its effect." The one-by-one judicialization of pharmaceutical access thus seems to open an additional tenuous space between treatment and research, a tenuousness that might well be replaced by standardized protocols and new regimens in the future. But we wondered to what extent parents were aware of the experimentality (Petryna 2009) that is going on in the bodies of their children-litigants. How can we facilitate a more informed public debate about the lived uncertainties of the science, effectiveness, and true costs of therapeutic advancements?

Parents at the hospital's genetic unit have crafted their own informal measures of the effectiveness of enzyme replacement therapies. Mirta, for example, mentions her children's increasing "alertness and dexterity" as well as minor details such as "the hair softening." Parents use various subjective criteria to index the negative impact that the legal odyssey is having on the children: "We know that this ongoing litigation is not good for their health. I can see the difference," Mirta continues. "When Jessica and Pedro don't have the therapy, they are compromised. They should take it continuously."

As families push through courts and medical-legal paperwork, their "biotechnical embrace" (DelVecchio Good 2007) strengthens. Meanwhile, the questionable efficacy that the doctors delivering the ERT are aware of becomes less and less an object of concern. When all goes well in this makeshift drug delivery system, Mirta adds, "The judge stamps our claim and we ourselves get the money and give it to the hospital which in turn buys the enzyme. The treatment costs 18,000 dollars per month, 36,000 dollars for both of them. It is a lot, right?"

Not even siblings with the same disease, like Pedro and Jessica, constitute a legitimate collective in this privatized and malleable right-to-health enterprise. Dr. Maria underscores the medical and juridical confusion: "One of the most difficult realities we face is that judges give different rulings for each MPS patient. Here we have the case of two siblings who both have MPS 6. They have different judges and each one gives treatment for different time periods." According to the lawyer, Mr. Moura, however, this is actually the best legal strategy: "I am against collective lawsuits. Each MPS patient is unique and takes different dosages, and their particularities might play against them if it were a collective case." For him, individual lawsuits could potentially circumvent the narrow criteria used in expert committee reviews and state prosecutors' appeals to "postpone treatment more and more." Arguably, the state and its legal surrogates are putting into circulation epistemic collectives that spring from a strategic deployment of evidence-based medicine. These virtual collectives (standing for a knowable population of needs that is no more) clash with the subject positions articulated by desperate patients and families within their temporary medical-legal and activist networks.

Pedro and Jessica did not have the right to clinical research, but they did have their constitutional right to health. As their mother puts it: "They should get the medicine *pra vida inteira* [for the whole life] so that we would not have to always activate the judiciary *pouco a pouco* [little by little]."

This family had a sense that their fight would only become more intense as right-to-health jurisprudence was evolving unpredictably. The state's highest court had recently ruled in favor of the government and held an MPS drug manufacturer responsible for the treatment costs of a child who had been in a clinical trial. State prosecutors requested and the court mandated that the manufacturer provide the patient with free treatment for life, even if this was not stipulated in the informed consent. To justify the decision, the State High Court wrote that "it is unacceptable for the manufacturer to use human beings as 'guinea pigs' in its studies and then leave people who were of vital importance helpless to obtain an extraordinarily expensive product, especially when health improvements were observed and patient expectations were raised" (Tribunal de Justiça do Estado do Rio Grande do Sul 2009).

Coda

With the global expansion of biomedical markets and their encroachment in public health care systems, we see significant institutional displacements and novel citizen-state-market formations. In the Brazilian case, the market finds utility in the government as a drug purchaser and distributor and in specific mobilized communities. These communities, cast as therapeutic market segments, use lawmaking and jurisprudence in order to be seen by the state and to make it act biopolitically. Government is thus geared less toward population health as a means of achieving productivity and control and more toward facilitating or triaging the relationship of rights-bearing subjects of interest to the biomedical market in the form of technology access.

People's life chances and health outcomes are overdetermined by what kind of market and juridical subjects they are able to become by appealing to the judiciary and government as well as to research and health industries. We have to attend to forms of statecraft (national and regional) and jurisprudence as well as to the political subjectivities that are built into this new apparatus of interests and rights if we are to understand both the possibilities that have opened up and the exclusionary dynamics at work in Brazil and elsewhere. Thus, from the perspective of judicialization, health in the time of global health is a painstaking work in progress by monadic juridical subjects in relation to therapeutic markets, ailing public health infrastructures, and fragile medical collectives. This essay has drawn attention to the precariousness of biopolitical interventions, showing how they are constantly entangled with and shaped by other (often economic) imperatives. The stories of patient-litigants and their families also point to the power of biotechnology to remake human and social worlds as it opens up new spaces of ethical problematization, desire, and political belonging. It is at the intersection of the therapeutic imperative, the biotechnical embrace, and the reason of the market that the intensity of survival becomes visible.

Notes

1. Retrieved 2/21/2011 from http://www.oestrangeiro.net/esquizoanalise/67-o-abecedario-de-gilles-deleuze.

2. An earlier version of this chapter appeared in *Social Research* (2011, 78[2]: 359–86).

3. We are deeply grateful for the research and editorial assistance of Mariana P. Socal, Roberta Grudzinski, Alex Gertner, Joshua Franklin, Jeferson Barbosa, Ramah McKay, and Peter Locke. We also acknowledge the support of the Ford Foundation and the Health Grand Challenges Initiative and the Woodrow Wilson School at Princeton University. Except in cases where individuals or institutions chose to be identified, we maintained their anonymity to the extent possible by using pseudonyms.

4. In discussing the pharmaceuticalization of health care and the judicialization of the right to health in Brazil, we draw from Biehl's book *Will to Live: AIDS Therapies and the Politics of Survival* (2007) and Petryna's book *When Experiments Travel: Clinical Trials and the Global Search for Human Subjects* (2009). We also draw from a multidisciplinary study on right-to-health litigation that is under way in southern Brazil and that is coordinated by Biehl.

5. The first MPS treatment was approved by the FDA in 2003 (laronidase for MPS I), followed by two other drugs approved in 2005 (galsulfase for MPS VI) and 2006 (idursulfase for MPS II). These drugs were approved by ANVISA in Brazil in 2006, 2009, and 2008 respectively.

6. The 1983 U.S. Orphan Drug Act provides incentives for the development of drugs to treat rare diseases affecting "less than 200,000 persons in the U.S." or "more than 200,000 persons in the U.S., but for which there is no reasonable expectation that the cost of developing and making available in the U.S. a drug for such disease or condition will be recovered from sales in the U.S. of such drug."

These incentives include tax credits for clinical research and seven years of market exclusivity for an FDA-approved drug.

7. The federal government acquired high-cost medicines in exceptional circumstances since the 1970s, but it was not until 1993 that an official program for the acquisition of these high-cost medicines (Programa de Medicamentos Excepcionais) was created (Ministry of Health 2010a). The federal government ceded the administrative responsibility of this program to state health secretariats, but without a well-defined cofinancing mechanism. Although many drugs were included in the program's initial formularies, only a few were effectively distributed to the population, due to erratic and irregular acquisition and distribution processes. In 2002, the Exceptional Medicines Program was extended to include ninety-two drugs and more precise criteria were formulated to inform their distribution (Souza 2002). Finally, in 2006, the Ministry of Health issued a Ministerial Decree (Portaria GM n° 2577 de 27 de Outubro de 2006) outlining the specific objectives and responsibilities of the States and the Federal government in regard to the Exceptional Medicines Program (Ministry of Health 2010). Currently, 110 therapeutic products (including medicines, biological products, and nutritional formulas) are included in the program, which is now called the "Specialized Component of Pharmaceutical Assistance" (Ministry of Health, 2010a).

8. In 2007, four drugs were responsible for 28 percent of the Health Ministry's drug expenditures: imiglucerase, epoetin alpha, human immune-globulin, and interferon alpha-2b.

9. See http://www.princeton.edu/grandchallenges/health/research-highlights/aids/.

10. For a detailed review of the public hearing, see: http://www.stf.jus.br/portal/cms/verTexto.asp?servico=processoAudienciaPublicaSaude.

11. In 2010, the Brazilian National Council of Justice issued a recommendation for judges to always verify at the National Commission of Research Ethics (Comissão Nacional de Ética em Pesquisas [CONEP]) if the requested drug was "part of experimental research programs" of the pharmaceutical industry and that, in that case, judges should mandate these industries to assume treatment continuity. (Recomendação n° 31, de 30 de Março de 2010. DJ-e n° 61/2010, em 07/04/2010, p. 4–6. Available at: http://www.cnj.jus.br/index.php?option=com_content&view=article&id=10547:recomendacao-no-31-de-30-de-marco-de-2010&catid=60:recomendas-do-conselho&Itemid=515.)

12. In his 1978–79 lectures at the Collège de France, Foucault argued that we can adequately analyze biopolitics only when we understand the economic reason within governmental reason: "Inasmuch as it enables production, need, supply, demand, value, and price, etcetera, to be linked together through exchange, the market constitutes a site of veridiction, I mean a site of veridiction-falsification for governmental practice. Consequently, the market determines that good government is no longer simply government that functions according to justice" (2008:32).

Afterword

The Peopling of Technologies

MICHAEL M. J. FISCHER

I want to explore the remarkable array of ethnographic case studies in this book by reading *for the people* and reading *for the bioecologies at play*. I use the term "ecologies" as a means of probing for the proper identifications and scales of interactions in global health, particularly at biochemical, molecular, computational, and informatics granularities that previously have not been accessible. We are arguably undergoing one or more epistemic revolutions, all too slow for the desperately ill, but stunningly fast in terms of the pedagogies in which we have been trained and in which we still too often think. Two indices for these epistemic changes—the molecular biology revolution and (bio)ecological imaginaries—may be sufficient to direct attention and to indicate the cascades, ramifications, and implications of paradigmatic shifts.

The expressions "when people come first" (and which ones) and "reading for the people" speak of power, stratification, inequality, structural violence, and incentives—the traditional social and political economy issues. The ecological perspective speaks of our nature—of how we fit into the webs of our habitats, and (with the largest number of cells in our bodies being bacteria, viruses, fungi, prions, and pheromones) our microbiomes, the barely discernible threads and signals within which we are constituted and which to variable degrees control how we change—our shifts in mood, the ways in which we age, and so on.

This is potent stuff—pervasive, diffuse, largely measurable only through instruments and indirect models, yet highly visceral, emotional, and capable of dividing us from one another politically and morally. It is the stuff of obdurately resistant reality and of imaginaries, partial understandings that grow and recompose.

I will use a series of orientations to make connections among the case studies in this book, as well as my own ethnographic research interviewing life scientists in India and the United States and doing ethnographic fieldwork in Singapore's Biopolis, to suggest how they may provide analytic insights into these epistemic shifts. Central is the peopling of biomedical technologies and the sciences involved. We should not view the biosciences and biotechnologies as magical black boxes to be dismissed as not solving all problems, or to be feared, but rather see them in their own right as rich ethnographic terrains in which to explore inventions of new kinds of social organizations; to observe struggles for moral worlds, psychocultural investments, and crosscultural scientific diplomacy and misunderstandings; and to search for solutions to the challenges of rebuilding or extending public health through new notions of rights, market tools, protection of commons, biopolitics, bioeconomies, and bioecologies. The series of orientations are: *mobile phone analogies* (as an image or metaphor of cheap, ubiquitous, and mobile high-tech genomics that saves lives, helps stop pandemics, and promises more personalized therapies); *translational research* (to make new biomedical knowledge therapeutically available); *shifts in moral culture and repairing the legacies of structural adjustment* (the political economy of public health); *forward-looking values* (entering into dialogue to build civil society foundations for public health); and *repetitions* (as new entry points).

II

Repetitions and Entry Points. We repeat ourselves: social medicine versus technology, holism versus instrumentalism, robust community versus cost-benefit. We rail against the narrow technological blinders of top-down policymakers, enthralled generation after new generation by similar fixes, solutions, statistical methods. We lament their failures to attend to politics, social systems, lives in flux, local sustainability, and health care as wellness rather than the mere reduction of disease burdens and health care costs. We remind everyone over and over that without attention to social conditions, technology is useless. We ask policymakers to historicize—"enter history and you will find the missing politics" of how priorities are set or abandoned (Biehl and Petryna, this volume)—or we show that "epidemics [and effects of floods, tsunamis, earthquakes] did not happen by accident" (Packard 2007:10; Fischer 2009: ch. 3) but are outcomes of development plans, agricultural expansion, the shifting of water flow, bad nutrition, wars, and migration, as well as the coevolution of our parasites, our genetic mutations—in short, of our bioecologies.

We have been repeating these dualisms and calls for the kind of historical depth and social analysis that Marcos Cueto describes in his incisive account of malaria eradication or containment since the 1950s. The sociopolitical structuring of the bilateral and multilateral system put in place by the First World to contain communism was justified as a "realistic humanism" that "should not be criticized or resisted." However, we should not forget the connections that were forged across the Cold War divide—for instance, how the Rockefeller Foundation's support for rural health in northern China in the 1930s "would later serve as a model for the famous barefoot doctor program under the communists" (Packard 2007:134).

We have also been calling for attention to historical, political-economic, and bioecological contexts since the bacteriological revolution and the drive to identify and root out pathogens in the late nineteenth and early twentieth centuries. Cueto focuses on a series of failed magic bullets, dating from 1955, when the malaria eradication campaign was announced in Mexico City: DDT, chloroquine, long-lasting insecticidal nets, mefloquine, and vaccines. In his 1900 textbook, *Malaria: According to the New Researches*, Angelo Celli insisted on the social and economic conditions that shape the habitats in which malaria invades, recurs, recedes, and reappears. Yet according to historian Randall Packard, Celli "contented himself with comparing two columns of figures, one showing increasing sales of state quinine and the other falling rates of death" (Packard 2007:126). Celli could not yet know that the reason quinine would only limit mortality (but not affect transmission or the endemic nature of malaria) was that quinine can do no more than interrupt the merozoite phase of the parasite's life cycle. Similarly, during the interwar period the International Labor Organization and the League of Nations Health Office focused on the "standardization of mortality statistics and providing a quantitative basis for chemotherapeutic drugs and vaccines" (Packard 2007:117). Social deprivation, diet, and overall health conditions of the population were "systematically eliminated . . . [and] malaria became a disease of parasites and mosquitoes" (Packard 2007:110).

As the quinine example makes clear, the failures of both social medicine solutions and vector control were due, in part, to the state of relative ignorance about what part of the parasite life cycle was vulnerable to what kind of control, and about the different feeding and breeding behaviors of the many species of *Anopheles* mosquitoes. More than twelve species of mosquito with different feeding and breeding behaviors and five or six different strains of malaria appear in Packard's review, not only *vivax* and *falciparum*, the two that recur in popular reviews. So the social medicine and medical anthropology brief of *When People Come First* cannot be *against* technology; rather, it must argue that scientific and technological knowledge can help, but not alone, and further that scientific and technical knowledges are chimerized with choices made through politics, funding, and community organizing.

History shows the benefits conferred by technology: lowland malaria clearance in Nepal, south of Rome, and in southern Africa. But these successes also had the effect of allowing higher-caste or wealthier populations to displace or subordinate the original inhabitants. In the Italian case, success under Mussolini after several earlier failures was achieved with little concern for the unprotected workers who made it happen. Technical success *for whom* becomes important as a question. Who gets displaced? Whose health is neglected in development projects that claim success? What have we learned ecologically about the interaction of habitat, pathogen, coevolving species, and unintended consequences (or intended ones) when water flow is redirected, of the effects of expanding agriculture and mining into new areas, and of the decline of malaria in maturing, more carefully cultivated landscapes? Indeed, declines in malaria due to maturing landscapes sometimes precede malaria control programs, mystifying the planners and public health assessors and adding to the cacophony of arguments about future public health strategies and expenditures.

Or, as anthropologist Michael Montoya—focusing on another contemporary epidemic, diabetes, a noncommunicable disease with extraordinary rates of growth globally—worries, echoing the title of this book: "Who are the people in these 'problem-oriented' approaches? We're the data points, we're the objects of our research, the objects of our well-intentioned interventions and sometimes our pity."[1] Montoya is working with poor communities in Santa Ana, California, and argues that the designation "lifestyle disease" for ailments like diabetes is a neoliberal way of blaming the victim, of insisting that only individuals are responsible for their own health care, downplaying, if not ignoring, the direct role played by the destruction of communities, indebtedness, pollution, violence, and other community dysfunctions. In this volume, Clara Han gives a similar powerful account of a poor community in Santiago, Chile, focusing on mental health, and Vincanne Adams provides a stunning confirmation of "we're [only] the data points" in cases from Nepal and New Orleans.

Who, and ecologically *what*, is the person in medicine? Consider a recent case of diabetes analyzed with genomic or multi-omic information along with molecular and physiological data that provides an extraordinary preview of personalized medicine. Michael Snyder, chair of Genetics and Director of Stanford's Center for Genomics and Personalized Medicine, sequenced his own "integrated Personal Omics Profile" or iPOP (his DNA, RNA, proteins, metabolites, and antibodies) and unexpectedly found a strong genetic predisposition for type 2 diabetes (Chen et al. 2012; Conger 2012). Serendipitously he developed the disease, apparently triggered by two common viruses (perhaps picked up from his young children), a rhinovirus and a respiratory syncytial virus. Because of the prior iPOP sequencing, he was able, probably for the first time in history, to identify the exact time of onset of the disease, to recognize how it was triggered (by an autoantibody targeting an insulin receptor binding protein), and to monitor how the disease developed and responded to countermeasures, tracking some four thousand genes and protein products that were being expressed at elevated or depressed levels.

Although such technology has dramatically resolved a handful of death's-door cases (e.g., Kolata 2012), it is out of reach for most. But its price will drop. Simplification and availability will come. In 2001, the first whole genome cost three billion dollars. Today's price is around US$1,000 and dropping fast. Interpretation, as with the first GPS systems, is complex, but today GPS systems are simple and available in many formats, even on cheap cameras and cell phones. I invoke this example not to hype high-tech medicine but to indicate the existence here of an emergent knowledge base that may well be transformative—and not just for the few, but for all, in the same way that the information technology revolution is changing life almost everywhere (hence the mobile phone analogy).

We need better terms of analysis than "technology versus the social"; we need to work at more granular and multiple scales of interactions. As the late Dr. Judah Folkman said, "translation to the clinic proceeds along a pathway strewn with obstacles and it's actually harder than making the discovery because it involves other people, and involves all their different views" (1999, quoted in Fischer 2010, 2012). By focusing on the peopling of technologies, this book's ethnographic case studies on HIV/AIDS, parasitic disease, and cancer in Africa (Reynolds Whyte et al., Moran-Thomas, Pfeiffer, and Livingston), multidrug-resistant tuberculosis in India (Ecks and Harper), and genetic and other diseases in the Caribbean and Brazil (Whitmarsh, Biehl and Petryna) are redefining the terms of research in global health and making global health a heuristic for understanding novel interactions among people, technoscience, environment, markets, and politics.

We are not quite done with malaria as a case study for global health care. I want to briefly invoke two more aspects of the malaria story from India, one having to do with India's 2012 announcement of the synthesis of a new antimalarial, Ranbaxy's Synriam, and the other with the travails of malaria vaccine innovation (Bhandari 2005). Both illustrate cross-national interactions in medical innovation that require "global health" analysis rather than merely nation-based bilateral and multilateral "international health." These terminological shifts accompanied the neoliberal interventionist agenda of the 1990s and early 2000s, which morphed into powerful mechanisms and modes of governance that prioritized technological magic bullets and formalistic (rather than real) "evidence-based" outcomes. In a recent recruiting drive to bring nonresident Indian scientists and engineers back to India, M. K. Bhan, pediatrician and the secretary of the Department of Biotechnology, suggested that the BRIC countries (Brazil, Russia, India, China) are poised to provide scalable solutions for the developing world. He cited the antimalarial Synriam: "We spent less than US$25m over three years (versus the $800 million to $1 billion figure that the pharmaceutical industry reckons as the cost of taking a new drug discovery through clinical trials to FDA approval) and provided a treatment at a cost of $1 per patient. This Ranbaxy product is a game changer." Synriam is a synthetic that can be scaled up more easily than plant-based artemisinin-based drugs, and one pill a day for three days is priced at 130 rupees ($2.47) for adults with "uncomplicated" *Plasmodium falciparum* malaria.

The story is layered. Synriam is hailed as the first new molecule to be devised and patented in India. (The component arterolane is the patent-able "new chemical entity.") When India joined the World Trade Organization it had to rewrite its patent laws, moving from protecting processes to instead protecting products. Ranbaxy was one of the more successful firms in making the transition to new drug discovery, albeit often by setting up labs and acquiring companies outside India. Synriam was developed in a joint venture with Medicines for Malaria Venture (MMV), a Geneva-based nonprofit foundation established in 1999. Ranbaxy will sell the drug at affordable prices to low- and middle-income countries in Africa, South America, and Asia.

Alongside this nation-based account, we should look at a different account of the same cross-national collaboration. Arterolane was discovered in 2003 by researchers from the United States, United Kingdom, Switzerland, and Australia, led by the University of Nebraska's Jonathan Vennerstrom. Ranbaxy was brought in for "translation," to take development through to the clinic. MMV invested some US$20 million, but it withdrew in 2007 and granted Ranbaxy a worldwide royalty-free license. Meanwhile, a majority stake in Ranbaxy was acquired by the Japanese firm Daiichi Sankyo in 2008, which wanted to consolidate its generics position globally, and drug discovery at Ranbaxy has been scaled back.

I tell this not to undermine the India-centric story, but to emphasize complementary narratives, alternatively focusing on: (1) institutional structures within India; (2) global market forces, crossnational research collaborations, and development pipelines; and (3) international organizations as charted by Cueto.

Developing malaria vaccines in India highlights the importance of not glossing over the peopling of the pipelines of biomedical technologies, and of not thinking of technologies as simple matters of implementation, but rather as the results of constant negotiation and invention within social organizations and networks. I have followed the work of malaria-vaccine scientist Chetan Chitnis since he was a postdoc at the NIH and identified a protein-binding interaction between malaria parasites and red blood cells. He then returned to New Delhi to set up a lab at the International Center for Genetic Engineering and Biotechnology (ICGEB), where he developed a recombinant DNA vaccine. At ICGEB, he solved the structure of the molecules, mapped the binding site, looked at polymorphisms (a major issue in making vaccines), and did fieldwork to show that people who make these antibodies are protected against malaria. He showed me the new GMP (good management practices, i.e., clean room and the like) fermenter he was learning to use and talked about the quality control scale-up required for clinical trial work, which cannot be done in an academic lab. In the beginning, it was learning by doing. There was no technology transfer office or project management expertise. Biotech was just starting in India: Shanta Biotech in Hyderabad had just produced a recombinant hepatitis B vaccine. Chitnis eventually found a company to help produce the vaccine, but he needed an adjuvant. The one he wanted was from GlaxoSmithKline (GSK). Because he had licensed the vaccine technology to an Indian company, GSK would not participate despite various proposed sensible-seeming royalty-sharing agreements, nor would the Indian company.

Translation, as Judah Folkman said, is not so easy. Similar patent and licensing issues have long prevented vitamin A–enhanced "golden rice" from being made available. After two years of frustrated negotiations, Chitnis restarted his project with an adjuvant from a nonprofit company in Seattle, but other roadblocks arose in the Indian regulatory system, which had experience with genetics but not with recombinant DNA products that would go into a "first in human" trial in India. At a loss, the regulatory bureaucracy turned hypercautious and began asking for toxicology not just in mice but in monkeys as well, something not required for vaccines (as opposed to drugs) in Europe and in the United States. Eventually approval was given, but with a proviso that regulators might require such trials later "because it is the law" (according to regulations for earlier technologies).

Chitnis narrated these problems of peopling the technological pipeline at a 2007 meeting about the setting up of a Translational Health Science and Technology Institute (THSTI) in New Delhi. He stressed the need for such a national-level center to take on both management and regulatory issues. Chitnis knew well from bitter experience that simply setting up a world-class academic center for basic and applied science does not create translation.

In sum, our growing ability to monitor (1) the life cycle of the malaria parasite in our bodies, habitats, and daily practices; (2) personalized medicine through the interactions of our genomes, proteomes, metabolomes, and antibodies, along with our parasites and companion species; and (3) translational pipelines for new therapies provide *ethnographic entry points* for assessing lively social worlds of translation amid science, medicine, ecology, and public health.

III

Translational Research. Evidence-based medicine for whom? Can we work the ethnographic evidence as corrective and complementary to evidence-based medicine and policy?

These questions follow on some of the rich discussion that Vincanne Adams sparked with her exquisite and maddening case examples of self-defeating formalist evidence-based medicine and its double discourses. The patient is missing: "It's not like medical researchers and public health professionals don't realize that something is missing. . . . The randomized controlled trial is a lot about validation within the profession," noted a doctoral student in public health. Public health goals precede data, and the mandate *to do* often supersedes self-aware reflection—"we know it doesn't work, but we have to do this" kind of thinking—among bureaucrats and consultants, notes Didier Fassin.

Just as the Brazilian patient-citizen-consumers presented by Biehl and Petryna do not wait for technology to trickle down, but have to become experts in legal and medical issues incorporating the need for "evidence-based" arguments, a different kind of case can illustrate some of the new frustrations faced even by highly educated "expert patients," who are trying to use patient-group organizing to forge changes in the ways evidence-based medicine is practiced. They ask—once again echoing the title of this book—how can we get a medical system that is focused on the patient? At issue here are not the divides between infectious and chronic diseases, between common and rare diseases, between biomedical research and translational clinical medicine, or between basic public health care and clinical medicine. Those are important, but the focus here is on the *peopling* of technologies, on the institutional infrastructures that facilitate or block action in these diverse arenas.

LAM (lymphangioleiomyomatosis) is a rare, progressive, and often fatal disease that affects young women in their childbearing years and kills by asphyxiation. Its cause is unknown, and there is no known remedy. The story of LAM can first of all highlight the painful shift in medicine from reductionism to something more holistic that can handle the multiple interacting ecosystems (from the fluctuations of the microbiome and epigenome to other levels of shuffling omics and changing habitats) that comprise allergies, asthma, autoimmune diseases, and cross-species pandemics, to name a few. Second, it can highlight the emotional healing arts, the high percentage of things not biomedical that nonetheless contribute to the feeling of wellness and to healing. Third, the LAM story can shine an "empirical lantern" on the dysfunctional institutional blockages, including legislative rules once thought of as (and still partly useful for) protections, especially of privacy and against discrimination by employers and insurers, such as HIPAA (the US Health Insurance Portability and Accountability Act).

The LAM Treatment Alliance (LTA), founded by Amy Farber, is a member of the Genetic Alliance founded by Sharon Terry, whose own organization PXE (pseudoxanthoma elasticum) International is another such patient-driven organization devoted to fighting a rare disease. While PXE International provides an important and much-cited intervention in intellectual property rights discussions, as well as a model for activist-consumer participation in the directing of medical research, the case of LAM exposes the current failure of biomedicine to live up to its aspirations and provides insights into the potential of patient-centered care, personalized medicine, and translational medicine. It is a pioneer in creative solutions.

Farber is a powerful speaker, fundraiser, convener of scientific workshops on LAM (along with her scientific board), and funder of fee-for-service work, as well as herself having experience as an NIH senior investigator and postdoctoral researcher. LTA collaborates with leading biomedical laboratories in Boston. With a PhD in anthropology, law-school training, and a thorough grounding in medical ethics, she provides an insider's account of the misalignments of the current medical system (with its intensive focus on evidence-based RCT methodologies) that stand in the way of truly patient-centered biomedical research. It is a double-bind: practical science is always a balance between the direct perception or experience-based understanding on the one hand and, on the other, statistical analysis and instrument-mediated evidence. Farber's account returns full circle to recover some of the common sense that has been lost in biomedicine's drive for reductionist causality, its focus on nonportable informed consent, such as privacy protections that prevent patients from accessing their own data, and its aggregation of clinical trial–sized populations. What is at issue, broadly speaking, is the continued disempowerment of the patient in favor of disciplinary specialists who are well-intentioned but misaligned and misincentivized to do serious personalized medicine. As her organization continues to engage diverse partners to achieve patient impact, Farber also invokes a modern form of complementary medicine, emphasizing the importance of paying attention to one's body and what one is doing on the good days and bad, a type of tracking pioneered by the "quantified self" movement, and the singularity of each person—in other words, an approach that is pragmatic, authentically personalized, and attends to what actually works for each life.

As she says of LTA, "We are not bringing a product to market. We are trying to move a field to truly benefit patients in the short term. There is no template for this work. The whole medical research drug development paradigm is frequently fraught for patients living today, unless you've got a single-gene-defect solid tumor that can be serially biopsied and/or monitored by one or more validated biomarkers." While whole genome sequencing, which surveys each person's whole genome and searches across databases (unlike earlier genome-wide association studies that selected only common variants across populations) is the latest potentially revolutionary tool promising future personalized medicine (as in the Michael Snyder story mentioned above), the problem is not just the overload of data. Importantly, it is hard to focus efforts within and across institutions; contractors (be they academic labs or companies) will make promises about what their technologies might be able to do, and it is impossible to hold them to account given uncertainties associated with the various steps involved and the unchartered nature of new initiatives in each disease area. Farber speaks about LTA's difficulties in working to help its patient population understand the challenges posed by the field's lack of good tools (i.e., cell lines, animal models, biomarkers) and by uncertainties and complexities around discovery-focused initiatives alongside the challenges of working against the clock to ensure that competition and data-sharing among academics and vendors work in patients' interests, and that those it funds deliver on obligations to share protocols and other information with one another or even simply with the LTA for internal use. Because of their size advantage, larger academic institutions may assume that any work they may do on the disease constitutes progress and that the LTA does not truly need access to the data generated by the research collaborations that it invests in cultivating and funding. Pragmatically, institutions may take administrative or data-sharing aspects of formal agreements they enter with the LTA less seriously than those with industry partners. Also, as a former NIH-funded researcher in her own right, Farber feels that partners trained by the culture surrounding NIH research may assume that organizations like the LTA are operating in a more traditional discovery mindset where deliverables need not, and in some cases should not, necessarily look like the aims agreed upon at the outset. While the LTA also hopes that research will be responsive to real-time developments in the lab or clinic and supports changes in direction when experiments are not fruitful, its objectives are not identical to those of a pure discovery paradigm that seeks knowledge for its own sake. Given the critical gaps in the LAM field, the LTA is constantly prioritizing so that it can direct the precious charitable dollars it raises for patients facing high-stakes races against time to where they can have the greatest impact. Without timely data-sharing with those it funds, the LTA cannot effectively deliver on its promise to patients, support partners' efficient progress, help troubleshoot delays, facilitate access to lung tissue or patient data, for example, or shift directions if research strays too far from a LAM focus.

Perhaps there are other ways of organizing pipelines; perhaps new social media and mobile phone–like platforms could provide ways through current bottlenecks. Even people like Don Berwick, former head of the Centers for Medicare and Medicaid, and management scholar Michael Porter are arguing that incentives for clinicians are often not aligned with outcomes for patients. Against a background of seven years' work to accelerate research within the traditional drug development paradigm, patients like Farber are trying to fast track research efforts to operationalize new mantras around the potential of personalized medicine, a new orthodoxy that rare diseases share pathways with other common diseases, that common diseases are bundles of rare diseases, even personalized diseases, and so on. Unfortunately, the facts of which tools exist, what is known and unknown in specific disease fields like LAM, do not neatly map onto the panacea templates for demo-ing personalized medicine. The whole hope, Farber says, is $N = 1$, using patients as their own controls and taking maximum advantage of the fact that there is no one more motivated than the patient herself to save her life. Meanwhile, clinicians seeing LAM patients at dispersed centers across the world may not be comfortable interacting with IRBs, or they may be unfamiliar with drugs being considered in clinical trials or simply and understandably too busy to report patient data in any detail. Researchers have been working for over ten years to define surrogate biomarkers or trial endpoints that would reliably indicate if a drug was effective in slowing or stopping disease progression. Given what we suspect about disease heterogeneity and the low likelihood that all LAM patients need the same intervention, there is great imperative to innovate, notwithstanding the statistical challenges.

Large randomized controlled trials are the gold standard of evidence-based medicine, but they are hard to fund, especially when it is a rare disease that is being studied. The LTA has, however, successfully recruited Novartis to sponsor a trial on LAM and has worked with other organizations to support the supposed "win" of other multiyear clinical trials. As it is difficult to do more than one or two trials in any five-year period due to low patient numbers and other resources, the LTA is working to find ways to implement a new dispersed $N = 1$ clinical trial paradigm. This may begin to address some of the structural misalignments and oversights. For example, the LTA is launching a virtual study using home spirometers and ovulation kits to explore a signal related to the relationship between breathing and the menstrual cycle that the majority of patients with LAM, a disease more sex-specific to women than breast cancer, have reported anecdotally for many years. Researchers, Farber says, have only recently started to explore this at the molecular level, but they have not leveraged clinical or translational insights because the "breathing folks" and the "hormone folks" do not naturally spend enough time learning or thinking together.

And so, finally, Farber has arrived at "the more radical thought": What would it be like to design a clinical trial around the patient's truly relevant quality of life outcomes? What would her own N = 1 clinical trial look like? It's not enough to just track and map breathing and hormone levels throughout the menstrual cycle against the subjective experience of breathing. Farber wants to track this and other variables against *her* "end points," the ones that really matter to her quality of life—to how she feels when she walks up the stairs in her house or carries her daughter up a particular hill to nursery school each day. Even the FDA takes self-reported measures of improvement in quality of life seriously. But to do this, you would need to start measuring. So Farber begins to track everything she does, breathes, eats, and feels with a special emphasis on lifestyle and environmental variables.

Some new technologies, ways of thinking, and connections help. An acquaintance of both Farber and Judah Folkman—an active member, before his death, of the LTA scientific advisory board—connected Farber with Linda Avey, among others, to explore this tracking space, building upon the LTA's earlier efforts to aggregate patient-reported and clinician-reported data, which were developed in partnership with the MIT Media Lab. Avey, who cofounded 23andMe, is now starting a new company, Curious, Inc., a platform for aggregating personal data, including tracking technology, that could prove insightful to Farber and other LAM patients. (23andMe gives individuals the ability to access their own genetic information and provides insights into their relative predispositions to diseases and conditions that have a genetic component. Its direct-to-consumer model challenges many existing regulatory constructs. Although at first the company did not claim that the information it was providing was medically actionable, but rather that it was intended only to educate the public in probabilistic thinking and to make genomics research more transparent, in 2012 it began to submit tests to the FDA as clinically relevant [AP 2012; Ray 2012]. 23andMe also gathers phenotypic data from its customers, has published several papers adding new discoveries to the genomics literature, and has received a first patent [Vorhaus 2012; Williams 2012; Wojcicki 2012].)

The Curious tracking technology includes a smartphone application that time stamps patient inputs and generates sophisticated graphs overlaying different variables over weeks, months, and years. The idea is to eventually overlay such data on genomic and other data sets generated by clinicians and bench researchers as well. The LTA will pilot this initial overlay experiment using one LAM patient's whole genome sequence. At the outset, the preponderance of the data for LAM will likely come from self-reporting by patients in LTA's global network or be obtained by importing aggregated datasets from patients and clinicians that the LTA has already collected.

One of the things that such patient-driven crowdsourcing can do is to get around the issue of nonportable informed consents to gain concrete insights into how individuals can modulate their disease course. Today, sharing data among centers and physicians is extremely difficult because of institutional bureaucracy and the HIPAA and other privacy and intellectual property "protections." As Farber puts it, bioscience and the biomedical system has come to be dominated by technical research and business protocols that encumber the kind of personalized patient-centered healing that is based on common sense and creatively leverages patient motivation and existing datasets within and across disease communities. Removing such roadblocks is vital, especially when aggregate knowledge about a disease is scarce and lifestyle and environmental choices that may impact patient outcomes have been underexplored. Even if only as a motivational frame to empower patients and free them from passively waiting, Farber asks LAM patients to think about what they are keeping in their lungs. It strikes them initially as a perplexing question, but she tells them to sit with it: "I'm not saying that you are causing your disease, but each of us is our own ecosystem, take what's going on in yours seriously, figure out what adjustments make you feel even a little bit better on certain days and worse on others, if you can—these may be different from person to person even with the same condition."

A doctor of Chinese medicine whom Farber has also involved in her care, and who draws on traditional Chinese healing traditions as well as biomedical-style experimentation, conducts classes at a hospital near Boston. He demonstrates simple movements, part of his own wellness regimen, that might help his students release physical pressure and increase flow. He sometimes uses cupping, acupuncture, herbs, mindfulness techniques, and the perspective that food is medicine. He has a class, she says, "full of people with stable tumors and cancers, who should already be dead." He helps some students address fears associated with frightening diagnoses and the consequences that fear may be creating in their bodies and minds. He sees Nobel laureates and Western-trained oncologists and helps them back to wellness and a healing lifestyle through new take-home practices. Complementary or alternative medical systems need not be about rejecting biomedicine; rather, they should make it possible to reconnect with larger worlds of thinking about health and wellness and ways to support one's body in the context of a life-threatening disease. Often, due to lack of formal data that has been generated so far in LAM research, the vast majority of clinicians seeing LAM patients, even at the world's best centers, either lack tools for partnering with LAM patients around these issues or may not be open to the idea that such adjustments may shift health outcomes. Too often, they simply say that there is no data, and they cannot professionally advise any action for which there are no conclusive clinical trial results. Farber recalls that when she was first diagnosed, she wanted to know what women with LAM whose breathing was still "normal" were doing and not doing—"perhaps there were insights into what might keep the disease from progressing in my own case." For HIPAA reasons (among other major overwhelming but purely technical barriers), there was no means of getting this type of data.

In sum, LTA's many problem-solving innovations are pioneering precisely because they focus attention on the peopling of technologies, mobile information access, and shifts in the moral-legal culture that emergent global and local medical and public health care systems will need if they are to have greater patient impact, especially in the realms of mental health and chronic progressive disorders.

IV

Shifts in Moral Culture and Repairing the Legacies of Structural Adjustment. Today there are shifting paradigms of institutional organization (patient-driven research coalitions, for example), of knowledge about bioecologies (such as Snyder's iPOP), and of marketing-shaped common sense (such as in the cases provided in this book by Clara Han's pragmatic savers and exchangers of pills, Ecks and Harper's medical representatives and doctors, Whitmarsh's ascetic consumers, and Biehl and Petryna's patient-litigants and activist judges; and more generally Dumit's [2012] unraveling of the logics of "drugs for life" for "patients in waiting" who can live better as drug "dependent-normals"). Given these shifts, perhaps there will be shifts as well in our moral cultures. This is the provocative implication of the chapters in this book on human rights by Joseph Amon and the uses of children in humanitarian discourse by Didier Fassin.

Following his larger explorations of contemporary moral economies (Fassin 2007, 2011, 2012), Fassin highlights a perfectly obvious but often overlooked ethnographic datum: children who lose their parents to AIDS are not necessarily abandoned. There are aunts and uncles and grandparents who may adopt them, and under a regime of humanitarian aid for children, they can become of economic value to those who take them in. To recognize this does not mean that aid is superfluous, but that a more community-based public health care approach might be appropriate. During the workshop discussion, Fassin reminded us that "the supposed exceptionality of AIDS . . . makes many Africans uncomfortable: What about other health issues? What about the other 'orphans,' of whom there are twice as many as from AIDS?"

Amon's account of rights language similarly reminds us that the moral terrain requires asking *who* is mobilizing the language of rights and for *what* ends: there are rights to know others' HIV status, rights to know one's own HIV status, rights to have access to information about AIDS and HIV, and there should be rights to not disclose when such disclosure could have poisonous or lethal effects. There is also in Brazil, as Biehl and Petryna show us, a "right to health" in an environment of pharmaceuticalized care. And there is as well the international community's gradual insistence on the right to intervene when governments fail in their "responsibility to protect" the health of their citizens and pose dangers to surrounding countries and global health. This was called for in 2008 by Zimbabwe health professionals, Physicians for Human Rights, and some within WHO, in response to cholera, TB, malaria, and AIDS crises that followed the closings of hospitals and a general breakdown in government services (Physicians for Human Rights 2008; Sollom 2009).

These disparate uses of rights language amount to a clear call for responsible ethnographic due diligence on the part of policymakers and funders, as well as humanitarian organizations and community organizers, to know how things actually work on the ground. It bears repeating (again and again): one size does not fit all. Consider Iran's highly regarded WHO Best Practices–awarded HIV/AIDS program. The national program could only be established by working out different semantics for different audiences—for provincial mullahs, the secular middle classes, and national bureaucrats. The country had denied the existence of AIDS on the grounds that it was a decadent Western disease that could not exist in an Islamic republic. The disease had to be coded, therefore, as a problem of needle use and addiction, and not as involving male-to-male transmission, not even in the prisons where the epidemic was too great to be ignored (Behrouzan 2010).

The workshop discussion around Fassin's chapter was particularly rich in its explorations of coded languages: There are "double-figures" of "mother/deviant sexworker and of grandmother taking care of orphans/ but resistant to Western medicine"—and each figure must be "cleaved from its shadow image" in order to be deployed. The "semantics of security, bioterrorism, epidemics on the one side and humanitarianism, solidarity, compassion on the other" are linked intimately and dialectically, and the logic of the innocence and purity of children makes invisible important complicities. There is, too, the ever-present problem of the non-recording of certain kinds of statistics in population-level analyses of the economic effects of investment in children's health.

Where people are captured or ignored by global health categories and interventions, they remain tethered to the politics of the state. And almost all the ethnographic cases in this book speak of a midlevel analytics of the state and of efforts to repair the destruction caused to public health systems by the structural adjustment programs in the 1980s and 1990s, repair that involves working within the vortex of new funding, interests, expertise, and technologies associated with global health: Han for Chile, Pfeiffer for Mozambique, Reynolds Whyte and colleagues for Uganda, Livingston for Botswana, Fassin for South Africa, Moran-Thomas for Ghana, Ecks and Harper for postsocialist India, Whitmarsh for Barbados and Trinidad and Tobago, and Biehl and Petryna for Brazil. At issue in these encounters and misencounters between global health and local public health are a variety of legal and regulatory mechanisms, as well as novel state-market formations and transitional social forms and moral orders for which ethnography can provide empirical lanterns and entry points for alternative evidence-making and policy framing. The chain of processes—"first destroy public health capacity through structural adjustment, then rebuild cost-effectively through consultancies, NGOs, and humanitarian aid"—can serve to place power in the hands of the international community, NGOs, donors, and consultants at the expense of local capacities (Fassin and Pandolfi 2010; Duffield 2001; Ghani and Lockhardt 2008). But the interventions and market mechanisms detailed in parts 2 and 3 of this book eloquently detail the slow revival and reinvention of these capacities, sometimes grimly and sometimes with real hope, often still under the constraints of structural adjustment programs, now called Poverty Reduction Strategy Papers or PRSPs (Pfeiffer, this volume).

The research led by Susan Reynolds Whyte (together with Danish and Ugandan colleagues) focuses attention on the double entendre of the neoliberal term "client" in Ugandan AIDS programs funded by international donors, including PEPFAR and the Global Fund. In practice, clients are both users of services and dependent for their lives on these services, which draw them into all kinds of "objective self-fashioning" (Dumit 1997) through medical paperwork and patron-client networks that attempt to remold their subjectivities as compliant patients. Clients, however, seek patrons in terms of friendship. It is a "lopsided friendship" in Julian Pitt-River's characterization (as Michael Whyte noted in the workshop) that inhabits hierarchical relationships in which clients use the idiom of friendship to solicit a patron's ability and obligation to redirect resources so as to make the client's social life viable. These are pervasive networks of social capital. Analogues elsewhere include our own use of "connections," Iranian *parti-bazi*, and Chinese *guanxi*. But a failure to understand how crucial these relationships become when there are not also reliably enforced rights can lead to misunderstandings among international donors (who stress contractual neoliberal relations) and local recipients (see also Shipton 2010). In this projectified and fragmented terrain, antiretroviral supply chains might form, in the words of Vincanne Adams, a "new kind of kinship chart." But as Michael Whyte pointed out, the multiple sources, actors, and treatment supply chains obfuscate and actively disenfranchise locals. Ethnographers and social media activists could help locals map out the sources, actors, and supply chains. This could be used in local political work directed at making local public health sustainable.

Ethnography, thus, is not merely descriptive. Once heard or read, the travails of patients and doctors in Botswana's only cancer ward, as presented by Livingston, will be hard to forget. The travails of the women in Santiago presented by Han leave a lasting impression as well, as do the Ugandan soldier-patients presented by Reynolds Whyte and colleagues, the mothers in Nepal presented by Adams, and the mucopolysaccharidosis (MPS) patients presented by Biehl and Petryna. Such is the force of the case studies in global health that this book espouses: descriptive, ethnographic, comparative, and acknowledging global network perfusion throughout local worlds. Ethnography can be an early warning system of problems that are just emerging, as with the emergent cancer epidemic in the wake of immune suppression resulting from HIV/AIDS treatments, which Livingston sees in Botswana and warns will spread throughout Africa. Ethnography is also, as Livingston remarked, "a humanist pursuit with a poetics" that can be a powerful tool for motivating policy without reducing people to two-dimensional victims or sufferers. What is it like to work in a cancer ward or public-sector HIV/AIDS clinic with broken machinery when there is a state-of-the-art Centers for Disease Control or Doris Duke Foundation clinic for HIV/AIDS nearby? Why does relatively rich Botswana have so little morphine available per capita (relative to, say, the United Kingdom)? Among these puzzles is the fact that morphine is very restrictively distributed through the International Narcotics Control Board. Where are the smugglers when we need them?

Ethnography can reveal on many scales how political economies and bioecologies align and misalign. James Pfeiffer's case study brings into sharp focus the trade-offs between the slow building of robust, public-sector health care systems and an emergency, vertically organized, limited-time-and-objectives mode of health care delivery that can operate swiftly because it circumvents bureaucratic and corrupt ministries of health. The drawbacks of the latter approach, Pfeiffer points out, include the need to invest heavily in expatriate salaries, logistics, and the building of parallel infrastructures. As in Mozambique, this approach often has the added disadvantage that it focuses on one disease and ignores the shadow epidemic of hunger and the disincentives that poverty enforces for other aspects of health. The guinea worm eradication program described by

Amy Moran-Thomas not only highlights the conflict of local priorities with those of a humanitarian intervention, but also shows how biology can be more wily than "the best laid plans of men." The guinea worm may yet continue as our companion species, if not as part of our immediate bodies. Similarly, Clara Han's account forcefully reminds us that medicines and public health care programs are absorbed and often refunctioned in the weave of everyday life, and that biomedicine and health are not the same.

Just as Reynolds Whyte and colleagues point to how an ethnography of supply chains can be mapped and made available in ways otherwise not locally accessible, so Ecks and Harper show ethnography bringing to light systemic lags in the global fight against multidrug-resistant tuberculosis. DOTS Plus, Ecks noted during workshop discussion, is only just being introduced in India, and medical representatives are convinced that government DOTS programs are enabling both the acceleration of resistance and a pile-up of resistant strains in the government DOTS clinics. The trade-offs on the macro-scale here are between market-driven pharmaceutical companies and public-sector clinics, rather than (as in Pfeiffer's case study) between PEPFAR, the Bill and Melinda Gates Foundation, and other humanitarian interventions on the one hand and public-sector clinics on the other. The temporalities are uncertain for donor interest, government financing, and companies alike. In the Indian case, Lupin's market dominance at the expense of previous leaders is a reminder that a new generation of therapies could again create new dominant players, and that given this state of affairs firms will remain ever vigilant about market share, what doctors prescribe, and control over public perceptions. The relations between political economy and public health are continually under construction.

V

Mobile Phone Analogies. The promises of new diagnostics and therapies—everything from multidisease, chip-based diagnostic screens; air and water quality monitors; home kits for testing for pesticides on vegetables (all cheap); to telemedical devices, genomic personalized medicines, stem-cell informed regenerative medicine, and perhaps even some do-it-yourself biology public education—all of these sometimes rest uneasily with demands for basic preventive medicine, access to care, disparities, and other issues of social medicine. But molecular biology and genomics (and, in a broader sense, all omics) are fundamental components of our changing epistemologies and of our knowledge about our bodies and ecological habitats, though they do not obviate our need to attend to other holistic components of health and healing.

The mobile phone analogy is adapted from George Church, Harvard Professor of Genetics, technology leader, and founder of the Personal Genome Project (PGP) through which he is trying to amass a large number of whole genomes, together with the medical and environmental records of volunteers, in hopes of making new approaches to disease and health widely available. As he once put it in a Harvard Medical School global health and social medicine class I coteach, it does no good to have one's own personal mobile phone and keep it to oneself—it is the connectivity that is functional. The same is true for genomes and other -omes. PGP volunteers must demonstrate both an understanding of molecular biology (this replaces formalistic informed consent) and a willingness to give up the privacy of their own genetic information (which is impossible to guarantee anyway, given the nature of digital technologies). Church wants to test what effects, if any, public availability of such information would or would not have.

Genomics is a tool not just for the singular body, but also for our emergent ecological consciousness. Church provokes a contemporary imaginary: when microscopes were new, people were shocked by the microorganisms they saw in the water; today we may be in for similar shocks when we realize that as we walk down the street we pass through clouds of genomes, not just a cloud of H1N1 here or multidrug-resistant tuberculosis there. No, if we constantly sampled our mouths we would find that they had taken in the genomes of all the people we just walked by. It raises the issue, he jokes, of whether you are entitled to sequence your own mouth when you are actually sequencing everybody else in your community at the same time, in real time.

We are exposed to allergens in air, water, and food, and to microorganisms and pathogens, he says, and our immune responses and our developmental or epigenomic biology responses to the environment can be measured. "So we have this cohort, we call it a kind of test cohort, to bring a test drive of personalized medicine . . . and in order to do this, to get the maximum feedback for the community, it needs to be shareable, ideally shareable globally, not just among top NIH researchers, but . . . really who knows . . . [among people] who [are] not in the NIH system."

A different peopling of technology is at stake in this political economy of sharing genomes and information. Consider emergent pandemics. Although much was made of SARS as a call for more robust global monitoring collaborations and systems, it was necessary to issue new calls when avian and swine flu arrived on the scene. Clearly, it takes more than one or two scares to motivate the global community to do the work that is needed: to improve global public health infrastructures, build trust among national health ministries, and devise bottom-up social infrastructures that actively involve frontline physicians, health care workers, and scientists (Fischer 2011). Indonesia to this day reserves the right to decline to share samples of its avian flu strains with Singapore and the international community, as it refused in 2005–6, on the defensible grounds that while it is expected to provide samples to the world, the vaccines and drugs that are developed using those samples are rarely made available to its population. Indonesia attacked the WHO system as attuned to the protection of capital rather than to the needs of the populations most at risk. And, as it turned out, the culling of backyard chickens (the focus of international agencies' strategy to battle the flu and an effort much resented by the people) was unwarranted, as the virus most probably came from large industrial chicken farms, not household chickens.

Among the paradigm shifts sparked by the SARS crisis was the role played by the Internet in forcing the WHO to change its policy of relying only on official state reports of epidemics (Fischer 2011). This and other uses of the digital media are shifting authority relations and creating new possibilities for civil society–based public health research, oversight, and policy. The idea of crowdsourcing, mentioned above in the context of patient-driven research endeavors, could also be tried in a research setting, as again India has pioneered. Samir Bhramachari, the director-general of India's Council of Scientific and Industrial Research (CSIR) launched an Open Source Drug Discovery Project (OSDD) in 2008, and in 2010 announced completion and publication on the Internet of an annotation of the four-thousand-gene tuberculosis genome, linking genes to their functions, which was accomplished by four hundred college students under senior OSDD scientists' supervision. Many in the genomics community objected that these amateurs could not be trusted, that the study was not in a peer-reviewed journal, that it had not been verified. Bhramachari responded that the data and analysis were publicly available and that people were free to perform further verification. Submission to a peer-reviewed publication was promised. Some leading scientists, including Gary Schoolnik of Stanford's TB Database and Richard Jefferson of Cambia, a company partnering with OSDD, expressed support for the experiment, saying that its primary failing so far was being "India-centric" and not yet having serious interaction with the Global Alliance for TB Drug Development (Jayaraman 2010; Bhramachari presentation, Human Genome Conference, Montpelier 2010).

Crowdsourcing and citizen science (or at least citizen oversight) is, like patient advocacy, increasingly on the to-do list when it comes to creating civil society–grounded robust public health. This is especially the case, as Whitmarsh says, in such environmental arenas as asthma research and analyses of carcinogenic toxic releases. New methods are being forged in arenas such as toxicogenomics, a response to the inadequacy of traditional toxicology's single-chemical testing protocols. It takes some effort to learn to deal with multiple large data sets informatically, in what Kim and Michael Fortun are calling "informatic environmentalism" as they ethnographically track both the emergence of these new fields and the struggles to keep some of this data from being sequestered on the grounds that it is corporate proprietary information or because its publication could endanger national security (K. Fortun 2004, 2012; K. and M. Fortun 2005, 2007).[2] Another tool being evaluated is the use of Google Flu Trends, a fast crowdsourcing tool, to help hospital emergency rooms prepare for influenza outbreaks instead of the slower traditional tracking methods of the Centers for Disease Control (Dugas et al. 2012; Ginsberg et al. 2009).

In this book, Cueto takes cognizance of the critical role of information technologies in improving public health in the area of infectious disease tracking; Biehl and Petryna of their role in the planning and logistics of fulfilling Brazil's promise of the right to health for all; Whitmarsh in epidemiological genetics public health policy; Pfeiffer of course in all the infrastructures of humanitarian aid delivery and public health sector rebuilding; and Ecks and Harper in pharmaceutical marketing. People too have their own ways of counting through their stories of life and death that run alongside those of governments and NGOs, operating as contextual critiques of international interventions. Moran-Thomas illustrates just this in her social history of guinea worm eradication.

In sum: (1) medical information kept private is much less useful than medical information shared; it is a community good (at the moment unequally appropriated); (2) genomic information is rapidly becoming cheap and having whole genomes available for quick and practical diagnostic use may be on the horizon; (3) we, both inside and out, are literally parts of our communities, and our understanding of this is rapidly expanding through the ecological imaginary that includes our microbiomes and epigenetics, our allergenic and inflammatory responses, all of which are involved in most diseases; and (4) social history is important to understanding the reworking of our human ecologies, health, and disease.

VI

Forward-Looking Values and Being in Dialogue. The final chapters in the book bring us back to questions of shifting epistemologies and bioecological imaginaries. And by focusing on cases of emergent transitions, these chapters also renew the question of how to pursue public health "when people come first."

Whitmarsh turns our attention to new epidemics of noninfectious chronic diseases (heart disease, diabetes, cancer, and asthma) that emerge as low-income countries increasingly take up the eating and living habits of the First World. No longer can it be said that these diseases are of low priority in the developing world. They are said to be diseases of affluence, but Whitmarsh's study shows that they require attention from public health systems as they can also ravage poor communities caught among shifting paradigms of common sense, epistemology, and morality.

There is an ongoing struggle between business models and public health commons (linked to state responsibility, international law, and labor regimes). A superb case to spark thinking about this struggle is Biehl and Petryna's look at the double bind in which Brazil finds itself as it tries to make good on its constitutional promise of a right to health (and access to medicines), while budgetary constraints make it impossible for supply to meet demand. The transitional solution is for patients to sue the state, and for judges to grant limited-period decisions mandating that prescriptions be filled and treatments provided. Even in relatively expensive and hopeless cases, patients are deemed to have the right to life and the right to avoid risk of death. The solution, which requires input from an unprecedented alliance of patient-litigants, activists, government reformers, pharmaceutical companies, and multilateral agencies, is "transitional" because it puts pressure on the state to find more permanent solutions to the contradictions of promise and capacity.

It is also transitional because gene therapies are now on the front lines, as AIDS drugs were in the 1990s. In 1996, Brazil made antiretroviral (ARV) drugs freely available to all in need. This required forcing the hands of multinational pharmaceutical companies by invoking the national medical crisis clauses of the WTO and TRIPS agreements, which allow domestic companies to produce generics of patented drugs or to mandate lower compulsory prices from multinationals. Another kind of institutional solution needs to be found to today's problems: "It is a new world," a doctor in Brazil's universal health care system says. This experiment in the judicialization of health care is remarkable for forcing the state to come up with solutions to scarcity without causing the collapse of the entire system. Informatics is not a trivial issue here.

Biehl and Petryna end, appropriately, with their focus on the struggle across these shifting paradigms of epistemologies, common sense, and moralities: "health in the time of global health is a painstaking work in progress." "By revealing the precariousness of biotechnical and biopolitical interventions," the stories of Brazil's patient-litigants and their families, like the stories of Amy Farber and of the patients that Julie Livingston, Reynolds Whyte and her colleagues, and the other ethnographers in this book present, point to how our human and social worlds are being remade, and they do this by opening up new spaces of contestation and new experimental solutions that people are already experiencing and testing, and that involve and implicate us all.

The lively debate that surrounded and animated these essays when they were being workshopped among people with varied experiences, disciplines, and geographical expertises mirrored the ethnographic ethos and ethics of active talking across situated perspectives and knowledges. Ethnographers need to seize these listening and early warning challenges and present them with all the analytic rigor and poetic vividness that ethnography at its best does so well. No less important, as many of these case studies argue, is that "critical global health studies," as well as health organizations and health research programs, and global health itself, require being in active continuing dialogue with all the people involved, not just producing "dialogues," policies, or ethical principles, but actually talking, exchanging, and involving one another, weaving the liveliness of the future.

Our health depends on it.

Notes

1. http://www.youtube.com/watch?v=r9hCq5AXmmw
2. Also on new citizen tools, web-supported platforms for creating open-source data based on groundwater contamination from fracking techniques of gas drilling, and illnesses people nearby are experiencing, see Wylie 2011.

Contributors

VINCANNE ADAMS is a professor of Medical Anthropology in the Department of Anthropology, History, and Social Medicine at the University of California, San Francisco. She is the author of *Tigers of the Snow and Other Virtual Sherpas* (1995), *Doctors for Democracy: Health Professionals in the Nepal Revolution* (1998), and *Markets of Sorrow, Labors of Faith: New Orleans in the Wake of Katrina* (2013). She is also the editor (with Stacy L. Pigg) of *Sex in Development: Science, Sexuality, and Morality in Global Perspective* (2005) and (with Mona Schrempf and Sienna R. Craig) of *Medicine Between Science and Religion: Explorations on Tibetan Grounds* (2010).

JOSEPH J. AMON is director of the Health and Human Rights Division at Human Rights Watch and a lecturer at the Woodrow Wilson School of Public and International Affairs at Princeton University. Trained in epidemiology, he is the author of more than three dozen peer-reviewed journal articles related to access to medicines, censorship and the denial of health information, arbitrary detention, and the role of civil society in the response to infectious disease outbreaks and environmental health threats.

JOÃO BIEHL is Susan Dod Brown Professor of Anthropology and Faculty Associate of the Woodrow Wilson School of Public and International Affairs at Princeton University. He is also the co-director of Princeton's Program in Global Health and Health Policy. Biehl is the author of *Vita: Life in a Zone of Social Abandonment* (2005) and *Will to Live: AIDS Therapies and the Politics of Survival* (2007). He is also the editor (with Byron Good and Arthur Kleinman) of *Subjectivity: Ethnographic Investigations* (2007).

MARCOS CUETO is a professor at the School of Public Health of the Universidad Peruano Cayetano Heredia and a researcher at the Instituto de Estudios Peruanos in Lima. He is currently a visiting professor at the Casa Oswaldo Cruz at FIOCRUZ, Brazil. A historian of medicine, he is the author of *Cold War, Deadly Fevers: Malaria Eradication in Mexico, 1955–1975* (2007) and is presently working on a history of global health and its impact on the World Health Organization.

STEFAN ECKS is a senior lecturer in the Department of Social Anthropology and director of the Medical Anthropology Programme at the University of Edinburgh. He is the author of *Eating Drugs: Psychopharmaceutical Pluralism in India* (2013) and has published articles on migration and health, medical pluralism, the anthropology of pharmaceuticals and food, and transcultural psychiatry in journals such as *BioSocieties*, the *Journal of the Royal Anthropological Institute*, and *Anthropology & Medicine*.

DIDIER FASSIN is James D. Wolfensohn Professor of Social Science at the Institute for Advanced Study and Director of Studies at the École des Hautes Études en Sciences Sociales in Paris. His books include *When Bodies Remember: Experiences and Politics of AIDS in South Africa* (2007), *The Empire of Trauma: An Inquiry into the Condition of Victimhood* (with Richard Rechtman, 2009), *Humanitarian Reason: A Moral History of the Present* (2011), and *La Force de l'Ordre: Une Anthropologie de la Police des Quartiers* (2012). He also edited (with Mariella Pandolfi) *Contemporary States of Emergency* (2010) and *A Companion to Moral Anthropology* (2012).

MICHAEL M. J. FISCHER is Andrew W. Mellon Professor in the Humanities and a professor of Anthropology and Science and Technology Studies at MIT, and a lecturer in the Department of Global Health and Social Medicine at Harvard Medical School. His books include *Anthropological Futures* (2009), *Emergent Forms of Life and the Anthropological Voice* (2003), *Anthropology as Cultural Critique* (with George E. Marcus, 1986, 1999), *Mute Dreams, Blind Owls, and Dispersed Knowledges* (2004), *Debating Muslims: Cultural Dialogues in Postmodernity and Tradition*

(1990), and *Iran: From Religious Dispute to Revolution* (1980). He is the editor (with Byron Good, Sarah Willen, and Mary Jo DelVecchio Good) of *A Medical Anthropology Reader: Theoretical Trajectories and Emergent Realities* (2010).

CLARA HAN is an assistant professor in the Department of Anthropology at Johns Hopkins University. She is the author of *Life in Debt: Times of Care and Violence in Neoliberal Chile* (2012) and has published articles in journals such as *Cultural Anthropology* and *Culture, Medicine, and Psychiatry*. Trained in medicine, she is conducting NSF-funded research on relatedness, incarceration, and the play of life and death in a neighborhood under police occupation in Santiago, Chile.

IAN HARPER is a senior lecturer and head of the Department of Social Anthropology at the University of Edinburgh. Trained in medicine, he is a Wellcome Trust Senior Investigator in Medical Humanities for the project "Understanding TB Control: Technologies, Ethics and Programmes," and has published on public health issues and pharmaceutical regulation and drug compliance and resistance in South Asia.

JULIE LIVINGSTON is a professor in the Department of History at Rutgers University. She is the author of *Improvising Medicine: An African Oncology Ward in an Emerging Cancer Epidemic* (2012) and *Debility and the Moral Imagination in Botswana* (2005). She is editor (with Jasbir Puar) of *Interspecies* (2011); (with Keith Wailoo, Steven Epstein, and Robert Aronowitz) of *Three Shots at Prevention: The HPV Vaccine and the Politics of Medicine's Simple Solutions* (2010); and (with Keith Wailoo and Peter Guarnaccia) of *A Death Retold: Jesica Santillan, the Bungled Transplant, and the Paradoxes of Medical Citizenship* (2006).

LOTTE MEINERT is a professor in the Department of Culture and Society at Aarhus University. She is the author of *Hopes in Friction: Schooling, Health, and Everyday Life in Uganda* (2008) and collaborated on the book *Second Chances: Living with ART in Uganda* (forthcoming). She is presently leading a research program on governance, trust, and land in postconflict northern Uganda.

AMY MORAN-THOMAS is a postdoctoral researcher at the Woodrow Wilson School of Public and International Affairs at Princeton University. Her work, appearing in publications such as the *Annual Review of Anthropology*, examines parasitic and metabolic disorders as windows into global health politics and ethics of care more broadly. Her current book project focuses on the global diabetes epidemic.

ADRIANA PETRYNA is Edmund J. and Louise W. Kahn Term Professor in the Department of Anthropology at the University of Pennsylvania. She is the author of *Life Exposed: Biological Citizens after Chernobyl* (2002, 2013) and *When Experiments Travel: Clinical Trials and the Global Search for Human Subjects* (2009). She also edited (with Andrew Lakoff and Arthur Kleinman) *Global Pharmaceuticals: Ethics, Markets, Practices* (2006).

JAMES PFEIFFER is an associate professor in the Department of Global Health with a joint appointment in the Department of Anthropology at the University of Washington in Seattle. He also directs the Mozambique Programs of Health Alliance International (a US-based nonprofit organization affiliated with the University of Washington) that focuses on strengthening primary health care in the public sector. He has published articles on NGOs and global health activism, HIV care and treatment scale-up, and Pentecostalism and Zionism in southern Africa in journals such as *Social Science & Medicine, American Anthropologist*, the *Journal of AIDS, Medical Anthropology Quarterly*, and the *American Journal of Public Health*.

JENIPHER TWEBAZE is a doctoral student in the Department of Anthropology at the University of Copenhagen. Her dissertation project "Medicines for Life" focuses on Ugandan health workers and clients of antiretroviral therapy. She collaborated on the book *Second Chances: Living with ART in Uganda* (forthcoming).

IAN WHITMARSH is an associate professor in the Department of Anthropology, History, and Social Medicine at the University of California, San Francisco. He is the author of *Biomedical Ambiguity: Race, Asthma, and the Contested Meaning of Genetic Research in the Caribbean* (2008) and editor (with David Jones) of *What's the Use of Race? Modern Governance and the Biology of Difference* (2010).

MICHAEL A. WHYTE is Emeritus Associate Professor of the Department of Anthropology at the University of Copenhagen. He led the first Danish anthropological study of AIDS in Africa during the early days of the epidemic and is currently involved in a study of land conflict in Uganda. He is editor (with Quentin Gausset and Torben Birch-Thomsen) of *Beyond Territory and Scarcity: Exploring Conflicts over Natural Resource Management* (2005) and collaborated on the book *Second Chances: Living with ART in Uganda* (forthcoming). He has coauthored numerous articles on food scarcity, land conflict, and AIDS.

SUSAN REYNOLDS WHYTE is a professor in the Department of Anthropology at the University of Copenhagen. She is the author of *Questioning Misfortune: The Pragmatics of Uncertainty in Eastern Uganda* (1998) and is lead author of *Second Chances: Living with ART in Uganda* (forthcoming). She edited (with Sjaak van der Geest and Anita Hardon) *Social Lives of Medicines* (2003) and (with Benedicte Ingstad) *Disability and Culture* (1995) and *Disability in Local and Global Worlds* (2007).

Acknowledgments

"And so each venture," T. S. Elliot writes, "is a new beginning, a raid on the inarticulate."

We loved doing this book. This is an effort to grapple with the worlds of global health today. To understand what is going on, to name what is missing, to try to find words for what is possible. To understand *with* people in the field, *with* students in the classroom, and *with* the case studies that colleagues and friends brought to this critical endeavor. Knowing that for us, "there is only the trying."

Thank you to all who helped to make this book possible. What a moving and gratifying experience it has been to engage the rich empirical materials and probing analytical work of all the book's contributors, and, through our colleagues and friends, to be brought into a larger ecology of comparative understanding and contact. We are fortunate to be part of this thoughtful chain, and we hope that the book will further expand what we can know and act on.

Princeton's Institute for International and Regional Studies (PIIRS) generously supported the April 2010 exploratory seminar in which the book's cases were initially presented and discussed. We are also grateful to Princeton's Health Grand Challenges Initiative, the Woodrow Wilson School for Public and International Affairs, and the Ford Foundation for supporting research and various events that helped build the book.

This project has greatly benefitted from intellectual exchanges with and assistance from a superb group of postdoctoral fellows and graduate and undergraduate students. We are particularly thankful to Amy Moran-Thomas, Erin Fitz-Henry, Peter Locke, Sebastian Ramirez, and Celeste Alexander for their terrific input and editorial help. We also thank Ramah McKay, Elizabeth Hallowell, Mariana P. Socal, Michael Joiner, Joshua

Franklin, Alex Gertner, Raphael Frankfurter, Courtney Crumpler, Naomi Zucker, Jessica Haley, Allison Daminger, Alyse Wheelock, Sonia T. Porter, Raaj Mehta, and Amy and Steven Porter.

Our academic institutions have been a source of continuous stimulation, and the human resources of both Princeton and Penn never cease to amaze us. We thank the engaging faculty and the wonderfully supportive staff of the departments, schools, and programs we are a part of: at Princeton, the Department of Anthropology, the Woodrow Wilson School of Public and International Affairs, the Center for Health and Wellbeing, the Program in Global Health and Health Policy, and the Program in Latin American Studies; and at Penn, the Department of Anthropology, the Department of the History and Sociology of Science, and the Benjamin Franklin Scholars Program. Special thanks to Shirley M. Tilghman and David P. Dobkin for all their support.

We learned much from discussions as we presented works-in-progress in our classes in medical anthropology, global health and health policy, cultures of medicine, globalization and health, and ethnography and social theory today. Over several years, the Science, Technology, and Medicine Interest Group of the Society for Medical Anthropology sponsored panels at the annual meetings of the American Anthropological Association that were incredibly productive.

Joseph J. Amon and Didier Fassin have been crucial interlocutors throughout, and we thank them for all their insights and help. We also owe a debt of gratitude to many scholars for their support and stimulating feedback, particularly Richard Parker, Nitsan Chorev, Christina Paxson, Ingo W. Sarlet, Laura B. Jardim, Michael E. Porter, Tom Vogl, Claudia W. Fonseca, Varun Gauri, Evan Lieberman, Nancy Scheper-Hughes, Arthur Kleinman, Paul Farmer, Angus Deaton, Anne Case, Steven Feierman, Deborah Thomas, Janet Monge, Philippe Bourgois, Marcia Inhorn, Kristina Graff, Lilia M. Schwarcz, and João Moreira Salles. Thank you also to Vik Muniz for his powerful artwork and to Claudia Warrak and Raul Loureiro for their beautiful design. The visionary work of Albert O. Hirschman has expanded our humanistic and critical horizons, as have keen conversations with Sarah Hirschman.

At Princeton University Press, we are deeply grateful to Peter Dougherty for his stalwart support of *When People Come First*. We also thank our editor Fred Appel for his editorial guidance, as well as Beth Clevenger, Mark Bellis, Maria Lindenfeldar, Lorraine Doneker, Eva Jaunzems, Lauren Lepow, Sylvia Coates, and Sarah David for their great help and fine work at every step.

Finally, we want to wholeheartedly thank our interlocutors in the field and our graduate and undergraduate students as well as our son Andre, for pushing boundaries and opening up new avenues for understanding and doing in this world.

References

Abbasi, Kamran. 1999. "The World Bank and World Health: Interview with Richard Feachem." *British Medical Journal* 318(7192): 1206–8.

Abebe, Taktek. 2010. "Beyond the 'Orphan Burden': Understanding Care for and by AIDS-Affected Children in Africa." *Geography Compass* 4(5): 460–74.

Actuarial Society of South Africa. 2006. "Orphans Statistics by Province." Accessed January 19, 2011: http://aids.actuarialsociety.org.za/default.asp?pageid=3165.

Adams, Vincanne. 2005. "Saving Tibet? An Inquiry into Modernity, Lies, Truths, and Belief." *Medical Anthropology* 24(1): 71–110.

Adams, Vincanne, Thomas Novotny, and Hannah Leslie. 2008. "Global Health Diplomacy." *Medical Anthropology* 27(4):315–23.

African Health. 1998. "Worldwide Battle against Malaria." *African Health* 20(5): 34.

Alvarado, Rubén, Jorge Vega, Gabriel Sanhueza, and María Graciela Muñoz. 2005. "Evaluación del Programa para la Detección, Diagnóstico y Tratamiento Integral de la Depresión en Atención Primaria, en Chile." *Pan American Journal of Public Health* 18(4/5): 278–86.

Amon, Joseph J. 2006. "Preventing the Further Spread of HIV/AIDS: The Essential Role of Human Rights." In *Human Rights Watch World Report 2006*. New York: Seven Stories Press.

———. 2008. "Dangerous Medicines: Unproven AIDS Cures and Counterfeit Antiretroviral Drugs." *Globalization and Health* 4(5).

Amon, Joseph J., Françoise Girard, and Salmaan Keshavjee. 2009. "Limitations on Human Rights in the Context of Drug-Resistant Tuberculosis: A Reply to Boggio et al." *Health and Human Rights: An International Journal* (Perspectives) 11(1): 1–10.

Amon, Joseph J., and Tiseke Kasambala. 2009. "Structural Barriers and Human Rights Related to HIV Prevention and Treatment in Zimbabwe." *Global Public Health* 4(6): 528–45.

Amon, Joseph J., and Katherine W. Todrys. 2008. "Fear of Foreigners: HIV-Related Restrictions on Entry, Stay, and Residence." *Journal of the International AIDS Society* 11: 8.

Anand, Sudhir, and Kara Hanson. 1997. "Disability-Adjusted Life Years: A Critical Perspective." *Journal of Health Economics* 16: 685–702.

Appiah, Kwame Anthony. 2008. *Experiments in Ethics.* Cambridge: Harvard University Press.

Applbaum, Kalman. 2010. "Marketing Global Health Care: The Practices of Big Pharma." In *The Socialist Register 2010: Morbid Symptoms: Health under Capitalism*, Leo Panitch, ed., 95–115. New York: Monthly Review Press.

Apter, Andrea J., Susan T. Reisine, Glenn Affleck, Erik Barrows, and Richard L. ZuWallack. 1998. "Adherence with Twice-Daily Dosing of Inhaled Steroids: Socioeconomic and Health-Belief Differences." *American Journal of Respiratory and Critical Care Medicine* 157(6): 1810–17.

Apter, Andrew. 1993. "Atinga Revisited: Yoruba Witchcraft and the Cocoa Economy." In *Modernity and Its Malcontents: Ritual Power in Postcolonial Africa*, J. Comaroff and J. L. Comaroff, eds., 111–29. Chicago: University of Chicago Press.

Araya, Ricardo. 1995. "Trastornos Mentales en la Atención Primaria Santiago, Chile." Santiago, Chile: Universidad de Chile, Departamento de Psiquiatría.

Araya, Ricardo, Rubén Alvarado, and Alberto Minoletti. 2009. "Chile: An Ongoing Mental Health Revolution." *Lancet* 374(9690): 597–98.

Araya, Ricardo, Graciela Rojas, Rosemarie Fritsch, Julia Acuña, and Glyn Lewis. 2001. "Common Mental Disorders in Santiago, Chile." *British Journal of Psychiatry* 176: 228–33.

———. 2003a. "Education and Income: Which Is More Important for Mental Health?" *Journal of Epidemiology and Community Health* 57: 501–5.

———. 2003b. "Treating Depression in Primary Care in Low-Income Women in Santiago, Chile: A Randomised Controlled Trial." *Lancet* 361: 995–1000.

———. 2006. "Inequities in Mental Health Care After Health Care System Reform in Chile." *American Journal of Public Health* 96(1): 109–113.

Ariès, Philippe. 1965. *Centuries of Childhood: A Social History of Family Life*. New York: Vintage (French edition 1960).

Arora, Vijay K., R. Sarin, and Knut Lonnroth. 2003. "Feasibility and Effectiveness of a Public-Private Mix Project for Improved TB Control in Delhi, India." *International Journal of Tuberculosis and Lung Disease* 7(12): 1131–38.

Arriagada, Irma. 2010. "La Crisis del Cuidado en Chile." In *Construyendo Redes: Mujeres Latinoamericanas en las Cadenas Globales de Cuidado*. Santiago: Centro de Estudios de la Mujer/INSTRAW.

Asad, Talal. 2003. *Formations of the Secular: Christianity, Islam, Modernity*. Palo Alto, CA: Stanford University Press.

Ashforth, Adam. 2005. *Witchcraft, Violence, and Democracy in South Africa*. Chicago: University of Chicago Press.

Associated Press. 2012. "23andMe Seeks FDA Approval for Personal DNA Test." *National Public Radio*. Accessed July 30, 2012: http://www.npr.org/templates/story/story.php?storyId=157598936.

Audibert, M. 1993. "Invalidité Temporaire et Production Agricole: Les Effets de la Dracunculose dans une Agriculture de Subsistence." *Revue d'Économie du Développement* 1: 23–26.

Austen, Ralph. 1993. "The Moral Economy of Witchcraft: An Essay in Comparative History." In *Modernity and Its Malcontents: Ritual Power in Postcolonial Africa*, J. Comaroff and J. L. Comaroff, eds. Chicago: University of Chicago Press.

Azevedo, S. 2007. "Remédios nos tribunais." Revista Época. December 12. http://revistaepoca.globo.com/Revista/Epoca/0,,EDG80696-8055-501,00-REMEDIOS+NOS+TRIBUNAIS.html.

Barrientos, Armando. 2000. "Getting Better after Neoliberalism: Shifts and Challenges of Health Policy in Chile." In *Health Reform and Poverty in Latin America*, Peter Lloyd-Sherlock, ed. London: Institute of Latin American Studies.

Barry, Michele. 2007. "The Tail End of Guinea Worm—Global Eradication without a Drug or a Vaccine." *New England Journal of Medicine* 356: 2561–64.

BASF Chemical Company. 2012. "Pharma Ingredients & Services." Accessed April 18, 2012: http://www.pharma-ingredients.basf.com/Home.aspx.

Bate, Roger. 2008. "Stifling Dissent on Malaria." *The American*, December 8. http://www.american.com/archive/2008/december-12-08/stifling-dissent-on-malaria.

Bayart, J. F. 1993. *The State in Africa: The Politics of the Belly*. New York: Longman.

Beck, Michael. 2007. "New Therapeutic Options for Lysosomal Storage Disorders: Enzyme Replacement, Small Molecules and Gene Therapy." *Human Genetics* 121: 1–22.

Beegle, Kathleen, Deon Filmer, Andrew Stokes, and Lucia Tiererova. 2010. "Orphanhood and the Living Arrangements of Children in Sub-Saharan Africa." *World Development* 38(2): 1727–46.

Behforouz, Heidi L., Paul Farmer, and Joia S. Muhkerjee. 2004. "From Directly Observed Therapy to Accompagnateurs: Enhancing AIDS Treatment Outcomes in Haiti and in Boston." *Clinical Infectious Diseases* 38: S429–36.

Behrouzan, Orkideh. 2011. "An Epidemic of Meanings: The Importance of Language, Gender, and History in HIV and AIDS Responses." In *The Fourth Wave: Violence, Gender, Culture and HIV in the 21st Century*, Vinh-Kim Nguyen and Jennifer Klot, eds. New York: UNESCO/Social Science Research Council.

Belcher, D. W., F. K. Wurapa, W. B. Ward, and I. M. Lourie. 1975. "Guinea Worm in Southern Ghana: Its Epidemiology and Impact on Agricultural Productivity." *American Journal of Tropical Medicine and Hygiene* 24(2): 243–49.

Bellingham, Bruce. 1988. "The History of Childhood Since the 'Invention of Childhood': Some Issues of the Eighties." *Journal of Family History* 13(2): 347–58.

Bender, Bruce G. 2002. "Overcoming Barriers to Nonadherence in Asthma Treatment." *Journal of Allergy and Clinical Immunology* 109(6 Suppl.): S554–59.

Berkman, Alan, Jonathan Garcia, Miguel Muñoz-Laboy, Vera Paiva, and Richard Parker. 2005. "A Critical Analysis of the Brazilian Response to HIV/AIDS: Lessons Learned for Controlling and Mitigating the Epidemic in Developing Countries." *American Journal of Public Health* 95(7): 1162–72.

Bhandari, Bhupesh. 2005. *The Ranbaxy Story: The Rise of an Indian Multinational*. New Delhi: Penguin.

Bhramachari, Samir. 2010. Presentation, Human Genome Conference, Montpelier.

Biehl, João. 2004. "The Activist State: Global Pharmaceuticals, AIDS, and Citizenship in Brazil." *Social Text* 80, 22(3): 105–32.

———. 2007. *Will to Live: AIDS Therapies and the Politics of Survival*. Princeton, NJ: Princeton University Press.

———. 2008. "Drugs for All: The Future of Global AIDS Treatment." *Medical Anthropology* 27(2): 99–105.

Biehl, João, Joseph J. Amon, Mariana P. Socal, and Adriana Petryna. 2012. "Between the Court and the Clinic: Lawsuits for Medicines and the Right to Health in Brazil." *Health and Human Rights: An International Journal* 14(1): 1–17.

Biehl, João, Adriana Petryna, Alex Gertner, Joseph J. Amon, and Paulo D. Picon. 2009. "Judicialisation of the Right to Health in Brazil." *Lancet* 373: 2182–84.

Bierlich, Bernhard. 1995. "Notions and Treatment of Guinea Worm in Northern Ghana." *Social Science and Medicine* 41(4): 501–9.

———. 2007. *The Problem of Money: African Agency and Western Medicine in Northern Ghana.* Oxford: Berghahn Books.

Bimi, L., A. R. Freeman, M. L. Eberhard, E. Ruiz-Tiben, and N. J. Pieniazek. 2005. "Differentiating *Dracunculus medinensis* from *D. insignis*, by the Sequence Analysis of the 18S rRNA Gene." *Annals of Tropical Medicine and Parasitology* 99: 511–17.

Birn, Anne-Emmanuelle. 2005a. "Uruguay on the World Stage: How Child Health Became an International Priority." *American Journal of Public Health* 95(9): 1506–17.

———. 2005b. "Gates's Grandest Challenge: Transcending Technology as Public Health Ideology." *Lancet* 366: 514–19.

Bloom, Barry R., David E. Bloom, Joel E. Cohen, and Jeffrey D. Sachs. 1999. "Investing in the World Health Organization." *Science* 284(5416): 911.

Bolnick, Deborah A., et al. 2007. "The Science and Business of Genetic Ancestry Testing." *Science* 318(5849): 399–400.

Bornstein, Erica, and Peter Redfield, eds. 2011. *Forces of Compassion: Humanitarianism between Ethics and Politics.* Santa Fe, NM: School of Advanced Research Press.

Boseley, Sarah. 2006. "Arata Kochi: Shaking up the Malaria World." *Lancet* 367(9527): 1973.

Botswana National Cancer Registry. 2006. *Analysis of Registered Cancer Patients 1986–2006.* Republic of Botswana Ministry of Health, Department of Public Health Disease Control Unit, Non-Communicable Diseases Programme. Draft copy.

Bourdieu, Pierre. 1998. "Neo-liberalism, the Utopia (Becoming Reality) of Unlimited Exploitation," 94–105. In *Acts of Resistance: Against the Tyranny of the Market.* New York: The New Press.

———. 2000. *Pascalian Meditations.* Cambridge, UK: Polity Press.

Bourne, Peter. 1982. "Global Eradication of Guinea Worm." *Journal of the Royal Society of Medicine* 75: 1–3.

Brada, Betsey. 2011. "'The World Is Our Clinic': Citizenship, Philanthropy, and the Logic of AIDS Treatment in Botswana." PhD dissertation, University of Chicago.

Braun, Lundy, Anne Fausto-Sterling, Duana Fullwiley, Evelynn M. Hammonds, Alondra Nelson, William Quivers, Susan M. Reverby, and Alexandra E. Shields. 2007. "Racial Categories in Medical Practice: How Useful Are They?" *PLoS Medicine* 4(9): e271.

Bray, Rachel. 2003. "Predicting the Social Consequences of Orphanhood in South Africa." *African Journal of AIDS Research* 2(1): 39–55.

Breman, Joel G., Wenceslaus L. Kilama, Brian Greenwood, Pierre Druilhe, David Nabarro, and Kamini Mendis. 2000. "Rolling Back Malaria: Action or Rhetoric." *Bulletin of the World Health Organization* 78(12): 1450–55.

Breman, J. G., and I. Arita. 2011. "The Certification of Smallpox Eradication and Implications for Guinea Worm, Poliomyelitis, and Other Diseases: Confirming and Maintaining a Negative." *Vaccine* 29(s4): D41–8.

Brhlikova, Petra, Ian Harper, Roger Jeffery, Nabin Rawal, Madhusudhan Subedi, and M. R. Santosh. 2011. "Trust and Regulation of Pharmaceuticals: South Asia in a Globalised World." *Global Health* 7(10): 1–13.

Brieger, William, Saubana A. Adekunle, Ganiyu A. Oke, and Azeez Adesope. 1996. "Culturally Perceived Illness and Guinea Worm Disease Surveillance." *Health Policy and Planning* 11(1): 101–6.

Brieger, William, Sakiru Otusanya, Joshua D. Adeniyi, Jamiyu Tijani, and Muyiwa Banjoko. 1997. "Eradicating Guinea Worm Disease without Wells: Unrealized Hopes of the Water Decade." *Health Policy and Planning* 12(4): 354–62.

Briss, Peter A., Ross C. Brownson, Jonathan Fielding, and Stephanie Zaza. 2004. "Developing and Using the Guide to Community Preventive Services: Lessons Learned about Evidence-Based Public Health." *Annual Review of Public Health* 25: 281–302.

Bristol, Nellie. 2008. "Donald R. Hopkins: Eradicating Guinea Worm Disease." *Lancet* 371: 1571.

Brody, Alan. 2006. "In One Country, AIDS on the Rampage." *New York Times*, August 12, http://www.nytimes.com/2006/08/12/opinion/12brody.html.

Brotherton, P. Sean. 2012. *Revolutionary Medicine: Health and the Body in Post-Soviet Cuba*. Durham, NC: Duke University Press.

Brown, Theodore M., Marcos Cueto, and Elizabeth Fee. 2006. "The World Health Organization and the Transition from 'International' to 'Global' Public Health." *American Journal of Public Health* 96(1): 62–72.

Brownson, Ross C., Elizabeth A. Baker, Terry L. Leet, and Kathleen N. Gillespie. 2003. *Evidence-Based Public Health*. Oxford: Oxford University Press.

Brownson, Ross C., James G. Gurney and Garland H. Land. 1999. "Evidence-Based Decision Making in Public Health." *Journal of Public Health Management Practice* 5(5): 86–97.

Bruce-Chwatt, Leonard Jan. 1980. "Need for New Weapons." *World Health Forum* 1: 23–24.

Brugha, Rauirí, Martine Donoghue, Mary Sterling, Phillimon Ndubani, Freddie Ssengooba, Benedita Fernandes, and Gill Walt. 2004. "The Global Fund: Managing Great Expectations." *Lancet* 364(9428): 95–100.

Burawoy, Michael. 1998. "The Extended Case Method." *Sociological Theory* 16(1): 4–33.

Burris, Scott, Leo Beletesky, Joseph A. Burleson, Patricia Case, and Zita Lazzarini. 2007. "Do Criminal Laws Influence HIV Risk Behavior? An Empirical Trial." *Arizona State Law Journal* 39(2): 467–519.

Buse, Ken, and Gill Walt. 2000. "Global Public-Private Partnerships. Part II: What Are the Health Issues for Global Governance?" *Bulletin of the World Health Organization* 78: 699–709.

Buss, Paulo M., and José R. Ferreira. 2010. "Health Diplomacy and South-South Cooperation: The Experiences of UNASUR Salud and CPLP's Strategic Plan for Cooperation in Health." *RECIIS Rev. Electron. Comun. Inf. Inov. Saúde* 4(1): 99–110; published online March. Accessed June 2012: http://www.revista.icict. fiocruz.br/index.php/reciis/article/view/351/520.

Butchart, Alexander. 1998. *The Anatomy of Power: European Constructions of the African Body*. London: Zed Books.

Cairncross, Sandy. 1995. "Victory over Guineaworm Disease: Partial or Pyrrhic?" *Lancet* 346(8988): 1440.

Cairncross, Sandy, Ralph Muller, and Nevio Zagaria. 2002. "Dracunculiasis (Guinea Worm Disease) and the Eradication Initiative." *Clinical Microbiology Reviews* 15(2): 223–46.

Cairncross, Sandy, Ahmed Taylor, and Andrew Seidu Korkor. 2012. "Why Is Dracunculiasis Eradication Taking So Long?" *Trends in Parasitology* 28(6): 225–30.

Campos, G.W.S. 2007. "O SUS entre a tradição dos Sistemas Nacionais e o modo liberal-privado para organizar o cuidado à saúde." *Ciência & Saúde Coletiva* 12: 1865–74.

Canguilhem, Georges. 1991. *The Normal and the Pathological*. New York: Zone Books.

———. 2008. *Knowledge of Life*. New York: Fordham University Press.

Carter, Jimmy. 2007. "Trip Report of Former US President Jimmy Carter: Africa Trip, Feb. 6–16, 2007." Accessed January 5, 2008: http://www.cartercenter.org/news/trip_reports/africa_2007.html.

Carter Center. 2002. "Q & A Session with Carter Center's Dr. Donald Hopkins on the Eradication of Smallpox." Accessed April 3, 2012: http://www.cartercenter.org/news/documents/doc1045.html.

———. 2004. "Final Reflections from Africa: February 3–5, Ghana." News & Publications. Accessed April 18, 2012: http://www.cartercenter.org/news/features/h/guinea_worm/miss_ghana.html.

———. 2006. "Miss Ghana Vows to Fight Guinea Worm Disease in Her Home Country." Accessed April 14, 2012: http://www.cartercenter.org/news/features/h/guinea_worm/miss_ghana.html.

———. 2011. "2011 Totals—Guinea Worm Countdown: The Road to Eradication, Countdown to Zero." Accessed April 26, 2012: http://www.cartercenter.org/health/guinea_worm/mini_site/current.html.

Cartwright, Nancy. 2011. "A Philosopher's View of the Long Road from RCTs to Effectiveness." *Lancet* 377(9775): 1400–1401.

Cartwright, Nancy, and Jeremy Hardie. 2012. *Evidence-Based Policy: A Practical Guide to Doing It Better*. New York: Oxford University Press.

Carvalho, Marcelo Felga, Ana Roberta Pati Pascom, Paulo Roberto Borges de Souza-Júnior, Giseli Nogueira Damacena, and Célia Landmann Szwarcwald. 2005. "Utilization of Medicines by the Brazilian Population, 2003." *Cadernos de Saúde Pública* 21, Suppl: 100–108.

Castel, Robert. 1991. "From Dangerousness to Risk." In *The Foucault Effect: Studies in Governmentality*. Graham Burchell, Colin Gordon, and Peter Miller, eds., 281–98. Chicago: University of Chicago Press.

Cavell, Stanley. 1979. *The World Viewed: Reflections on the Ontology of Film*. Cambridge, MA: Harvard University Press.

———. 1997. "Comments on Veena Das's Essay, 'Language and Body: Transactions in the Construction of Pain.' " In *Social Suffering*, Arthur Kleinman, Veena Das, and Margaret Lock, eds., 93–99. Berkeley: University of California Press.

Centers for Disease Control [CDC]. 2011a. "Parasites—Dracunculiasis (Also Known as Guinea Worm Disease): Eradication Program." Accessed April 29, 2012: http://www.cdc.gov/parasites/guineaworm/gwep.html.

———. 2011b. "Progress toward Global Eradication of Dracunculiasis, January 2010–June 2011." *Morbidity and Mortality Weekly Report* 60(42): 1450–53.

Cernea, Michael. 1991. *Putting People First: Sociological Variables in Rural Development*. Washington, DC: A World Bank Publication.

Chabal, Patrick, and Jean Paul Daloz. 1999. *Africa Works: Disorder as Political Instrument*. Bloomington: Indiana University Press.

Chaganti, Subba R. 2007. *Pharmaceutical Marketing in India*. New Delhi: Excel Books.

Chapman, Rachel. 2003. "Endangering Safe Motherhood in Mozambique: Prenatal Care as Pregnancy Risk." *Social Science and Medicine* 57(2): 355–74.

Chaudhuri, Sudip. 2005. *The WTO and India's Pharmaceuticals Industry*. New Delhi: Oxford University Press.

Chen, Rui, et al. 2012. "Personal Omics Profiling Reveals Dynamic Molecular and Medical Phenotypes." *Cell* 148(6): 1293–1307.

Chieffi, A. L., and R. B. Barata. 2009. "Judicialização da política pública de assistência farmacêutica e eqüidade." *Cadernos de Saúde Pública* 25(8): 1839–49.

Clarke, Lorne A. 2007. "Mucopolysaccharidosis Type I." *GeneReviews*, September 21. http://www.ncbi.nlm.nih.gov/books/NBK1162/.

———. 2008. "The Mucopolysaccharidoses: A Success of Molecular Medicine." *Expert Reviews in Molecular Medicine* 10: e1.

Cleland, Charles S., Yoshio Nakamura, Tito R. Mendoza, Katherine R. Edwards, Jeff Douglas, and Ronald C. Serlin. 1996. "Dimensions of the Impact of Cancer Pain in a Four Country Sample: New Information from Multidimensional Scaling." *Pain* 67(2–3): 267–73.

Cliff, Julie. 1991. "The War on Women in Mozambique: Health Consequences of South African Destabilization, Economic Crisis, and Structural Adjustment." In *Women and Health in Africa*, Meredith Turshen, ed., 15–33. Trenton, NJ: Africa World Press.

———. 1993. "Donor Dependence or Donor Control? The Case of Mozambique." *Community Development Journal* 28(3): 237–44.

Coetzee, David, Katherine Hilderbrand, Eric Goemaere, Francine Matthys, and Marleen Boelaert. 2004. "Integrating Tuberculosis and HIV Care in the Primary Care Setting in South Africa." *Tropical Medicine and International Health* 9(6): A11–A15.

Cohen, Jon. 2006. "The New World of Global Health." *Science* 311(5758): 162–67.

Coll-Seck, Awa Marie, Tedros Ghebreyesus, and Alan Court. 2008. "Malaria: Efforts Starting to Show Widespread Results." *Nature* 452(718): 810.

Collins, Francis S., and Victor A. McKusick. 2001. "Implications of the Human Genome Project for Medical Science." *Journal of the American Medical Association* 285(5): 540–44.

Collucci, C. 2009. "Triplicam as ações judiciais para obter medicamentos." Folha de São Paulo, Jan 9, 2009. Accessed August 10, 2010: http://proquest.umi.com/pqdweb?did=1653546171&sid=2&Fmt=3&clientId=17210&RQT=309&VName=PQD.

Comacchio, Cynthia. 1998. *Nations Are Built of Babies: Saving Ontario's Mothers and Children, 1900–1940*. Montreal: McGill-Queen's University Press.

Comaroff, Jean. 2007. "Beyond Bare Life: AIDS, (Bio)politics, and the Neoliberal Order." *Public Culture* 19(1): 197–219.

Comaroff, Jean, and John Comaroff. 1991. *Of Revelation and Revolution: Christianity, Colonialism, and Consciousness in South Africa*. Chicago: University of Chicago Press.

———. 2001. *Millennial Capitalism and the Culture of Neoliberalism*. Durham, NC: Duke University Press.

———. 2006. "Law and Disorder in the Postcolony: An Introduction." In *Law and Disorder in the Postcolony*, Jean Comaroff and John Comaroff, eds., 1–56. Chicago: University of Chicago Press.

Conger, Krista. 2012. "Revolution in Personalized Medicine: First-Ever Integrative 'Omics' Profile Lets Scientist Discover, Track His Diabetes Onset." Stanford School of Medicine, 15 March. http://med.stanford.edu/ism/2012/march/snyder.html.

Connor, Edward, et al. 1994. "Reduction of Maternal-Infant Transmission of Human Immunodeficiency Virus Type 1 with Zidovudine Treatment." *New England Journal of Medicine* 331(18): 1173–80.

Conrad, Peter. 2007. *The Medicalization of Society: On the Transformation of Human Conditions into Treatable Disorders*. Baltimore, MD: Johns Hopkins University Press.

Constituição Federal do Brasil. 1988. http://dtr2004.saude.gov.br/susdeaz/legislacao/arquivo/01_Constituicao.pdf.

Crossette, Barbara. 1998a. "New Leader of WHO Gets Big Grant to Hire Experts." *New York Times*, July 21.

———. 1998b. "2 Physicians Lead the Race for Top Job." *New York Times*, January 11.

———. 1998c. "UN and World Bank Unite to Wage War on Malaria." *New York Times*, October 13.

Cueto, Marcos. 2007. *Cold War, Deadly Fevers: Malaria Eradication in Mexico, 1955–1975*. Baltimore, MD: Johns Hopkins University Press.

Cunningham, Hugh. 1995. *Children and Childhood in Western Society Since 1500*. New York: Longman.

Cutler, David, Angus Deaton, and Adriana Lleras-Muney. 2006. "The Determinants of Mortality." *Journal of Economic Perspectives* 20(3): 97–120.

Cutler, David M., and Mark McClellan. 2001. "Is Technological Change in Medicine Worth It?" *Health Affairs* 20(5): 11–29.

Dannreuther, Charles, and Jasmine Gideon. 2008. "Entitled to Health? Social Protection in Chile's Plan AUGE." *Development and Change* 39(5): 845–64.

Das, Veena. 1997. "Language and the Body: Transactions in the Construction of Pain." In *Social Suffering*, Arthur Kleinman, Veena Das, and Margaret Lock, eds., 67–93. Berkeley: University of California Press.

Das, Veena, and Ranendra K. Das. 2006. "Pharmaceuticals in Urban Ecologies: The Register of the Local." In *Global Pharmaceuticals: Ethics, Markets, Practices*, Adriana Petryna, Andrew Lakoff, and Arthur Kleinman, eds., 171–205. Durham, NC: Duke University Press.

———. 2007. "How the Body Speaks: Illness and the Lifeworld among the Urban Poor." In *Subjectivity: Ethnographic Investigations*, João Biehl, Byron Good, and Arthur Kleinman, eds., 66–97. Berkeley: University of California Press.

Da Silva, V. A., and F. V. Terrazas. 2011. "Claiming the Right to Health in Brazilian Courts: The Exclusion of the Already Excluded." *Law and Social Inquiry* 36(4): 825–53.

Daston, Lorraine. 1995. "The Moral Economy of Science." *Osiris* 10: 2–24.

Daut, R. L., and Charles S. Cleland. 1982. "The Prevalence and Severity of Pain in Cancer." *Cancer* 50(9): 1913–18.

Davis, Angela. 1981. *Women, Race and Class*. New York: Random House.

Deaton, Angus. 2008. "Income, Health, and Well-Being around the World." *Journal of Economic Perspectives* 22(2): 53–72.

———. 2010. "Instruments, Randomization, and Learning about Development." *Journal of Economic Literature* 48: 424–55.

———. 2012. Lecture: "How Can We Learn What Works in Health and Development?" Global Health Colloquium, Princeton University, October 5.

DECIT (Departamento de Ciência e Tecnologia, Secretaria de Ciência e Tecnologia e Insumos Estratégicos do Ministério da Saúde). 2006. "Avaliação de tecnologias em saúde: Institucionalização das ações no Ministério da Saúde." *Revista de Saúde Pública* 40(4): 743–47.

De Cock, Kevin M., and Anne M. Johnson. 1998. "From Exceptionalism to Normalization: A Reappraisal of Attitudes and Practice around HIV Testing." *British Medical Journal* 316: 290–93.

De Cock, Kevin M., Dorothy Mbori-Ngacha, and Elizabeth Marum. 2002. "Shadow on the Continent: Public Health and HIV/AIDS in Africa in the 21st Century." *Lancet* 360: 67–72.

De Cock, Kevin M., et al. 2000. "Prevention of Mother-to-Child HIV Transmission in Resource-Poor Countries: Translating Research into Policy and Practice." *Journal of the American Medical Association* 283(9): 1175–82.

DelVecchio Good, Mary-Jo, Paul Brodwin, Arthur Kleinman, and Byron Good, eds. 1992. *Pain as Human Experience: Anthropological Perspectives on the Lived Worlds of Chronic Pain Patients in North America*. Berkeley: University of California Press.

DelVecchio Good, Mary-Jo. 2007. "The Medical Imaginary and the Biotechnical Embrace: Subjective Experiences of Clinical Scientists and Patients." In *Subjectivity: Ethnographic Investigations*, João Biehl, Byron Good, and Arthur Kleinman, eds., 362–380. Berkeley: University of California Press.

DelVecchio Good, Mary-Jo, Byron Good, and Jesse Grayman. 2010. "Complex Engagements: Responding to Violence in Postconflict Aceh." In *Contemporary States of Emergency: The Politics of Military and Humanitarian Interventions*, Didier Fassin and Mariella Pandolfi, eds., 241–68. New York: Zone Books.

Denzter, Susan. 2009. "The Devilish Details of Delivering on Global Health." *Health Affairs* 28: 946–47.

Derrida, Jacques. 1978. "Structure, Sign, and Play in the Discourse of the Human Sciences." In *Writing and Difference*, Alan Bass, trans. Chicago: University of Chicago Press.

Desowitz, Robert S. 2000. "The Malaria Vaccine: Seventy Years of the Great Immune Hope." *Parassitologia* 42: 173–82.

de Waal, Alex, and Alan Whiteside. 2003. "New Variant Famine: AIDS and Food Crisis in Southern Africa. *Lancet* 362: 1234–37.

Díaz, Ximena. 2009. "Calidad de Trabajo. Nuevos Riesgos para la Salud Mental de Trabajadores y Trabajadoras." *Cuadernos de Investigación* 4: 1–25.

Díaz, Ximena, and Amalia Mauro. 2010. *Reflexiones sobre Salud Mental y Trabajo en Chile: Analisis de Siete Casos desde una Perspectiva de Género*. Santiago, Chile: Centro de Estudios de la Mujer.

Dobson, Mary J., Maureen Malowany, and Robert W. Snow. 2000. "Malaria Control in East Africa: The Kampala Conference and the Pare-Taveta Scheme: A Meeting of Common and High Ground." *Parassitologia* 42(1–2): 149–66.

Donzelot, Jacques. 1979. *The Policing of Families*. New York: Random House (French edition 1977).

Douglas, Mary. 1966. *Purity and Danger: An Analysis of the Concepts of Pollution and Taboo*. London: Routledge and Kegan Paul.

Duffield, Mark. 2001. *Global Governance and the New Wars: The Merging of Development and Security*. London: Zed Books.

Duflo, Esther, and Michael Kremer. 2008. "Use of Randomization in the Evaluation of Development Effectiveness." In *Reinventing Foreign Aid*, William R. Easterly, ed., 93–120. Cambridge, MA: MIT Press.

Dugas, A. F., Y.-H. Hsieh, S. R. Levin, J. M. Pines, D. P. Mareiniss, A. Mohareb, C. A. Gaydos, T. M. Perl, and R. E. Rothman. 2012. "Google Flu Trends: Correlation with Emergency Department Influenza Rates and Crowding Metrics." *Clinical Infectious Diseases*, 54(4): 463–69.

Dumit, Joseph. 1997. "A Digital Image of the Category of the Person." In *Cyborgs and Citadels: Anthropological Interventions in Emerging Sciences and Technologies*, Gary Lee Downey and Joseph Dumit, eds., 83–102. Santa Fe, NM: School of American Research Press. Reprinted in 2004 in *Picturing Personhood: Brain Scans and Biomedical Identity*. Princeton, NJ: Princeton University Press.

———. 2012. *Drugs for Life: How Pharmaceutical Companies Define Our Health*. Durham, NC: Duke University Press.

Dumit, Joseph, and Nathan Greenslit. 2006. "Informed Health and Ethical Identity Management." *Culture, Medicine and Psychiatry* 30: 127–34.

Duster, Troy. 2005. "Buried Alive: The Concept of Race in Science." In *Genetic Nature/Culture: Anthropology and Science beyond the Two Culture Divide*, Alan H. Goodman, Deborah Heath, and M. Susan Lindee, eds., 258–77. Berkeley: University of California Press.

Dwork, Deborah. 1987. *War Is Good for Babies and Other Children: A History of the Infant and Child Welfare Movement in England, 1898–1918*. London: Tavistock.

Easterly, William R. 2006. *The White Man's Burden: Why the West's Efforts to Aid the Rest Have Done So Much Ill and So Little Good*. New York: Penguin.

Ecks, Stefan. 2005. "Pharmaceutical Citizenship: Antidepressant Marketing and the Promise of Demarginalization in India." *Anthropology and Medicine* 12(3): 239–54.

———. 2008. "Three Propositions for an Evidence-Based Medical Anthropology." *Journal of the Royal Anthropological Institute* (14 supp): S77–S92.

———. 2010. "Near-Liberalism: Global Corporate Citizenship and Pharmaceutical Marketing in India." In *Asian Biotech: Ethics and Communities of Fate*, Aihwa Ong and Nancy Chen, eds., 144–63. Durham, NC: Duke University Press.

Editorial. 2004. "Roll Back Malaria: A Failing Global Health Campaign." *British Medical Journal* 328 (7448): 1086–87.

Eisenstadt, Shmuel N., and Louis Roniger. 1980. "Patron-Client Relations as a Model of Structuring Social Exchange." *Comparative Studies in Society and History* 22(1): 42–77.

England, Roger. 2007. "The Dangers of Disease Specific Programmes for Developing Countries." *British Medical Journal* 335: 565.

Engle, Patrice, Sarah Castle, and Purnima Menon. 1996. "Child Development: Vulnerability and Resilience." *Social Science and Medicine* 43(5): 621–35.

Enserink, Martin, and Leslie Roberts. 2007. "Did They Really Say . . . Eradication?" *Science* 318(5856): 1544–45. http://www.sciencemag.org/cgi/content/full/318/5856/1544.

Epstein, Helen. 2007. *The Invisible Cure: Africa, the West, and the Fight against AIDS*. New York: Farrar, Straus and Giroux.

Epstein, Steve. 1996. *Impure Science: AIDS Activism and the Politics of Knowledge*. Berkeley: University of California Press.

———. 2009. *Inclusion: The Politics of Difference in Medical Research*. Chicago: University of Chicago Press.

European Journal of Cancer. 2007. "News: Cancer Control in Africa." *European Journal of Cancer* 43(10): 1493–97.

Evans-Pritchard, Edward E. 1937. *Witchcraft, Oracles and Magic among the Azande*. Oxford: Clarendon Press.

Evidence-Based Medicine Working Group. 1992. "Evidence-Based Medicine: A New Approach to Teaching the Practice of Medicine." *Journal of the American Medical Association* 268(17): 2420–25.

Farmer, Paul. 2000. "The Consumption of the Poor: Tuberculosis in the 21st Century." *Ethnography* 1(2): 183–216.

———. 2001. *Infections and Inequalities: The Modern Plagues*. Berkeley: University of California Press.

———. 2004. *Pathologies of Power: Health, Human Rights, and the New War on the Poor*. Berkeley: University of California Press.

Farmer, Paul. 2005. "Never Again? Reflections on Human Values and Human Rights." The Tanner Lecture on Human Values, delivered at the University of

Utah, May. http://www.pih.org/inforesources/news/Farmer-Tanner-Lecture 2005.pdf.

———. 2008. "Challenging Orthodoxies: The Road Ahead for Health and Human Rights." *Health and Human Rights: An International Journal* 10(1): 5–19.

———. 2011. *Haiti after the Earthquake.* New York: Public Affairs.

Fassin, Didier. 2003. "The Embodiment of Inequality: AIDS as Social Condition and Historical Experience in South Africa." *EMBO Reports* 4: S4–S9.

———. 2004. "Crise Epidémiologique et Drame Social." In *Afflictions. L'Afrique du Sud, de l'Apartheid au Sida,* Didier Fassin, ed., 9–19. Paris: Karthala.

———. 2007. *When Bodies Remember: Experiences and Politics of AIDS in South Africa.* Berkeley: University of California Press.

———. 2008. "AIDS Orphans, Raped Babies, and Suffering Children: The Moral Construction of Childhood in Post-Apartheid South Africa." In *Healing the World's Children,* Cynthia Comacchio, Janet Golden, and George Weisz, eds., 111–24. Montreal: McGill-Queen's University Press.

———. 2009a. "Les Économies Morales Revisitées." *Annales. Histoire, Sciences Sociales* 64(2): 1237–66.

———. 2009b. "A Violence of History: Accounting for AIDS in Post-Apartheid South Africa." In *Global Health in Times of Violence,* Barbara Rylko-Bauer, Linda Whiteford, and Paul Farmer, eds., 113–35. Santa Fe, NM: School of Advanced Research Press.

———. 2010. "Noli Me Tangere: The Moral Untouchability of Humanitarianism." In *Forces of Compassion: Humanitarianism between Ethics and Politics,* Erica Bornstein and Peter Redfield, eds., 35–52. Santa Fe, NM: School for Advanced Research Press.

———. 2011. *Humanitarian Reason: A Moral History of the Present.* Berkeley: University of California Press.

———. 2012. "That Obscure Object of Global Health." In *Medical Anthropology at the Intersections: Histories, Activisms, and Futures,* Marcia C. Inhorn and Emily A. Wentzell, eds. Durham, NC: Duke University Press.

———. Forthcoming. "Adventures of African Nevirapine: The Political Biography of a Magic Bullet." *In Changing States of Science: Ethnographic and Historical Perspectives on Government, Citizenship and Medical Research in Contemporary Africa,* Paul Wenzel Geissler, ed. Durham, NC: Duke University Press.

Fassin, Didier, Frédéric le Marcis, and Todd Lethata. 2008. "Life and Times of Magda A.: Telling a Story of Violence in South Africa." *Current Anthropology* 49(2): 225–46.

Fassin, Didier, and Mariella Pandolfi, eds. 2010. *Contemporary States of Emergency: The Politics of Military and Humanitarian Interventions.* New York: Zone Books.

Fauvet, Paul. 2000. "Mozambique: Growth with Poverty, a Difficult Transition from Prolonged War to Peace and Development." *Africa Recovery* 14(3): 12–19.

Feierman, Elizabeth Karlin. 1981. "Alternative Medical Services in Rural Tanzania: A Physician's View." *Social Science and Medicine Part B* 15(3): 399–404.

Feierman, Steven. 1985. "Struggles for Control: The Social Roots of Health and Healing in Modern Africa." *African Studies Review* 28(2–3): 73–145.

Feierman, Steven, Arthur Kleinman, Kathleen Stewart, Paul Farmer, and Veena Das. 2010. "Anthropology, Knowledge-Flows and Global Health." *Global Public Health* 5(2): 122–28.

Feldman, Ilana, and Miriam Ticktin, eds. 2010. *In the Name of Humanity: The Government of Threat and Care.* Durham, NC: Duke University Press.

Ferguson, James. 1994. *The Anti-Politics Machine: "Development," Depoliticization and Bureaucratic Power in Lesotho.* Minneapolis: University of Minnesota Press.

———. 2006. *Global Shadows: Africa in the Neoliberal World Order.* Durham, NC: Duke University Press.

Ferraz, O.L.M. 2009. "The Right to Health in the Courts of Brazil: Worsening Health Inequities?" *Health and Human Rights: An International Journal* 11(2): 33–45.

Ferzacca, Steve. 2000. "'Actually I Don't Feel That Bad': Managing Diabetes and the Clinical Encounter." *Medical Anthropology Quarterly* 14(1): 28–50.

Fidler, David. 2007. "Architecture amidst Anarchy: Global Health's Quest for Governance." *Global Health Governance* 1(1): 1–17. http://diplomacy.shu.edu/academics/global health/journal/PDF/Fidler-article.pdf.

———. 2008. "Global Health Jurisprudence: A Time of Reckoning." *Georgetown Law Journal* 96(2): 393–412.

Finkler, Kaja, Cynthia Hunter, and Rick Idema. 2008. "What Is Going On? Ethnography in Hospital Spaces." *Journal of Contemporary Ethnography* 37(2): 246–50.

Fischer, Michael M. J. 2003. *Emergent Forms of Life and the Anthropological Voice.* Durham, NC: Duke University Press.

———. 2009. *Anthropological Futures.* Durham, NC: Duke University Press.

———. 2010. "Dr. Folkman's Decalogue and Network Analysis." In *A Medical Anthropology Reader: Theoretical Trajectories and Emergent Realities,* B. Good, M.M.J. Fischer, S. Willen, and M.J.D. Good, eds., Malden, MA: Wiley-Blackwell.

———. 2011. "Biopolis: Asian Science in the Global Circuitry." Paper presented at the National University of Singapore Workshop on Biopolis.

———. 2012. "Lively Capital and Translational Medicine." in *Biotechnologies, Ethics and Governance in Global Markets,* K. Sunder Rajan, ed. Durham, NC: Duke University Press.

Foley, K. M. 1979. "Pain Syndromes in Patients with Cancer." In *Advances in Pain Research and Therapy,* K. M. Foley, John J. Bonica, and Vittorio Ventafridda, eds., 59–75. New York: Raven Press.

Fortun, Kim. 2004. "From Bhopal to the Informating of Environmental Health: Risk Communication in Historical Perspective." *OSIRIS* 19/1 (Special Issue, "Landscapes of Exposure: Knowledge and Illness in Modern Environments," Gregg Mitman, Michelle Murphy, and Christopher Sellers, eds.): 283–96.

———. 2012. "Biopolitics and the Informating of Environmentalism." In *Lively Capital: Biotechnologies, Ethics, and Governance in Global Markets,* Kaushik Sunder Rajan, ed. Durham, NC: Duke University Press.

Fortun, Kim, and Michael Fortun. 2005. "Scientific Imaginaries and Ethical Plateaus in Contemporary U.S. Toxicology." *American Anthropologist* 107(1): 43–54.

————. 2007. "Experimenting with the Asthma Files." Paper presented at the Experimental Systems Workshop, University of California, Irvine, 13–14 April.

Fortun, Michael. 2008. *Promising Genomics: Iceland and deCODE Genetics in a World of Speculation*. Berkeley: University of California Press.

Foucault, Michel. 1980. *The History of Sexuality*, vol. 1. New York: Vintage Books.

————. 1994a (1973). *The Birth of the Clinic: An Archaeology of Medical Perception*. New York: Vintage Books.

————. 1994b. "Technologies of the Self." In *Ethics: Subjectivity and Truth*, Paul Rabinow, ed., 223–52. New York: The New Press.

————. 2001. "Le Souci de la Vérité." In *Dits et Écrits II, 1976–1988*, 1487–97. Paris: Gallimard.

————. 2007. *Security, Territory, Population: Lectures at the Collège de France, 1977–1978*. New York: Picador.

————. 2008. *The Birth of Biopolitics: Lectures at the Collège de France, 1978–1979*. New York: Palgrave Macmillan.

Frank, Volker. 2004. "Politics without Policy: The Failure of Social Concertation in Democratic Chile, 1990–2000." In *Victims of the Chilean Miracle: Workers and Neoliberalism in the Pinochet Era, 1972–2002*, Peter Winn, ed., 71–124. Durham, NC: Duke University Press.

Freedman, Lynn. 2005. "Achieving the MDGs: Health Systems as Core Social Institutions." *Development* 48(1): 19–24.

French-Davis, Ricardo. 2004. "Entre el Neoliberalismo y el Crecimiento con Equidad: Tres Décadas de Política Económica en Chile." Buenos Aires: Fundación OSDE, Siglo Veintiuno Editores Argentina.

Frenk, Julio. 2006. "Bridging the Divide: Comprehensive Reform to Improve Health in Mexico." In *Lecture for WHO Commission on Social Determinants of Health*. Nairobi: WHO.

————. 2010. "The Global Health System: Strengthening National Health Systems as the Next Step for Global Progress." *PLoS Med* 7(1). Online: http://www.plosmedicine.org/article/info%3Adoi%2F10.1371%2Fjournal.pmed.1000089.

Fullwiley, Duana. 2006. "Biosocial Suffering: Order and Illness in Urban West Africa." *BioSocieties* 1(4): 421–38.

————. 2007. "The Molecularization of Race: Institutionalizing Human Difference in Pharmacogenetics Practice." *Science as Culture* 16: 1–30.

Gallup, John L., and Jeffrey D. Sachs. 2001. "The Economic Burden of Malaria." *American Journal of Tropical Medicine and Hygiene* 64(1 suppl): 85–96.

Galvão, Jane. 2002. "Access to Antiretroviral Drugs in Brazil." *Lancet* 360(9348): 1862–65.

Garabrant, David H., Janetta Held, Bryan Langholz, John M. Peters, and Thomas M. Mack. 1994. "DDT and Related Compounds and Risk of Pancreatic Cancer." *Journal of the National Cancer Institute* 84: 764–71.

Garcés, Mario. 1997. *Historia de la Comuna de Huechuraba: Memoria y Oralidad Popular Urbana*. Santiago, Chile: ECO Educación y Comunicaciones.

Garcia, Angela. 2008. "The Elegiac Addict: History, Chronicity, and the Melancholic Subject." *Cultural Anthropology* 23(4): 718–46.

Gardenour, Brenda, and Misha Tadd, eds. 2012. *Worms, Parasites, and the Human Body in Religion and Culture*. New York: Peter Lang.

Garrett, Laurie. 2007. "The Challenge of Global Health." *Foreign Affairs* Jan/Feb. Online: http://www.foreignaffairs.com/articles/62268/laurie-garrett/the-challenge-of-global health.

Gauri, Varun, and Daniel M. Brinks, eds. 2008. *Courting Social Justice: Judicial Enforcement of Social and Economic Rights in the Developing World*. Cambridge: Cambridge University Press.

Geertz, Clifford. 2007. "'To Exist Is to Have Confidence in One's Way of Being': Rituals as Model Systems." In *Science without Laws: Model Systems, Cases, Exemplary Narratives*, Angela N. H. Creager, Elizabeth Lunbeck, and M. Norton Wise, eds., 212–24. Durham, NC: Duke University Press.

Geissler, P. Wenzel. 1998a. "Worms Are Our Life, part 1: Understandings of Worms and the Body among the Luo of Western Kenya." *Anthropology and Medicine* 5(1): 63–79.

———. 1998b. "Worms Are Our Life, part 2: Luo Children's Thoughts about Worms and Illness." *Anthropology and Medicine* 5(2): 133–44.

Geschiere, Peter. 1997. *The Modernity of Witchcraft: Politics and the Occult in Postcolonial Africa*. Charlottesville: University of Virginia Press.

Ghani, Ashraf, and Clare Lockhardt. 2008. *Fixing Failed States: A Framework for Rebuilding a Fractured World*. Oxford: Oxford University Press.

Giacomini, Mira K., and Deborah J. Cook, for the Evidence-Based Medicine Working Group. 2000. "Users' Guide to the Medical Literature, XXIII. Qualitative Research in Health Care: Are the Results of the Study Valid?" *Journal of the American Medical Association* 284(3): 357–62.

Gibb, Diana, and Beatriz Tess. 1999. "Interventions to Reduce Mother-to-Child Transmission of HIV Infection: New Developments and Current Controversies." *AIDS* 13 (suppl. A): S93–S102.

Gideon, Jasmine. 2001. "The Decentralization of Primary Health Care Delivery in Chile." *Public Administration and Development* 21: 223–31.

Ginsberg J., M. H. Mohebbi, R. S. Patel, L. Brammer, M. S. Smolinski, and L. Brilliant. 2009. "Detecting Influenza Epidemics Using Search Engine Query Data." *Nature* 457(7232): 1012–14.

Glauber, James H., and Anne L. Fuhlbrigge. 2002. "Stratifying Asthma Populations by Medication Use." *Annals of Allergy, Asthma, and Immunology* 88: 451–56.

Global Development Advisors. 2009. *Independent Evaluation of the Roll Back Malaria Partnership, 2004–2008*. September 30.

Global Fund for AIDS, Tuberculosis and Malaria. 2010. Accessed June 27, 2010: http://www.theglobalfund.org/en/about/.

Global Health Chronicles. 2009. "Guinea Worm Chronicle." Centers for Disease Control, Emory Global Health Institute, and Robert Wood Johnson Foundation. Accessed January 12, 2012: http://globalhealthchronicles.org/guineaworm.

Global Partnership to Roll Back Malaria. 2001. *Roll Back Malaria Country Strategies & Resource Requirements*. Geneva: World Health Organization.

Goldstone, Brian. 2012. "The Miraculous Life." PhD dissertation, Duke University.

Goody, Ester. 1973. *Contexts of Kinship*. Cambridge: Cambridge University Press.

Goody, Jack. 1962. *Death, Property and the Ancestors: A Study of the Mortuary Customs of the LoDagga of West Africa.* Palo Alto, CA: Stanford University Press.

Gordon, Deborah R. 1988. "Clinical Science and Clinical Expertise: Changing Boundaries between Art and Science in Medicine." In *Biomedicine Examined,* Margaret Lock and Deborah Gordon, eds., 257–98. Dordrecht: Kluwer Academic Press.

Grady, Denise. 2005. "Experts to Consider Withdrawal of Asthma Drugs." *New York Times,* July 13.

Gray, Natasha. 2005. "Independent Spirits: The Politics of Policing Anti-Witchcraft Movements in Colonial Ghana, 1908–1927." *Journal of Religion in Africa* 35(2): 139–58.

Green, Edward C. 1997. "Purity, Pollution and the Invisible Snake in Southern Africa." *Medical Anthropology* 17(2): 83–100.

Greene, Jeremy A. 2008. *Prescribing by Numbers: Drugs and the Definition of Disease.* Baltimore, MD: Johns Hopkins University Press.

Greenway, Chris. 2004. "Dracunculiasis (Guinea Worm Disease)." *Canadian Medical Association Journal* 170(4): 495–500.

Grosse, Scott D., Coleen A. Boyle, Aileen Kenneson, Muin J. Khoury, and Benjamin S. Wilfond. 2006. "From Public Health Emergency to Public Health Service: The Implications of Evolving Criteria for Newborn Screening Panels." *Pediatrics* 117(3): 923–29.

Grove, David. 1994. *A History of Human Helminthology.* Oxon, UK: CAB International.

Guay, Laura, et al. 1999. "Intrapartum and Neonatal Single-dose Nevirapine Compared with Zidovudine for Prevention of Mother-to-Child Transmission of HIV-1 in Kampala, Uganda: HIVNET 012 Randomised Trial." *Lancet* 354: 795–802.

Guimarães, R. 2004. "Bases para uma política nacional de ciência, tecnologia e inovação em saúde." *Ciência & Saúde Coletiva* 9(2): 375–87.

Hacking, Ian. 1991. "The Making and Molding of Child Abuse." *Critical Inquiry* 17: 253–88.

———. 1995. "The Looping Effects of Human Kinds." In *Causal Cognition: A Multidisciplinary Debate,* Ann Sperber, Dan Premack, and James Premack, eds., 351–83. Oxford: Clarendon Press.

Hahn, Robert A., and Marcia C. Inhorn. 2008. *Anthropology and Public Health: Bridging Differences in Culture and Society,* 2nd edition. New York: Oxford University Press.

Hammer, Jeffrey S., and Peter A. Berman. 1995. "Ends and Means in Public Health Policy in Developing Countries." In *Health Sector Reform in Developing Countries: Making Health Development Sustainable,* Peter Berman, ed., 37–58. Boston: Harvard University Press.

Han, Clara. 2012. *Life in Debt: Times of Care and Violence in Neoliberal Chile.* Berkeley: University of California Press.

Hanlon, Joseph. 1996. *Mozambique: Who Calls the Shots?* London: James Currey.

———. 2010. Mozambique 156, news reports and clippings, 22 February 2010, Open University, United Kingdom.

Harper, Ian. 2005. "Interconnected and Interinfected: DOTS and the Stabilisation of the Tuberculosis Control Programme in Nepal." In *The Aid Effect: Giving and Governing in International Development*, David Mosse and David Lewis, eds. London: Pluto.

Harper, Ian, Nabin Rawal, and Madhusudan Subedi. 2011. "Disputing Distribution: Ethics and Pharmaceutical Regulation in Nepal." *Studies in Nepali History and Society* 16(1): 1–39.

Harper, Richard. 2000. "The Social Organization of the IMF's Mission Work: The Examination of International Auditing." In *Audit Cultures: Anthropological Studies in Accountability, Ethics and the Academy*, Marilyn Strathern, ed. New York: Routledge.

Harris, Gardner. 2009. "Pfizer Pays $2.3 Billion to Settle Marketing Case." *New York Times*, Sept. 2. http://www.nytimes.com/2009/09/03/business/03health.html.

Harvey, David. 2007. *A Brief History of Neoliberalism*. New York: Oxford University Press.

Hawkins, Sean. 2002. *Writing and Colonialism in Northern Ghana: The Encounter between the LoDagga and the 'World of Paper.'* Toronto: University of Toronto Press.

Hayden, Cori. 2007. "A Generic Solution? Pharmaceuticals and the Politics of the Similar in Mexico." *Current Anthropology* 48(4): 475–95.

Henderson, Donald. 2009. *Smallpox: The Death of a Disease*. New York: Prometheus Books.

———. 2012. "A History of Eradication—Successes, Failures, and Controversies." *Lancet* 379(9819): 884–85.

Herzfeld, Michael. 1992. *The Social Production of Indifference: Exploring the Symbolic Roots of Western Bureaucracy*. Chicago: University of Chicago Press.

Hinterberger, Amy. 2010. "Disparate Biosocialities: 'Race' in Canada's National Genomics Strategy." In *What's the Use of Race? Modern Governance and the Biology of Difference*, Ian Whitmarsh and David S. Jones, eds., 246–83. Cambridge, MA: MIT Press.

Hirschfeld, Lawrence. 2002. "Why Don't Anthropologists Like Children?" *American Anthropologist* 104(2): 611–27.

Hirschman, Albert O. 1970. "The Search for Paradigms as a Hindrance to Understanding." *World Politics* 22(3): 329–43.

———. 1971. *A Bias for Hope: Essays on Development and Latin America*. New Haven, CT: Yale University Press.

———. 1998. *Crossing Boundaries: Selected Writings*. New York: Zone Books.

Hoeppli, Reinhard. 1959. *Parasites and Parasitic Infection in Early Medicine and Science*. Singapore: University of Malaya Press.

Hoffmann, F., and F. Bentes. 2008. "Accountability for Economic and Social Rights in Brazil." In *Courting Social Justice: Judicial Enforcement of Social and Economic Rights in the Developing World*, V. Gauri and D. Brinks, eds., 100–145. New York: Cambridge University Press.

Homedes, Núria, and Antonio Ugalde. 2005. "Why Neoliberal Health Reforms Have Failed in Latin America." *Health Policy* 71: 83–96.

Hopkins, Donald. 1992. "Honing in on Helminths." *American Journal of Tropical Medicine and Hygiene* 46: 626–34.

———. 2002 [1982]. *The Greatest Killer: Smallpox in History.* Chicago: University of Chicago Press.

Hopkins, Donald R., Ernesto Ruiz-Tiben, Robert L. Kaiser, Andrew N. Agle, and P. Craig Withers. 1993. "Dracunculiasis Eradication: Beginning of the End." *American Journal of Tropical Medicine and Hygiene* 49: 281–89.

Hopkins, Donald, and Ernestine Hopkins. 1992. "Guinea Worm: The End in Sight." In *Medical and Health Annual*, E. Bernstein, ed. Chicago: Encyclopedia Britannica.

Hopkins, Donald, and Ernesto Ruiz-Tiben. 2011. "Dracunculiasis (Guinea Worm Disease): Case Study of the Effort to Eradicate Guinea Worm." In *Water Sanitation–Related Diseases and the Environment: Challenges, Interventions, and Preventative Measures*, Janine Selendy, ed. New York: John Wiley & Sons.

Hopkins, D. R., E. Ruiz-Tiben, P. Downs, P. C. Withers, and J. H. Maguire. 2005. "Dracunculiasis Eradication: The Final Inch." *American Journal of Tropical Medicine and Hygiene* 73(4): 669–75.

Hopkins, D. R., E. Ruiz-Tiben, T. K. Ruebush, N. Diallo, A. Agle, and P. C. Withers. 2000. "Dracunculiasis Eradication: Delayed, Not Denied." *American Journal of Tropical Medicine and Hygiene* 62(2): 163–68.

Hopkins, Donald, and Craig Withers. 2002. "Sudan's War and Eradication of Dracunculiasis." *Lancet* 360(s1): s21–2.

HPG (Health Partners Group). 2007. "Mapping of Vertical Funding," presentation and report to health SWAP partners, December, 2007, Maputo, Mozambique.

Human Rights Watch. 2002. *Ignorance Only: HIV/AIDS, Human Rights and Federally Funded Abstinence-Only Programs in the United States.* New York: Human Rights Watch.

———. 2005. *The Less They Know, the Better: Abstinence-Only HIV/AIDS Programs in Uganda.* New York: Human Rights Watch.

———. 2006. *No Bright Future: Government Failures, Human Rights Abuses and Squandered Progress in the Fight against AIDS in Zimbabwe.* New York: Human Rights Watch.

———. 2008a. *Neighbors in Need: Zimbabweans Seeking Refuge in South Africa.* New York: Human Rights Watch. http://www.hrw.org/en/reports/2008/06/18/neighbors-need-0.

———. 2008b. *An Unbreakable Cycle: Drug Dependency Treatment, Mandatory Confinement, and HIV/AIDS in China's Guangxi Province.* New York: Human Rights Watch.

———. 2009. *Unbearable Pain: India's Obligation to Ensure Palliative Care.* New York: Human Rights Watch.

———. 2012. *Sex Workers at Risk: Condoms as Evidence of Prostitution in Four US Cities.* New York: Human Rights Watch.

Human Rights Watch, Deutsche AIDS-Hilfe, the European AIDS Treatment Group, and the African HIV Policy Network. 2009. *Returned to Risk: Deportation of HIV-Positive Migrants.* New York: Human Rights Watch.

Human Rights Watch and Thai AIDS Treatment Action Group. 2007. *Deadly Denial: Barriers to HIV/AIDS Treatment for People Who Use Drugs in Thailand.* New York: Human Rights Watch.

Hunter, John. 1999. "An Introduction to Guinea Worm on the Eve of Its Departure." *Social Science and Medicine* 43(9): 1399–1425.

Huttly, Sharon R.A., Deborah Blum, Betty R. Kirkwood, Robert N. Emeh, Ngozi Okeke, Michael Ajala, Gordon S. Smith, Deborah C. Carson, Oladeinade Dosunmu-Ogunbi, and Richard G. Feachem. 1990. "The Imo State (Nigeria) Drinking Water Supply and Sanitation Project 2: Impact on Dracunculiasis, Diarrhoea and Nutritional Status." *Transactions of the Royal Society of Tropical Medicine and Hygiene* 73: 669–75.

Hyatt, Harry Middleton. 1978. *Hoodoo Conjuration Witchcraft Rootwork.* Cambridge, MD: Memoirs of the Alma Egan Hyatt Foundation, v. 1–5.

Imbens, Guido W. 2010. "Better LATE than Nothing: Some Comments on Deaton (2009) and Heckman and Urzua (2009)." *Journal of Economic Literature* 48(2): 399–423.

Inhorn, Marcia C., and Emily A. Wentzell, eds. 2012. *Medical Anthropology at the Intersections: Histories, Activisms, and Futures.* Durham, NC: Duke University Press.

Instituto Nacional de Estatistica (INE). 1998. *Inquérito Nacional aos Agregados Familiares Sobre Condições de Vida: 1996–1997* (National Family Survey on Living Conditions). Maputo: Government of Mozambique.

International Agency for Research on Cancer (IARC). 2010. Global fact sheets. Accessed June 14, 2010: http://globocan.iarc.fr/.

International AIDS Society. n.d. "Share Your Stories of How HIV-Related Travel Restrictions Affected You, Your Colleagues or Your Relatives." http://www.iasociety.org/Default.aspx?pageId=157.

"International Commission for the Certification of Dracunculiasis Eradication: Report and Recommendations." 2005. World Health Organization Fifth Meeting. Geneva.

International Narcotics Control Board. 2005. *Report of the International Narcotics Control Board for 2004.* New York: United Nations.

International Planned Parenthood Federation, Global Network of People Living with HIV/AIDS, International Community of Women Living with HIV/AIDS. n.d. "Verdict on a Virus." http://www.gnpplus.net/images/stories/2008_verdict_on_a_virus.pdf.

Iriemenam, N. C., W. A. Oyibo, and A. F. Fagbenro-Beyioku. 2008. "Dracunculiasis—The Saddle Is Virtually Ended." *Parasitology Research* 102(3): 343–47.

Jackson, Jean. 1999. *Camp Pain: Talking with Chronic Pain Patients.* Philadelphia: University of Pennsylvania Press.

James, Erica. 2010. *Democratic Insecurities: Violence, Trauma, and Intervention in Haiti.* Berkeley: University of California Press.

Janes, Craig R., and Kitty K. Corbett. 2009. "Anthropology and Global Health." *Annual Review of Anthropology* 38: 167–83.

Janzen, John M. 1978. *The Quest for Therapy in Lower Zaire.* Berkeley: University of California Press.

Jayaraman, K. S. 2010. "India's Tuberculosis Genome Project Under Fire." *Nture,* June 15. http://www.nature.com/news/2010/100609/full/news.2010.285.html.

Jewkes, Rachel, and Naeemah Abrahams. 2002. "The Epidemiology of Rape and Sexual Coercion in South Africa: An Overview." *Social Science and Medicine* 55(7): 1231–44.

Jewkes, Rachel, Naeemah Abrahams, and Zodumo Mvo. 1998. "Why Do Nurses Abuse Patients? Reflections from South African Obstetric Services." *Social Science and Medicine* 47(11): 1781–95.

Jewkes, Rachel, Martin Lorna, and Penn-Kekana Loveday. 2002. "The Virgin Cleansing Myth: Cases of Child Rape Are Not Exotic." *Lancet* 359(937): 711.

Jones, David S., and Roy H. Perlis. 2006. "Pharmacogenetics, Race, and Psychiatry: Prospects and Challenges." *Harvard Review: Psychiatry* 14(2): 92–108.

Justice, Judith. 1989. *Policies, Plans and People: Foreign Aid and Health Development.* Berkeley: University of California Press.

Kahn, Jonathan. 2004. "How a Drug Becomes 'Ethnic': Law, Commerce, and the Production of Racial Categories in Medicine." *Yale Journal of Health Policy, Law, and Ethics* 4(1): 1–46.

Kaler, Amy, and Susan Cotts Watkins. 2001. "Disobedient Distributors: Street-Level Bureaucrats and Would-Be Patrons in Community-Based Family Planning Programs in Rural Kenya." *Studies in Family Planning* 32(3): 254–69.

Kaljee, Linda M., and Robert Beardsley. 1992. "Psychotropic Drugs and Concepts of Compliance in a Rural Mental Health Clinic." *Medical Anthropology Quarterly* 6(3): 271–87.

Kapferer, Bruce. 2005. "Situations, Crisis and the Anthropology of the Concrete: The Contribution of Max Gluckman." *Social Analysis* 49(3): 85–122.

Kamat, Vinay R., and Mark Nichter. 1998. "Pharmacies, Self-Medication and Pharmaceutical Marketing in Bombay, India." *Social Science and Medicine* 47(6): 779–94.

Kaufman, Jay S., and Susan A. Hall. 2003. "The Slavery Hypertension Hypothesis: Dissemination and Appeal of a Modern Race Theory." *Epidemiology* 14(1): 111–18.

Kelkar-Khambete, A., K. Kielmann, S. Pawar, J. Porter, V. Inamdar, A Datye, and S. Rangan. 2008. "India's Revised National Tuberculosis Control Programme: Looking Beyond Detection and Cure." *International Journal of Tuberculosis and Lung Disease* 12(1): 87–92.

Keusch G. T., W. L. Kilama, S. Moon, N. A. Szlezak, and C. M. Michaud. 2010. "The Global Health System: Linking Knowledge with Action—Learning from Malaria." *PLoS Med* 7(1). Online: http://www.plosmedicine.org/arZcle/info%3Adoi%2F10.1371%2Fjournal.pmed.1000089.

Khoury, Muin J. 2003. "Genetics and Genomics in Practice: The Continuum from Genetic Disease to Genetic Information in Health and Disease." *Genetics in Medicine* 5(4): 261–63.

Kim, Aehyung, Ajay Tandon, and Ernesto Ruiz-Tiben. July 1997. "Cost-Benefit Analysis of the Global Dracunculiasis Eradication Campaign." Accessed October 30, 2012: http://cartercenter.org/documents/2101.pdf.

Kim, Jim Yong. 2004. "Scaling Up Access to Care in Resource Constrained Settings: What Is Needed?" XV International AIDS Conference, Bangkok Plenary Address. Accessed July 9, 2009: http://www.who.int/3by5/plenaryspeech/en.

Kim, Jim Yong, and Paul Farmer. 2006. "AIDS in 2006—Moving toward One World, One Hope?" *New England Journal of Medicine* 355: 645–47.

Kim, Jim Yong, and Michael E. Porter. n.d. "Redefining Global Health Care Delivery." Unpublished paper.

Kim, Jim Yong, J. Rhatigan, S. H. Jain, R. Weintraub, and M. E. Porter. 2010. "From a Declaration of Values to the Creation of Value in Global Health: A Report from Harvard University's Global Health Delivery Project." *Global Public Health: An International Journal for Research, Policy and Practice* 5(2):181–88.

Kleinman, Arthur. 1980. *Patients and Healers in the Context of Culture: An Exploration of the Borderland between Anthropology, Medicine, and Psychiatry.* Berkeley: University of California Press.

———. 2010. "Four Social Theories for Global Health." *Lancet 375:* 1518–19.

Knight, Kelly. 2010. "Tricky: Evidence, Facts, and Reproduction among Homeless Women Addicts in California." University of California, San Francisco, Program in Medical Anthropology. PhD dissertation.

Koenig, Barbara A., Sandra Soo-Jin Lee, and S. Richardson, eds. 2008. *Revisiting Race in the Age of Genomics.* New Brunswick, NJ: Rutgers University Press.

Koenig, Serena P., Fernet Leandre, and Paul Farmer. 2004. "Scaling-Up HIV Treatment Programmes in Resource-Limited Settings: The Rural Haiti Experience." *AIDS* 18:S21–S25.

Kolata, Gina. 2012. "In Leukemia Treatment, Glimpses of the Future." *New York Times,* July 8, A1, 9.

Koshy, Rachel C., Deborah Rhodes, Saraswathi Devi, and S. A. Grossman. 1998. "Cancer Pain Management in Developing Countries: A Mosaic of Complex Issues Resulting in Inadequate Analgesia." *Supportive Care in Cancer* 6: 430–37.

Kremer, Michael, and Edward Miguel. 2007. "The Illusion of Sustainability." *The Quarterly Journal of Economics,* 1007–65.

Krieger, Nancy. 2011. *Epidemiology and the People's Health: Theory and Context.* New York: Oxford University Press.

Krishna, R. Jai, and Rumman Ahmed. 2012. "Ranbaxy Launches Novel Anti-Malaria Drug." *Wall Street Journal,* April 25. http://online.wsj.com/article/SB1 0001424052702304811304577365641151741560.html.

Kristof, Nicholas D. 2007. "Attack of the Worms." *New York Times* (Op-Ed), July 2.

Kutin, K., T. F. Kruppa, R. Brenya, and R. Garms. 2004. "Efficiency of *Simulium sanctipauli* as a Vector of *Onchocerca volvulus* in the Forest Zone of Ghana." *Medical and Veterinary Entomology* 18(2): 167–73.

Kwasi Sarpong, Peter. 2004. "Witchcraft, Magic, and Dreams." In *Witchcraft Mentality Seminars: Applications to Ministry and Development,* 9–13. Tamale, Ghana: Tamale Institute of Cross Cultural Studies.

Lakoff, Andrew. 2004. "The Anxieties of Globalization: Antidepressant Sales and Economic Crisis in Argentina." *Social Studies of Science* 34(2): 247–69.

———. 2006. *Pharmaceutical Reason: Knowledge and Value in Global Psychiatry.* Cambridge: Cambridge University Press.

Lakoff, Andrew, and Stephen J. Collier, eds. 2008. *Biosecurity Interventions: Global Health and Security in Question.* New York: Columbia University Press.

Lalitha, C. M., and R. Anandan. 1980. "Guinea Worm Infections in Dogs: Tamil Nadu, India." *Cheiron* 9: 198–99.

Lallemant, Marc, and Gonzague Jourdain. 2010. "Preventing Mother to Child Transmission of HIV: Protecting This Generation and the Next." *New England Journal of Medicine* 363(16): 1570–72.

Lancet. 1975. "Epitaph for Global Malaria Eradication?" *Lancet* 306(7923): 15–16.

———. 1983. "After Smallpox, Guinea Worm?" *Lancet* 321(8317): 161–62.

———. 1992. "Guinea Worm: Good News from Ghana." *Lancet* 340(8831): 1322–23.

———. 2000. "Donor Responsibilities in Rolling Back Malaria." *Lancet* 356(9229): 521.

———. 2005. "Reversing the Failures of Roll Back Malaria." *Lancet* 365(9469): 1439.

———. 2007. "Is Malaria Eradication Possible?" *Lancet* 370(9597): 1459.

Landau, Paul. 1996. "Explaining Surgical Evangelism in Colonial Southern Africa: Teeth, Pain and Faith." *Journal of African History* 37(2): 261–81.

Lara, Joseph. 2009. "Exploratory Analysis of the Facility-Level Factors Associated with HAART Abandonment in Central Mozambique." MPH thesis, University of Washington, Seattle.

Larson, H. J. 2011. "Addressing the Vaccine Confidence Gap." *Lancet* 378: 526–35.

Latour, Bruno. 1987. *Science in Action: How to Follow Scientists and Engineers through Society*. Cambridge, MA: Harvard University Press.

———. 1993. *We Have Never Been Modern*, Catherine Porter, trans. Cambridge, MA: Harvard University Press.

———. 2005. *Reassembling the Social: An Introduction to Actor-Network-Theory*. Oxford: Oxford University Press.

Leclerc-Madlala, Suzanne. 2002. "On the Virgin-Cleansing Myth: Gendered Bodies, AIDS, and Ethnomedicine." *African Journal of AIDS Research* 1(1): 87–95.

Lemarchand, Rene, and Keith Legg. 1972. "Political Clientelism and Development: A Preliminary Analysis." *Comparative Politics* 4(2): 149–78.

Lerer, Leonard, and Richard Matzopoulos. 2001. "The Worst of Both Worlds: The Management Reform of the World Health Organization." *International Journal of Health Services* 31: 2415–38.

LeVine, Robert. 2007. "Ethnographic Studies of Childhood: A Historical Overview." *American Anthropologist* 109(2): 247–60.

Lévi-Strauss, Claude. 1963. *Structural Anthropology*. New York: Basic Books.

Litvinov, V. F., and V. P. Litvinov. 1981. "Helminths of Predatory Mammals from Azerbaijan, SSR, USSR." *Parazitologiya* 13: 210–23.

Litvinov, V. F., and A. Lysenko. 1982. "Dracunculiasis: History of the Discovery of the Intermediate Host and the Eradication of Foci of Invasion." *Proceedings of a Workshop on Opportunities for Control of Dracunculiasis, 16–19 June*. Washington, DC: National Research Council.

Livingston, Julie. 2008. "Disgust, Bodily Aesthetics, and the Ethic of Being Human in Botswana." *Africa* 78(2): 288–307.

———. 2012. *Improvising Medicine: An African Oncology Ward in an Emerging Cancer Epidemic*. Durham, NC: Duke University Press.

Lock, Margaret. 2003. "Medicalization and the Naturalization of Social Control." In *Encyclopedia of Medical Anthropology*, vol. 1: *Health and Illness in the*

World's Cultures, Carol R. Ember and Marvin Ember, eds., 116–25. New York: Springer Publishing Company.

Loewenberg, Samuel. 2007. "The US President's Malaria Initiative: 2 Years On." *Lancet* 370(9603): 1893–94.

Loewenson, Rene, and David McCoy. 2004. "Access to Antiretroviral Treatment in Africa: New Resources and Sustainable Health Systems Are Needed." *British Medical Journal* 328: 241–42.

Logie, Dorothy, and Mhoira Leng. 2007. "Africans Die in Pain Because of Fears of Opiate Addiction." *British Medical Journal* 335(7622): 685.

Long, Debi, Cynthia L. Hunter, and Sjaak van der Geest. 2008. "Introduction: When the Field Is a Ward or Clinic: Hospital Ethnography." *Anthropology and Medicine* 15(2): 71–78.

Lu, Chunling, Catherine M. Michaud, Kashif Khan, and Christopher J. L. Murray. 2006. "Absorptive Capacity and Disbursements by the Global Fund to Fight AIDS, Tuberculosis and Malaria: Analysis of Grant Implementation." *Lancet* 368(9534): 483–88.

Lupin. 2009. Annual Report 2008–2009. "Mumbai: Lupin Limited." Accessed June 27, 2010: http://www.lupinworld.com.

Lynch, Katherine. 2000. "Infant Mortality, Child Neglect, and Child Abandonment in European History: A Comparative Analysis." In *Population and Economy: From Hunger to Modern Economic Growth*, Tommy Bengtsson and Osamu Saito, eds. 133–64. Oxford: Oxford University Press.

MacGaffey, Wyatt. 2006. "Death of a King, Death of a Kingdom? Social Pluralism and Succession to High Office in Dagbon, Northern Ghana." *Journal of Modern African Studies* 44(1): 79–99.

Madon, Temina, Karen J. Hofman, Linda Kupfer, and Roger I. Glass. 2007. "Implementation Science." *Science* 318: 1728–29.

Maeseneer, Jan D., Chris van Weel, David Egilman, Khaya Mfenyana, Arthur Kaufman, and Nelson Sewankambo. 2008. "Strengthening Primary Care: Addressing the Disparity between Vertical and Horizontal Investment." *British Journal of General Practice* 58: 3–4.

Mahmoud, Adel. 2004. "The Global Vaccination Gap." *Science* 305: 147.

Mair, Lucy P. 1961. "Clientship in East Africa." *Cahiers d'Études Africaines* 2(6): 315–25.

Malaria Consortium. 2002. *Achieving impact: Roll Back Malaria in the next phase: final report of the external evaluation of Roll Back Malaria.* Liverpool: Malaria Consortium.

Manderson, Lenore, and Carolyn Smith-Morris, eds. 2010. *Chronic Conditions, Fluid States: Chronicity and the Anthropology of Illness.* New Brunswick, NJ: Rutgers University Press.

Manyere, Irene. 1996. "The Uses of the Pain Assessment Tools by Nurses in Botswana in Assessing and Managing Pain." B.Ed. Nursing thesis, University of Botswana.

Marchal, Bruno, Anna Cavalli, and Guy Kegels. 2009. "Global Health Actors Claim to Support Health System Strengthening—Is This Reality or Rhetoric?" *PLoS Medicine* 6(4).

Maskovsky, Jeff. 2005. "Do People Fail Drugs, or Do Drugs Fail People? The Discourse of Adherence." *Transforming Anthropology* 13(2): 136–42.

Maslove, David M., Anisa Mnyusiwalla, Edward J. Mills, Jessie McGowan, Amir Attaran, and Kumanan Wilson. 2009. "Barriers to the Effective Treatment and Prevention of Malaria in Africa: A Systematic Review of Qualitative Studies." *BMC International Health and Human Rights* 9: 26. http://www.biomedcentral.com/1472-698X/9/26.

Masquelier, Adeline. 1999. "'Money and Serpents, Their Remedy Is Killing': The Pathology of Consumption in Southern Niger." *Research in Economic Anthropology* 20: 97–115.

Mayo Clinic Staff. "Bone Marrow Biopsy and Aspiration: Definition." http://www.mayoclinic.com/health/bone-marrow-biopsy/CA00068.

Mbembe, Achille. 2003. "Necropolitics." *Public Culture* 15(1): 11–40.

McNeil, Donald G. 2002. "U.N. Disease Fund Opens Way to Generics." *New York Times*, October 16.

———. 2006. "Dose of Tenacity Wears Down Ancient Horror." *New York Times*, March 26.

———. 2007. "Drugs Banned, World's Poor Suffer in Pain." *New York Times*, September 10. http://nytimes.com/2007/09/10/health/10pain.html.

Meckel, Richard. 1990. *Save the Babies: American Public Health Reform and the Prevention of Infant Mortality, 1850–1929*. Baltimore, MD: Johns Hopkins University Press.

Meinert, Lotte, Michael Whyte, Susan R. Whyte, and Betty Kyaddondo. 2004. "Faces of Globalization: AIDS and ARV Medicine in Uganda." *Folk* 45:105–123.

Meinert, Lotte, Hanne O. Mogensen, and Jenipher Twebaze. 2009. "Tests for Life Chances: CD4 Miracles and Obstacles in Uganda." *Anthropology & Medicine* 16(2): 195–209.

Meintjes, Helen, and Sonja Giese. 2006. "Spinning the Epidemic: The Making of Mythologies of Orphanhood in the Context of AIDS." *Childhood* 13(3): 407–30.

Meintjes, Helen, Katharine Hall, Double-Hugh Marera, and Andrew Boulle. 2010. "Orphans of the AIDS Epidemic? The Extent, Nature and Circumstances of Child-Headed Households in South Africa." *AIDS Care* 22(1): 40–49.

Mendis, Kamini, Aafje Rietveld, Marian Warsame, Andrea Bosman, Brian Greenwood, and Walther H. Wernsdorfer. 2009. "From Malaria Control to Eradication: The WHO Perspective." *Tropical Medicine and International Health* 14(7): 802–9.

Mendive, Susana. 2004. "Entrevista al Dr. Juan Marconi, Creador de la Psiquiatría Intracomunitaria. Reflexiones Acerca de su Legado Para la Psicología Comunitaria Chilena." *Psykhe* 13(2): 187–99.

Merleau-Ponty, Maurice. 1962. *Phenomenology of Perception*. New York: Humanities Press.

Messeder, Ana Márcia, Claudia Garcia Osorio-de-Castro, and Vera Lucia Luiza. 2005. "Mandados judiciais como ferramenta para garantia do acesso a medicamentos no setor público: a experiência do Estado do Rio de Janeiro, Brasil." *Cad. Saúde Pública* 21(2): 525–34.

Meyer, Birgit. 1998. "Commodities and the Power of Prayer: Pentecostalist Attitudes towards Consumption in Contemporary Ghana." *Development and Change* 29(4): 751–76.

MIDEPLAN. 2006. Encuesta de Caracterización Socioeconómica Nacional (CASEN). G.d.C.M.d.P. Nacional, ed. Santiago.

Miguel, Edward, and Michael Kremer. 2004. "Worms: Identifying Impacts on Education and Health in the Presence of Treatment Externalities." *Econometrica* 72(1): 159–217.

Ministerio de Trabajo y Previsión Social, Chile. 2003. *Fija el texto refundido, coordinado y sistemizado del Código del Trabajo*. Santiago: Gobierno de Chile. http://www.leychile.cl/N?i=207436&f=2012-08-08&p=

Ministry of Health (Brazil). 2010a. "Histórico do Componente de Medicamentos de Dispensação Excepcional." Accessed July 2, 2010: http://portal.saude.gov.br/portal/saude/profissional/visualizar_texto.cfm?idtxt=34014&janela=1.

———. 2010b. "Elenco de Medicamentos do Componente Especializado da Assistência Farmacêutica." Accessed December 30, 2010: http://portal.saude.gov.br/portal/saude/profissional/visualizar_texto.cfm?idtxt=34029&janela=1.

Ministry of Planning and Development (Mozambique). 2010. National Directorate of Studies and Policy Analysis. Poverty and Wellbeing in Mozambique: Third National Poverty Assessment. Maputo: Government of Mozambique.

Ministry of Planning and Finance, Mozambique. 1998. Understanding Poverty and Well-Being in Mozambique: The First National Assessment (1996–97). Maputo: Government of Mozambique.

Minkler, Meredith. 2004. *Community Organizing and Community Building for Health*. New Brunswick, NJ: Rutgers Press.

MINSAL. 2000. Plan Nacional de Salud Mental y Psiquiatría. G.d.C. Ministerio de Salud, ed., 1–232. Gobierno de Chile.

Mitchell, Clyde. 1983. "Case Study and Situational Analysis." *Sociological Review* 31(2): 187–211.

Molyneux, David. 2010. "Eradicating Guinea Worm Disease—A Prelude to NTD Elimination." *Lancet* 376(9745): 947–48.

Molyneux, David, and Vinand M. Nantulya. 2004. "Linking Disease Control Programmes in Rural Africa: A Pro-Poor Strategy to Reach Abuja Targets and Millennium Development Goals." *British Medical Journal* 328(7449): 1129–32.

Montoya, Michael J. 2007. "Bioethnic Conscription: Genes, Race, and Mexicana/o Ethnicity in Diabetes Research." *Cultural Anthropology* 22(1): 94–128.

———. 2011. *Making the Mexican Diabetic: Race, Science, and the Genetics of Inequality*. Berkeley: University of California Press.

Morenikeji, O., and A. Asiatu. 2010. "Progress in Dracunculiasis Eradication in Oyo State, Southwest Nigeria: A Case Study." *African Health Science* 10(3): 297–301.

Morris, Kelly. 2003. "Cancer? In Africa?" *Lancet Oncology* 4: 5.

Mosweunyane, Tjantilili. 1994. "The Knowledge of Nurses Working in Botswana Health Care Settings in Regard to Pain Control," B.Ed. Nursing thesis, University of Botswana.

Moyo, J. M. 1994. "The Extent to Which Nurses Meet Clients' Needs for Pain Management within the First 48 Hours Post C-section." B.Ed. Nursing thesis, University of Botswana.

Mozambique Ministry of Health. 2009. *Inquérito Nacional de Prevalência, Riscos Comportamentais e Informação sobre o HIV e SIDA em Moçambique (IN-SIDA)*. MOH and INS: Maputo.

Mugyenyi, Peter. 2008. *Genocide by Denial: How Profiteering from HIV/AIDS Killed Millions*. Kampala, Uganda: Fountain.

———. 2009. "Flat-Line Funding for PEPFAR: A Recipe for Chaos." *Lancet* 374: 292.

Muhammad, G., M. Z. Khan, M. Athar, and M. Saqib. 2005. "Dracunculus Infection in a Dog during the 'Post-Eradication' Period: The Need for a Longer Period of Surveillance." *Annals of Tropical Medicine and Parasitology* 99: 105–107.

Mukherjee, Joia S., and Fr. Eddy Eustache. 2007. "Community Health Workers as a Cornerstone for Integrating HIV and Primary Healthcare." *AIDS Care* 19: 73–82.

Mulemi, B. A. 2010. "Coping with Cancer and Adversity: Hospital Ethnography in Kenya." PhD dissertation, University of Amsterdam.

Muller, Ralph. 2005. "Guinea Worm Disease: The Final Chapter?" *Trends in Parasitology* 21: 521–24.

Multisectoral Technical Working Group for HIV/AIDS. 2008. *2007 HIV/AIDS epidemiologic report*. Maputo, Mozambique: National HIV/AIDS Control Program.

Muraskin, William. 1996. "Origins of the Children's Vaccine Initiative: The Political Foundations." *Social Science and Medicine* 42(12): 1721–34.

Murdoch, Lydia. 2006. *Imagined Orphans: Poor Families, Child Welfare, and Contested Citizenship in London*. New Brunswick, NJ: Rutgers University Press.

Murphy, Edward L. 2007. "A Home of One's Own: Finding a Place in the Fractured Landscapes of Urban Chile." PhD dissertation, University of Michigan.

Murray, Laura, and Gilbert Burnham. 2009. "Understanding Childhood Sexual Abuse in Africa." *Lancet* 373: 1924–26.

Murray, Scott A., Elizabeth Grant, Angus Grant, and Marilyn Kendall. 2003. "Dying from Cancer in Developed and Developing Countries: Lessons from Two Qualitative Interview Studies of Patients and Their Careers." *British Medical Journal* 326(7385): 368.

Mussa, Abdul. 2009. "Mozambican Health Workers' Perspectives on International Aid." MPH thesis, University of Washington, Seattle.

Nabarro, David N., and Kamini Mendis. 2000. "Roll Back Malaria Is Unarguably Both Necessary and Possible." *Bulletin of the World Health Organization* 78(12): 1454–55.

Nabarro, David N., and Elizabeth M. Tayle. 1998. "The 'Roll Back Malaria' Campaign." *Science* 280(5372): 2067–68.

Nájera, José. 1989. "Malaria and the Work of WHO." *Bulletin of the World Health Organization* 67(3): 229–43.

Narasimhan, Vasant, and Amir Attaran. 2003. "Roll Back Malaria? The Scarcity of International Aid for Malaria Control." *Malaria Journal* 2(8): 1–8.

National Library of Medicine. 2011. "Hazardous Substances Data Bank: Temephos." U.S. National Institutes of Health. Accessed October 24, 2011: http://toxnet.nlm.nih.gov/cgi-bin/sis/search/f?./temp/~iCSiGB:1.

Natterson-Horowitz, Barbara, and Kathryn Bowers. 2012. *Zoobiquity: What Animals Can Teach Us about Health and the Science of Healing.* New York: Knopf.

Nelson, Barbara. 1984. *Making an Issue of Child Abuse: Political Agenda Setting for Social Problems.* Chicago: University of Chicago Press.

New York Times. 1969. "Malaria Campaign to Be Reappraised." *New York Times,* March 16.

———. 2005. Editorial: "How Not to Roll Back Malaria." *New York Times,* October 16.

Nguyen, Vinh-Kim. 2004. "Antiretroviral Globalism, Biopolitics, and Therapeutic Citizenship." In *Global Assemblages,* Aihwa Ong and Stephen Collier, eds. London: Blackwell.

———. 2010. *The Republic of Therapy: Triage and Sovereignty in West Africa's Time of AIDS.* Durham, NC: Duke University Press.

Nguyen, Vinh-Kim, Cyriaque Yapo Ako, Pascal Niamba, Aliou Sylla, and Issoufou Tiendrébéogo. 2007. "Adherence as Therapeutic Citizenship: Impact of the History of Access to Antiretroviral Drugs on Adherence to Treatment." *AIDS* 21 (Suppl 5): S31–S35.

Nichter, Mark. 1989. *Anthropology and International Health: South Asian Case Studies.* New York: Springer.

———. 2008. *Global Health: Why Cultural Perceptions, Social Representations and Biopolitics Matter.* Tucson: University of Arizona Press.

Nóbrega, Otávia de Tolêdo, André Ricardo Marques, Ana Cleire Gomes de Araújo, Margô Gomes de Oliveira Karnikowski, Janeth de Oliveira Silva Naves, and Lynn Dee Silver. 2007. "Retail Prices of Essential Drugs in Brazil: An International Comparison." *Revista Panamericana de Salud Pública* 22(2): 118–23.

Nordstrom, Carolyn. 1997. *A Different Kind of War Story.* Philadelphia: University of Pennsylvania Press.

Nunn, Amy Stewart, Elize Massard da Fonseca, Francisco I. Bastos, and Sofia Gruskin. 2009. "AIDS Treatment in Brazil: Impacts and Challenges." *Health Affairs* 28(4): 1103–13.

Offen, Naphtali, Elizabeth A. Smith, and Ruth E. Malone. 2008. "Is Tobacco a Gay Issue? Interviews with Leaders of the LGBT Community." *Culture, Health and Sexuality* 10(2): 143–57.

Okie, Susan. 2006. "Fighting HIV—Lessons from Brazil." *New England Journal of Medicine* 354(19): 1977–81.

Olson, Elizabeth. 1998. "Ex-Prime Minister of Norway Wins Top Job at WHO." *New York Times,* January 28.

Ooms, Gorik, Wim van Damme, Brook K. Baker, Paul Zeitz, and Ted Schrecker. 2008. "The 'Diagonal' Approach to Global Fund Financing: A Cure for the Broader Malaise of Health Systems?" *Globalization and Health* 4: 6.

Osei-Atweneboana, M. Y., M. D. Wilson, R. J. Post, and D. A. Boakye. 2001. "Temephos-Resistant Larvae of *Simulium sanctipauli* Associated with a Distinctive New Chromosome Inversion in Untreated Rivers of South-Western Ghana." *Medical and Veterinary Entomology* 15(1): 113–16.

Packard, Randall. 2007. *The Making of a Tropical Disease: A Short History of Malaria.* Baltimore. MD: Johns Hopkins University Press.

Packard, Randall, and Paul Epstein. 1991. "Epidemiologists, Social Scientists, and the Structure of Medical Research on AIDS in Africa." *Social Science and Medicine* 33(7): 771–83.

Padian, Nancy S., Sandra I. McCoy, Jennifer E. Balkus, and Judith N. Wasserheit. 2010. "Weighing the Gold in the Gold Standard: Challenges in HIV Prevention Research." *AIDS* 24: 621–35.

Palmer, Karen. 2010. *Spellbound: Inside West Africa's Witch Camps*. New York: Free Press.

Pálsson, Gísli, and Paul Rabinow. 1999. "Iceland: The Case of a National Human Genome Project." *Anthropology Today* 15(2): 14–18.

Paluzzi, Joan E., and Fernando A. Garcia. 2008. "Health for All: Alma Ata Is Alive and Well in Venezuela." *Social Medicine* 3(4): 217–20.

Panter-Brick, Catherine. 2000. "Nobody's Children? A Reconsideration of Child Abandonment." In *Abandoned Children*, Catherine Panter-Brick and Malcolm Smith, eds., 1–26. Cambridge: Cambridge University Press.

Parish, Jane. 2000. "From the Body to the Wallet: Conceptualizing Akan Witchcraft at Home and Abroad." *Journal of the Royal Anthropological Institute* 6(3): 487–500.

Parker, John. 2006. "Northern Gothic: Witches, Ghosts and Werewolves in the Savannah Hinterland of the Gold Coast, 1900–1950s." *Africa* 76(3): 352–80.

Parker, Richard G. 2009. "Civil Society, Political Mobilization, and the Impact of HIV Scale-Up on Health Systems in Brazil." *Journal of Acquired Immune Deficiency Syndromes* 52 (Suppl 1): S49–S51.

Parkhurst, Justin O. 2002. "The Ugandan Success Story? Evidence and Claims of HIV1 Prevention." *Lancet* 360: 78–80.

Parkhurst, Justin O., and Louisiana Lush. 2004. "The Political Environment of HIV: Lessons from a Comparison of Uganda and South Africa." *Social Science and Medicine* 59: 1913–24.

Parkin, D. Max, Freddy Sitas, Mike Chirenje, Lara Stein, Raymond Abratt, and Henry Wabinga. 2008. "Part I: Cancer in Indigenous Africans: Burden, Distribution, and Trends." *Lancet Oncology* 9(7): 683–92.

Patel, Vikram, Preston Garrison, Jair de Jesus Mari, Harry Minas, Martin Prince, and Shekhar Saxena. 2008. "The *Lancet*'s Series on Global Mental Health: 1 Year On." *Lancet* 372: 1354–57.

———. 2009. "Packages of Care for Depression in Low- and Middle-Income Countries." *PLoS Medicine* 6(10): 1–7.

Patterson, Amy. 2003. "AIDS, Orphans, and the Future of Democracy in Africa." In *The Children of Africa Confront AIDS*, Arvind Singhal and Stephen Howard, eds., 13–39. Athens: Ohio University Press.

Patton, Michael Quinn. 2004. "A Microcosm of Global Challenges Facing the Field: Commentary on HIV/AIDS Monitoring and Evaluation." *New Directions for Evaluation* 103: 163–71.

Paul, J. E. 1988. "A Field Test Report of Implementation Planning and a Cost-Benefit Model for Guinea Worm Eradication in Pakistan." WASH field report no. 231. Water and Sanitation for Health Project. Washington, DC: USAID.

Pavignani, E., and J. R Durão. 1999. "Managing External Resources in Mozambique: Building New Aid Relationships on Shifting Sands?" *Health Policy and Planning* 14(3): 243–53.

PBS. 2006. "Global Health Champions: Donald R. Hopkins." [Episode 4: "Deadly Messengers."] *Rx for Survival*. Accessed April 27, 2012: http://www.pbs.org/wgbh/rxforsurvival/series/champions/donald_r_hopkins.html.

Peck, Robert, et al. 2003. "The Feasibility, Demand, and Effect of Integrating Primary Care Services with HIV Voluntary Counseling and Testing: Evaluation of a 15-Year Experience in Haiti, 1985–2000." *Journal of Acquired Immune Deficiency Syndromes* 33(4): 470–75.

Pellow, Deborah. 2011. "Internal Transmigrations: A Dagomba Diaspora." *American Ethnologist* 38(1): 132–47.

Pepe, Vera Lucia Edais, Miriam Ventura, João Maurício Brambati Sant'ana, Tatiana Aragão Figueiredo, Vanessa dos Reis de Souza, Luciana Simas, and Claudia Garcia Serpa Osorio-de-Castro. 2010. "Caracterização de demandas judiciais de fornecimento de medicamentos 'essenciais' no Estado do Rio de Janeiro, Brasil." *Cadernos de Saúde Pública* 26(3): 461–71.

Perrone, Matthew. 2012. "23andMe Seeks FDA Approval for Personal DNA Test." *Sci-Tech*. Accessed July 30, 2012: http://today.msnbc.msn.com/.

Petras, James F., and Fernando Ignacio Leiva. 1994. *Democracy and Poverty in Chile: The Limits to Electoral Politics*. Boulder, CO: Westview Press.

Petryna, Adriana. 2009. *When Experiments Travel: Clinical Trials and the Global Search for Human Subjects*. Princeton, NJ: Princeton University Press.

Petryna, Adriana, Andrew Lakoff, and Arthur Kleinman, eds. 2006. *Global Pharmaceuticals: Ethics, Markets and Practices*. Durham, NC: Duke University Press.

Pfeiffer, James. 2003. "International NGOs and Primary Health Care in Mozambique: The Need for a New Model of Collaboration." *Social Science and Medicine* 56(4): 725–38.

Pfeiffer, James, Wendy Johnson, Meredith Fort, Aaron Shakow, Amy Hagopian, Steve Gloyd, and Kenneth Gimbel-Sherr. 2008. "Strengthening Health Systems in Poor Countries: A Code of Conduct for Nongovernmental Organizations." *American Journal of Public Health* 98(12): 2134–40.

Pfeiffer, James, and Rachel Chapman. 2010. "Anthropological Perspectives on Structural Adjustment and Public Health." *Annual Review of Anthropology* 39: 149–65.

Physicians for Human Rights. 2008. "Zimbabwean Health Workers Call for Crisis Response." Cambridge, MA. Press Release, November 19.

Pitcher, Anne M. 2002. *Transforming Mozambique: The Politics of Privatization, 1975–2000*. Cambridge: Cambridge University Press.

Pitcher, Graeme, and Douglas Bowley. 2002. "Infant Rape in South Africa." *Lancet* 359: 274–75.

Pogge, Thomas. 2010. "The Health Impact Fund: Better Pharmaceutical Innovations at Much Lower Prices." In *Incentives for Global Health: Patent Law and Access to Essential Medicines*, Thomas Pogge, Matt Rimmer, and Kim Rubenstein, eds. Cambridge: Cambridge University Press.

Pollock, Linda. 1983. *Forgotten Children. Parent-Child Relations from 1500 to 1900*. Cambridge: Cambridge University Press.

Polson, K. A., S. C. Rawlins, W. G. Brogdon, and D. D. Chadee. 2010. "Organophosphate Resistance in Trinidad and Tobago Strains of *Aedes aegypti.*" *Journal of the American Mosquito Control Association* 26(4): 403–10.

Portenoy, Russell, and Pauline Lesage. 1999. "Management of Cancer Pain." *Lancet* 353(9165): 1695–1700.

Porter, Michael E. 2009. "A Strategy for Health Care Reform—Toward a Value-Based System." *New England Journal of Medicine* 361(2): 109–112.

———. 2010. "Redefining Global Health Delivery." Lecture at the Global Health Colloquium, Princeton University, September 24.

Porter, Michael E., and Elizabeth O. Teisberg. 2006. *Redefining Health Care: Creating Value-Based Competition on Results.* Cambridge, MA: Harvard Business School Press.

Posel, Deborah. 2005. "The Scandal of Manhood: 'Baby Rape' and the Politicization of Sexual Violence in Post-Apartheid South Africa." *Culture, Health and Sexuality* 7(3): 239–52.

Prasad, R., R. G. Nautiyal, P. K. Mukherji, A. Jain, K. Singh, and R. C. Ahuja. 2002. "Treatment of New Pulmonary Tuberculosis Patients: What Do Allopathic Doctors Do in India?" *International Journal of Tuberculosis and Lung Disease* 6: 1845–53.

Progress toward Global Eradication of Dracunculiasis. 2007. *MWWR Weekly.* Centers for Disease Control. Accessed December 10, 2007: http://www.cdc.gov/mmwr/preview/mmwrhtml/mm5632al.htm.

Rabinow, Paul. 1992. "Artificiality to Enlightenment: From Sociobiology to Biosociality." In *Incorporations*, Jonathan Crary and Sanford Kwinter, eds., 234–52. New York: Zone.

Raikhel, Eugene. 2010. "Post-Soviet Placebos: Epistemology and Authority in Russian Treatments for Alcoholism." *Culture, Medicine, and Psychiatry* 34(1): 132–68.

Ramiah, Ilavenil, and Michael R. Reich. 2005. "Public-Private Partnerships and Antiretroviral Drugs for HIV/AIDS: Lessons from Botswana." *Health Affairs* 24(2): 545–51.

Rasmussen, Sonja A., and Cynthia A. Moore. 2004. "Public Health Approach to Birth Defects, Developmental Disabilities and Conditions." *American Journal of Medical Genetics* C 125(1): 1–3.

Rathi, Akshat. 2012. "Ranbaxy Launches New Anti-Malarial Synriam." *Chemistry World.* Accessed May 3: http://www.rsc.org/chemistryworld/2012/05/ranbaxy-launches.

Ray, Turna. 2012. "Seeking 510(k) Clearance for Genomic Testing Service, 23andMe Maintains Direct-to-Consumer Ethos." *Pharmaceutical Intelligence*, July 31: http://pharmaceuticalintelligence.com/2012/08/01/23andme-takes-first-step-toward-fda-clearance/.

Real Academia. 2010. "Real Academia Española." In *Diccionario de la Lengua Española.*

Redfield, Peter. 2005. "Doctors, Borders, and Life in Crisis." *Cultural Anthropology* 20(3): 328–61.

Reeves, William C. 1972. "Can the War to Contain Infectious Disease Be Lost?" *American Journal of Tropical Medicine and Hygiene* 21(3): 251–59.

Rehwagen, Christiane. 2006. "WHO Recommends DDT to Control Malaria." *British Medical Journal* 333(7569): 622.

Reinhardt, Uwe, Peter S. Hussey, and Gerard F. Anderson. 2004. "U.S. Health Care Spending in an International Context." *Health Affairs* 23(3): 10–25.

Reis, R. 1994. "Evil in the Body, Disorder in the Brain: Interpretations of Epilepsy and the Treatment Gag in Swaziland." *Tropical and Geographic Medicine* 46: S40–3.

Reynolds, Pamela. 2000. "The Ground of All Making: State Violence, the Family and Political Activists." In *Violence and Subjectivity*, Veena Das, Arthur Kleinman, Mamphela Ramphele, and Pamela Reynolds, eds., 141–70. Berkeley: University of California Press.

Richards, Frank, Ernesto Ruiz-Tiben, and Donald Hopkins. 2011. "Dracunculiasis Eradication and the Legacy of the Smallpox Campaign: What's New and Innovative? What's Old and Principled?" *Vaccine* 29(s4): D86–90.

Riesco, Manuel. 2005. "Trabajo y Previsión Social en el Gobierno de Lagos." In *Gobierno de Lagos: Balance Crítico*, G. Salazar Vergara, ed., 43–70. Santiago, Chile: LOM Ediciones.

Rinaldi, A. 2009. "Free, At Last! The Progress of New Disease Eradication Campaigns for Guinea Worm Disease and Polio, and the Prospect of Tackling Other Diseases." *Science and Society* 10(3): 215–21.

Rodríguez, M. M., J. Bisset, M. Ruiz, and A. Soca. 2002. "Cross-Resistance to Pyrethriod and Organophosphorous Insecticides Induced by Selection with Temephos in *Aedes aegypti* (Diptera: Culicidae) from Cuba." *Journal of Medical Entomology* 39(6): 882–88.

Rojas, Graciela, Ricardo Araya, and Glyn Lewis. 2005. "Comparing Sex Inequalities in Common Affective Disorders across Countries: Great Britain and Chile." *Social Science and Medicine* 60: 1693–1703.

Roll Back Malaria Partnership. 2008. "Global Malaria Action Plan, Part I Section 4: Funding for Malaria Today." Accessed July, 2010: http://www.rollbackmalaria.org/gmap/1-4.html.

Rollet, Catherine. 1990. *La Politique à l'Egard de la Petite Enfance sous la Troisième République*. Paris: Presses Universitaires de France.

Román, Oscar, and Félix Muñoz. 2008. "Una Mirada Crítica en Torno al Plan AUGE: Algunos Aspectos Generales y Valóricos." *Revista Médica de Chile* 136: 1599–1603.

Rose, Nikolas. 2007. *The Politics of Life Itself: Biomedicine, Power, and Subjectivity in the 21st Century*. Princeton, NJ: Princeton University Press.

Rosenberg, Tina. 2012. "In Rwanda, Health Care Coverage that Eludes the U.S." *New York Times*, July 3. http://opinionator.blogs.nytimes.com/2012/07/03/rwandas-health care-miracle.

Rouse, Carolyn. 2009. *Uncertain Suffering: Racial Health Disparities and Sickle Cell Disease*. Berkeley: University of California Press.

Rowden, Rick. 2009. *The Deadly Ideas of Neoliberalism: How the IMF Has Undermined Public Health and the Fight against AIDS*. London: Zed Books.

Ruiz-Tiben, Ernesto, and Donald R. Hopkins. 2006. "Dracunculiasis (Guinea Worm Disease) Eradication." *Advances in Parasitology* 61: 275–309.

Rwakimari, John, Donald R. Hopkins, and Ernesto Ruiz-Tiben. 2006."Uganda's Successful Guinea Worm Eradication Program." *American Journal of Tropical Medicine and Hygiene* 75: 3–8.

Ryan, Frank. 1992. *Tuberculosis: The Greatest Story Never Told*. Bromsgrove, UK: Swift Publishers.

Rylko-Bauer, Barbara, Linda Whiteford, and Paul Farmer, eds. 2009. *Global Health in Times of Violence*. Santa Fe, NM: School for Advanced Research Press.

Sachs, Jeffrey D. 2002. "A New Global Effort to Control Malaria." *Science* 298(5591): 122–24.

Sackett, David L., William Rosenberg, J. A. Muir Gray, R. Brian Haynes, and W. Scott Richardson. 1996. "Evidence-Based Medicine: What It Is and What It Isn't." *British Medical Journal* 312(13): 71–72.

Sackett, David L., Sharon E. Straus, E. Scott Richardson, William Rosenberg, and R. Brian Haynes. 2000. *Evidence-Based Medicine: How to Practice and Teach EBM*. New York: Churchill Livingstone.

Salazar Vergara, Gabriel. 2005. "Ricardo Lagos, 2000–2005: Perfíl Histórico, Trasfondo Popular." In *Gobierno de Lagos: Balance Crítico*, G. Salazar Vergara, ed., 71–100. Santiago, Chile: LOM Ediciones.

Samsky, Ari. 2011. "'Since We Are Taking the Drugs': Labor and Value in Two International Drug Donation Programs." *Journal of Cultural Economy* 4(1): 27–43.

Save the Guinea Worm Foundation. 2007. "Defending the World's Most Endangered Species." Accessed September 15, 2009: http://www.deadlysins.com/guineaworm/index.htm.

Scarry, Elaine. 1985. *The Body in Pain: The Making and Unmaking of the World*. Oxford: Oxford University Press.

Scheffer, Mário, Andrea Lazzarini Salazar, and Karina Bozola Grou. 2005. "O remédio via justiça: um estudo sobre o acesso a novos medicamentos e exames em HIV/AIDS no Brasil por meio de ações judiciais." Brasília, DF: Ministério da Saúde.

Scheper-Hughes, Nancy. 1987. "The Cultural Politics of Child Survival." In *Child Survival*, Nancy Scheper-Hughes, ed., 1–29. Dordrecht: Kluwer.

———. 1992. *Death without Weeping: The Violence of Everyday Life in Brazil*. Berkeley: University of California Press.

Schieber, George J., Pablo Gottret, Lisa K. Fleisher, and Adam A. Leive. 2007. "Financing Global Health: Mission Unaccomplished." *Health Affairs* 26(4): 921–34.

Schild, Verónica. 2000. "Neo-Liberalism's New Gendered Market Citizens: The 'Civilizing' Dimension of Social Programmes in Chile." *Citizenship Studies* 4(3): 275–305.

Schmidt, Michael S., and Katie Thomas. 2012. "Abbot Settles Marketing Lawsuit." *New York Times*, May 7. http://www.nytimes.com/2012/05/08/business/abbott-to-pay-1-6-billion-over-illegal-marketing.html?partner=rssnyt&emc=rss.

Schmoll, Pamela. 1993. "Black Stomachs, Beautiful Stones: Soul-Eating among Hausa in Niger." *Modernity and Its Malcontents: Ritual and Power in Post-colonial Africa*, J. Comaroff and J. L. Comaroff, eds. Chicago: University of Chicago Press.

Schneider, Helen. 2002. "On the Fault-Line: The Politics of AIDS Policy in Contemporary South Africa." *African Studies* 61: 145–67.

Schönteich, Martin. 1999. "AIDS and Age: South Africa's Crime Time Bomb?" *AIDS Analysis Africa* 10(2): 3–4.

Schull, Natasha Dow. 2006. "Machines, Medication, Modulation: Circuits of Dependency and Self-Care in Las Vegas." *Culture, Medicine, and Psychiatry* 30: 223–247.

Schwartz, Hillel. 1986. *Never Satisfied: A Cultural History of Diets, Fantasies and Fat*. New York: Free Press.

Scott, James. 1976. *The Moral Economy of the Peasant: Rebellion and Subsistence in Southeast Asia*. New Haven: Yale University Press.

Seidu Korkor, Andrew, and Mawusi Afele. 2009. "Countdown to Wipe Out Guinea-Worm in Ghana." *Bulletin of the World Health Organization* 87: 649–50.

Serres, Michel. 1982. *The Parasite*. Minneapolis: University of Minnesota Press.

Shapin, Steven, and Simon Schaffer. 1986. *Leviathan and the Air-Pump: Hobbes, Boyle and the Experimental Life*. Princeton, NJ: Princeton University Press.

Shields, Alexandra E., Michael Fortun, Evelynn M. Hammonds, Patricia A. King, Caryn Lerman, Rayna Rapp, and Patrick E. Sullivan. 2005. "The Use of Race Variables in Genetic Studies of Complex Traits and the Goal of Reducing Health Disparities: A Transdisciplinary Perspective." *American Psychologist* 60(1): 77–103.

Shim, Janet K. 2005. "Constructing 'Race" Across the Science-Lay Divide: Racial Formation in the Epidemiology and Experience of Cardiovascular Disease." *Social Studies of Science* 35(3): 405–36.

Shipton, Parker. 2010. *Credit between Cultures: Farmers, Financiers, and Misunderstanding in Africa*. New Haven, CT: Yale University Press.

Shorter, Edward. 1976. *The Making of the Modern Family*. New York: Basic Books.

Sierra Leone. 2007. The Prevention and Control of HIV and AIDS Act. June 15. http://www.sierra-leone.org/Laws/2007-8p.pdf.

Singer, Merrill, and G. Derrick Hodge, eds. 2010. *The War Machine and Global Health*. Lanham, MD: AltaMira Press.

Singla, Neeta, P. P. Sharma, R. Singla, and R. C. Jain. 1998. "Survey of Knowledge, Attitudes and Practices for Tuberculosis among General Practitioners in Delhi, India." *International Journal of Tuberculosis* 2(5): 284–389.

Sodemann, Morten, S. Biai, M. S. Jakobsen, and P. Aaby. 2006. "Knowing a Medical Doctor Is Associated with Reduced Mortality among Sick Children Consulting a Paediatric Ward in Guinea-Bissau, West Africa." *Tropical Medicine and International Health* 11(12): 1868–77.

Sollom, Richard. 2009. *Health in Ruins: A Man-Made Disaster in Zimbabwe*. (A Physicians for Human Rights Report). http://physiciansforhumanrights.org/library/reports/zimbabwe-health-in-ruins-2009.html.

Souza, R. R. de. 2002. "O programa de medicamentos excepcionais." In *Protocolos Clínicos e Diretrizes Terapêuticas – Medicamentos Excepcionais*, P. D. Picon and A. Beltrame, eds., 11–12. Brasília, DF: Ministério da Saúde.

Staniland, Martin. 1975. *Lions of Dagbon: Political Change in Northern Ghana*. Cambridge: Cambridge University Press.

Stearns, Peter N. 2002. *Fat History: Bodies and Beauty in the Modern West*. New York: New York University Press.

Stepan, Nancy Leys. 2011. *Eradication: Ridding the World of Diseases Forever?* Ithaca, NY: Cornell University Press.

Stephens, Sharon. 1995. "Children and the Politics of Culture in 'Late Capitalism.'" In *Children and the Politics of Culture*, Sharon Stephens, ed., 3–48. Princeton, NJ: Princeton University Press.

Strathern, Marilyn, ed. 2000. *Audit Cultures: Anthropological Studies in Accountability, Ethics and the Academy*. New York: Routledge.

Stubbs, S. G., and E. W. Bligh. 1931. *Sixty Centuries of Health and Physick*. London: Sampson, Low, Marston & Co.

Sunder Rajan, Kaushik. 2006. *Biocapital: The Constitution of Postgenomic Life*. Durham, NC: Duke University Press.

Susser, Mervyn, and Ezra Susser. 1996. "Choosing a Future for Epidemiology: II." *American Journal of Public Health* 86(5): 674–77.

Swidler, Ann. 2009a. "Dialectics of Patronage: Logics of Accountability at the African AIDS-NGO Interface." In *Globalization, Philanthropy, and Civil Society*, David C. Hammack and Steven Heydemann, eds., 192–220. Bloomington: Indiana University Press.

———. 2009b. "Responding to AIDS in Sub-Saharan Africa: Culture, Institutions, and Health." In *Successful Societies: How Institutions and Culture Affect Health*, Peter Hall and Michèle Lamont, eds., 128–50. Cambridge: Cambridge University Press.

Swidler, Ann, and Susan Cotts Watkins. 2009. "'Teach a Man to Fish': The Sustainability Doctrine and Its Social Consequences." *World Development* 37(7): 1182–96.

Tait, David. 1963. "A Sorcery Hunt in Dagbon." *Africa: Journal of the International African Institute* 33(2): 136–47.

Tanner, Marcel, and Marcel Hommel. 2010. "Towards Malaria Elimination—A New Thematic Series." *Malaria Journal* 20(9): 24.

Tanner, Marcel, and Don de Savignya. 2008. "Malaria Eradication Back on the Table." *Bulletin of the World Health Organization* 86(2): 82–83.

Tayeh, A., S. Cairncross, and G. Maude. 1996. "The Impact of Health Education to Promote Cloth Filters on Dracunculiasis Prevalence in the Northern Region, Ghana." *Social Science and Medicine* 43: 1205–11.

TB Alliance. 2007. *Pathway to Patients: Charting the Dynamics of the Global TB Drug Market*. New York: TB Alliance.

———. 2009. *Accelerating the Pace: Annual Report 2009*. New York: TB Alliance.

Thomas, Katie. 2012. "J. & J. Fined $2 Billion in Drug Case." *New York Times*, April 11. http://www.nytimes.com/2012/04/12/business/drug-giant-is-fined-1-2-billion-in-arkansas.html?_r=1&emc=tnt&tntemail0=y.

Thomas, Katie, and Michael S. Schmidt. 2012. "Glaxco Agrees to Pay $3 Billion in Fraud Settlement." *New York Times*, July 7: http://www.nytimes.com/2012/07/03/business/glaxosmithkline-agrees-to-pay-3-billion-in-fraud-settlement.html?pagewanted=all.

Thome, B. 2010. "Pregnancy, HIV, and Prevention of Mother to Child Transmission (PMTCT) in Central Mozambique: Community Influences on Loss to Follow Up." MPH thesis, University of Washington, Seattle.

Thompson, Edward Palmer. 1971. "The Moral Economy of the English Crowd in the Eighteenth Century." *Past and Present* 50: 76–136.

———. 1991. "The Moral Economy Reviewed." In *Customs in Common*, E. P. Thompson, ed., 259–351. London: The Merlin Press.

Tikar, S. N., A. Kumar, G. B. Prasad, and S. Prakash. 2009. "Temephos-Induced Resistance in *Aedes aegypti* and Its Cross-Resistance Studies to Certain Insecticides from India." *Parasitology Research* 105: 57–63.

Timmermans, Stefan, and E. S. Kolker. 2004. "Evidence-Based Medicine and the Reconfiguration of Medical Knowledge." *Journal of Health and Social Behavior* 45(suppl): 177–93.

Timmermans, Stefan, and Aaron Mauck. 2005. "The Promise and Pitfalls of Evidence-Based Medicine." *Health Affairs* 24(1): 18–28.

Todrys, Katherine W., and Joseph J. Amon. 2012. "Criminal Justice Reform as HIV and TB Prevention in African Prisons." *PLoS Medicine* 9(5): e1001215.

Townsend, Peter, and Nick Davidson. 1982. *Inequalities in Health: The Black Report*. Report by Sir Douglas Black, Professor J. N. Morris, Dr. Cyril Smith, and Professor Peter Townsend. Harmondsworth: Penguin Books.

Travis, Kate. 2007. "Cancer in Africa: Health Experts Aim to Curb Potential Epidemic." *Journal of the National Cancer Institute* 99(15): 1146–47.

Treichler, Paula. 1999. *How to Have Theory in an Epidemic: Cultural Chronicles of AIDS*. Durham, NC: Duke University Press.

Tribunal de Justiça do Estado do Rio Grande do Sul, Sétima Câmara Cível. 2009. Apelação Cível Nº 70031235633. Accessed February 21, 2010: http://www.es-pacovital.com.br/noticia_complemento_ler.php?id=1690&noticia_id=17087.

Trostle, James. 1996. "Introduction: Inappropriate Distribution of Medicines by Professionals in Developing Countries." *Social Science and Medicine* 42(8): 1117–20.

———. 2005. *Epidemiology and Culture*. New York: Cambridge University Press.

UBOS, Uganda Bureau of Statistics, and Macro International Inc. 2007. *Uganda Demographic and Health Survey 2006*. Calverton, MD: UBOS and Macro International Inc.

UNAIDS. 2009. "Guidance Note on HIV and Sex Work." http://europeandcis.undp.org/hivaids/show/BA9B818E-F203-1EE9-B2F77C61A3A4F37F.

———. 2010. "Non-discrimination in HIV Responses." 26th Meeting of the UNAIDS Programme Coordinating Board, 22-24 June, Geneva. http://data.unaids.org/pub/BaseDocument/2010/20100526_non_discrimination_in_hiv_en.pdf.

UNAIDS, African Union, and World Health Organization. 2006. "Brazzaville Commitment on Scaling Up Towards Universal Access to HIV and AIDS Prevention, Treatment, Care and Support in Africa by 2010." Brazzaville, Republic of Congo, March 8. http://www.afro.who.int/en/divisions-a-programmes/atm/ acquired-immune-deficiency-syndrome/aids-publications/doc_download/3780-brazzaville-commitment-on-universal-access-to-hiv-and-aids-prevention-treatment-care-and-support.html.

UN Committee on Economic, Social and Cultural Rights. 2000. "Substantive Issues Arising in the Implementation of the International Covenant on Economic, Social and Cultural Rights." General Comment No. 14, The Right to the Highest Attainable Standard of Health. Geneva: Office of the UN High Commissioner for Human Rights.

UNICEF. 2004. *A Framework for Protection: Care and Support of Orphans and Vulnerable Children Living in a World with HIV and AIDS*. Geneva: UNICEF.

United Nations. 2000. "United Nations Millennium Declaration." New York, Fifty-fifth session (Agenda item 60b), September 18. Accessed March 11, 2013: http://www.un.org/millennium/declaration/ares552e.pdf.

University of Wisconsin Pain and Policy Studies Group. 2006. *Availability of Morphine and Pethidine in the World and Africa*. Madison: University of Wisconsin.

Uplekar, Mukund W., and D. S. Shepard. 1991. "Treatment of Tuberculosis by Private General Practitioners in India." *Tubercle* 72: 284–90.

US Congress. 2003. *HIV/AIDS, TB and Malaria: Combating a Global Pandemic: Hearing before the Subcommittee on Health of the Committee on Energy and Commerce, House of Representatives, One Hundred and Eighth Congress, first session, 20 March, 2003*. Washington: US Government Printing Office.

Utzinger, Jurg, Yesim Tozan, Fadi Doumani, and Burton H. Singer. 2002. "The Economic Payoffs of Integrated Malaria Control in the Zambian Copperbelt between 1930 and 1950." *Tropical Medicine and International Health* 7(8): 657–77.

van der Geest, Sjaak, and Kaja Finkler. 2004. "Hospital Ethnography: Introduction." *Social Science and Medicine* 59(10): 1995–2001.

Vecchiato, Norbert. 1997. "'Digestive Worms': Ethnomedical Approaches to Intestinal Parasitism in Southern Ethiopia." In *The Anthropology of Infectious Disease*, Marcia Inhorn and Peter Brown, eds. Amsterdam: Gordon and Breach Publishers.

Vianna, L. W., and M. B. Burgos. 2005. "Entre princípios e regras: Cinco estudos de caso de ação cível público." *Dados* 48(4): 777–843.

Vieira, Fabiola Sulpino. 2009. "Ministry of Health's Spending on Drugs: Program Trends from 2002 to 2007." *Rev. Saúde Pública* 43(4): 674–81.

Vieira, Fabiola Sulpino, and Paola Zucchi. 2007. "Distorções causadas pelas ações judiciais à política de medicamentos no Brasil." *Rev. Saúde Pública* 41(2): 214–22.

Voelker, Rebecca. 2007. "Persistence Pays Off in Guinea Worm Fight." *Journal of the American Medical Association* 298(16): 1856–57.

Vorhaus, Dan. 2012. "Patenting and Personal Genomics: 23andMe Receives Its First Patent, and Plenty of Questions." Genomics Law Report. June 1: http://www.genomicslawreport.com/index.php/2012/06/01/patenting-and-personal-genomics-23andme-receives-its-first-patent-and-plenty-of-questions/.

Wailoo, Keith. 2010. "The Politics of Pain: Liberal Medicine, Conservative Care, and the Governance of Relief in America since the 1950s." The Fielding Garrison Lecture, American Association for the History of Medicine Annual Meeting, April 30, Rochester, MN.

Waitzkin, Howard, Celia Iriat, Alfredo Estrada, and Silvia Lamadrid. 2001. "Social Medicine Then and Now: Lessons from Latin America." *American Journal of Public Health* 91(10): 1592–1601.

Walt, Gina, and Angela Melamed. 1983. *Mozambique: Towards a People's Health Service*. London: Zed Books.

Walter, Nicholas D., Thomas Lyimo, Jacek Skarbinski, Emmy Metta, Elizeus Kahigwa, Brendan Flannery, Scott F. Dowell, Salim Abdulla, and S. Patrick Kachur. 2009. "Why First-Level Health Workers Fail to Follow Guidelines for Managing Severe Disease in Children in the Coast Region, the United Republic of Tanzania." *Bulletin of the World Health Organization* 87(2): 99–107.

Walton, David A., Paul Farmer, Wesler Lambert, F. Leandre, Serena P. Koenig, and Joia S. Mukherjee. 2004. "Integrated HIV Prevention and Care Strengthens Primary Health Care: Lessons from Rural Haiti." *Journal of Public Health Policy* 25: 137–58.

Watts, Susan. 1998. "Perceptions and Priorities in Disease Eradication: Dracunculiasis Eradication in Africa." *Social Science and Medicine* 46: 799–810.

WebMD. "Cancer Health Center: Bone Marrow Aspiration and Biopsy." http://www.webmd.com/a-to-z-guides/bone-marrow-aspiration-and-biopsy?page=3.

Weinstein, Andrew G., et al. n.d. "Achieving Adherence to Asthma Therapy." AAAAI Quality of Care for Asthma Committee Paper. Milwaukee, WI: American Academy of Allergy, Asthma and Immunology. Unpublished.

West, Harry, and Todd Sanders. 2003. *Transparency and Conspiracy: Ethnographies of Suspicion in the New World Order*. Durham, NC: Duke University Press.

Whiteside, Alan, and Clem Sunter. 2000. *AIDS: The Challenge for South Africa*. Cape Town: Human and Rousseau-Tafelberg.

Whitmarsh, Ian. 2008a. *Biomedical Ambiguity: Race, Asthma, and the Contested Meaning of Genetic Research in the Caribbean*. Ithaca, NY: Cornell University Press.

———. 2008b. "Biomedical Ambivalence: Asthma Diagnosis, the Pharmaceutical, and Other Contradictions in Barbados." *American Ethnologist* 35(1): 49–63.

———. 2009a. "Hyperdiagnostics: Postcolonial Utopics of Race-Based Biomedicine." *Medical Anthropology* 28(3): 285–315.

———. 2009b. "Medical Schismogenics: Compliance and 'Culture' in Caribbean Biomedicine." *Anthropological Quarterly* 82(2): 453–82.

WHO. See "World Health Organization"

Whyte, Susan Reynolds. 2009. "At Home with Antiretroviral Therapy in Uganda." In *Theory and Action: Essays for an Anthropologist*, Marian Tankink and Sjaak van der Geest, eds., 238–45. Diemen: Uitgeverij AMB.

———. 2011. "Writing Knowledge and Acknowledgement: Possibilities in Medical Research." In *Evidence, Ethos and Experiment: The Anthropology and History of Medical Research in Africa*, Wenzel Geissler, ed. Oxford: Berghahn.

Whyte, Susan Reynolds, Sjaak van der Geest, and Anita Hardon. 2002. *Social Lives of Medicines*. Cambridge: Cambridge University Press.

Whyte, Susan Reynolds, Michael A. Whyte, and David Kyaddondo. 2010. "Health Workers Entangled: Confidentiality and Certification." In *Morality, Hope and Grief: Anthropologies of AIDS in Africa*, Hansjörg Dilger and Ute Luig, eds., 80–101. New York: Berghahn.

Whyte, Susan R., Michael A. Whyte, Lotte Meinert, and Betty Kyaddondo. 2004. "Treating AIDS: Dilemmas of Unequal Access in Uganda." *Journal of Social Aspects of HIV/AIDS* 1(1): 14–26.

Williams, Patricia. 2012. "Whose Body Is It Anyway?" *The Nation*, June 25, 9.

Wilson, Duff. 2010. "Novartis Settles Off-Label Marketing Case over 6 Drugs for $422.5 Million." *New York Times*, September 30. http://www.nytimes.com/2010/10/01/health/policy/01novartis.html.

Wojcicki, Anne. 2012. "Announcing 23andMe's First Patent." May 28, amended June 1: http://spittoon.23andme.com/news/announcing-23andmes-first-patent/.

Wolf, Eric R. 1966. "Kinship, Friendship and Patron-Client Relations." In *The Social Anthropology of Complex Societies*, Michael Banton, ed., 1–22. London: Tavistock.

Wolff, Mary S. 1993. "Blood Levels of Organochlorine and Risk of Breast Cancer." *Journal of the National Cancer Institute* 85: 648–52.

World Bank. 2002. *Improving Health for the Poor in Mozambique: The Fight Continues*. African Region Human Development, Working Paper Series 23789. Washington, D.C.: World Bank.

———. 2009. Brazil Country Brief. http://go.worldbank.org/UW8ODN2SV0.

———. 2011. "Republic of Ghana: Tackling Poverty in Northern Ghana." PREM 4/AFTAR Africa Region. Accra, Ghana.

World Commission on Environment and Development. 1987. *Our Common Future*. New York: Oxford University Press.

World Health Organization. 1969. *Twenty-Second World Health Assembly, Boston, Massachusetts, 8–25 July 1969, Part II, Plenary Meetings, Committees, Summary Records and Reports*. Geneva: World Health Organization.

———. 1992. *Report of the Ministerial Conference on Malaria, Amsterdam, 26–27 October 1992*. Geneva: World Health Organization.

———. 1993a. *A Global Strategy for Malaria Control*. Geneva: World Health Organization.

———. 1993b. *Implementation of the Global Malaria Control Strategy*. Geneva: World Health Organization.

———. 1994. *The Work of WHO 1992–1993: Biennial Report of the Director-General to the World Health Assembly and to the United Nations*. Geneva: World Health Organization.

———. 1998. "Dr. Gro Harlem Brundtland Elected Director-General of the World Health Organization." WHO Press Release, May 17. Accessed August 19, 2007: http://www.malaria.org/NEWS5_15.HTM.

———. 2002a. "Increasing Access to Knowledge of HIV Status: Conclusions of a WHO Consultation, 3–4 December, 2001." http://www.who.int/hiv/pub/vct/en/hiv_2002_09_en.pdf.

————. 2002b. *Operational Guide for National Tuberculosis Control Programmes on the Introduction and Use of Fixed-Dose Combination Drugs*. (WHO/CDS/TB/2002.308 – WHO/EDM/PAR/2002.6).

————. 2002c. *World Health Report: Reducing Risks, Promoting Healthy Life*. Geneva: World Health Organization.

————. 2003. *A Community Health Approach to Palliative Care for HIV/AIDS and Cancer Patients*. Geneva: World Health Organization.

————. 2006. *World Health Report: Working Together for Health*. Geneva: World Health Organization.

————. 2009a. "Death and DALY Estimates for 2004 by Cause for WHO Member States: Persons, All Ages." Department of Measurement and Health Information, Disease and Injury Country Estimates. Accessed March 27 2012: http://www.who.int/healthinfo/global_burden_disease/estimates_country/en/index.html.

————. 2009b. *Global Development Advisors, Independent Evaluation of the Roll Back Malaria Partnership, 2004–2008*. Geneva: World Health Organization.

————. 2009c. *Global Tuberculosis Control: Epidemiology, Strategy, Financing: WHO Report 2009*. Geneva: World Health Organization.

————. 2010a. *Stop TB Strategy*: http://www.who.int/tb/strategy/stop_tb_strategy/en/index.html.

————. 2010b. *India: National Health System Profile*: http://searo.who.int/EN/Section313/Section1519.htm.

————. 2012. "Dracunculiasis Eradication: Global Surveillance Summary, 2011." *Weekly Epidemiological Record* 87: 177–88.

World Health Organization Collaborating Center for Research, Training and Eradication of Dracunculiasis. 2011. "Guinea Worm Wrap-Up, #202." Atlanta, GA: Centers for Disease Control and Prevention.

World Health Organization Global Malaria Programme. 2007. "The Use of DDT in Malaria Vector Control." WHO Position Statement. Geneva: World Health Organization.

World Health Organization International Agency for Research on Cancer. n.d. "Fact Sheets." Accessed June 14, 2010: http://globocan.iarc.fr/.

World Health Organization Study Group on Malaria Control as Part of Primary Health Care. 1983. *Malaria Control as Part of Primary Health Care: Report of a WHO Study Group*. Geneva: World Health Organization.

World Health Organization and UNAIDS. 2010. "Technical Guidance Note for Global Fund HIV Proposals: Human Rights and Law." http://www.who.int/hiv/pub/toolkits/HRandLaw_Technical_Guidance_GlobalFundR10_June2010.pdf.

Wylie, Sara. 2011. "Corporate Bodies and Chemical Bonds: An STS Analysis of the American Natural Gas Industry". PhD dissertation, MIT.

Yacoob, Mary, William Brieger, and Susan Watts. 1989. "Primary Health Care: Why Has Water Been Neglected?" *Health Policy and Planning* 4: 328–33.

Yamey, Gavin. 2004. "Roll Back Malaria: A Failing Global Health Campaign." *British Medical Journal* 328: 1086–87.

Yamin, Alicia Ely, and Oscar Parra-Vera. 2010. "Judicial Protection of the Right to Health in Colombia: From Social Demands to Individual Claims to Public Debates." *Hastings International and Comparative Law Review* 33(2): 101–130.

Yu, Dongbao, Yves Souteyrand, Mazuwa A. Banda, Joan Kaufman, and Joseph H. Perriëns. 2008. "Investment in HIV/AIDS Programs: Does It Help Strengthen Health Systems in Developing Countries?" *Globalization and Health* 4(8).

Zelizer, Viviana. 1985. *Pricing the Priceless Child: The Changing Social Value of Children*. Princeton, NJ: Princeton University Press.

Zondi, M., and J. D. Kvalsvig. 1996. *Traditional Medicine and Parasite Infections: Perceptions about Worms among Traditional Healers in KwaZulu-Natal*. Durban, South Africa: Child Development Program.

Index

ABATE chemical, 226–27, 228–29

ABC approach (Uganda), 104, 105

accountability: advocacy and, 97, 181–83, 339; EBM seen as solution to demands for public health, 84; evidence-based medicine (EBM) audit culture of, 67, 76–79; government service, 182, 330; illness and individual, 325; increasing demands for NGO, 77; infused into heart of the research methodology, 78–79; major aid flows to Africa and, 170; medicinal access and, 330

Adams, Vincanne, 25–26, 54, 134, 351, 355, 365, 366

Africa: Booster Program for Malaria Control in Africa work in, 48; brief history of Ghana guinea worm in West, 210–15; Ghana Guinea Worm Eradication Program success in, 138–39, 207–36; human rights controversy over HIV testing in, 99; marginalization of pain in clinical medicine in, 188–91; Mozambique's ART programs, 168–81; Namibian High Court forced sterilization order (2012), 106; Nigerian guinea worm eradication, 214–15, 217, 221; People's Republic of Congo, 36; personalistic patron-client systems in, 151. *See also* malaria eradication programs; South Africa; Uganda

African-Americans: chronic racial disparities and public health genetics, 318–22; metabolic syndrome and, 321; women targeted as at-risk population, 320–22

African palliative care movement, 188

Afro-Caribbean population, 318

AIDS "exceptionalism," 94, 98

AIDS journal, 83

AIDS Law Project (now Section 27), 103

AIDS orphanhood: comparing 1993 and 2002 surveys on South African, 125–26; controversies over AIDS in South Africa and role of, 126–28; increasing rates of, 112, 113; "moral economies" concept to address, 27–29; "problematization" of, 111, 127–29; projections of, 125; "Survival Guide for AIDS Orphans" (*Mail & Guardian*) on, 125. *See also* HIV/AIDS epidemic

AIDS-related Kaposi's sarcoma *See*. Botswana cancer epidemic

AIDS Support Organization (TASO) [Uganda], 141, 142, 153–54, 156, 161–62

áimo (vital energy), 287, 292, 299

Alvarado, Rubén, 280, 283

American biomedicine: chronic disease focus of, 303; as critical to Barbados government health interventions, 304; public health shift toward genetic predisposition, 316–18; statistics mapping used in, 305. *See also* United States

American Diabetes Association, 320

American Heart Association, 320

Amon, Joseph J., 26–27, 91, 363

Annan, Kofi, 42

Anopheles mosquitoes, 350

antidepressants: as "adaptation" medicine, 292; used to restore *áimo* (vital energy), 287, 292, 299; Violeta's story on using, 276–78. *See also* depression

antimalarial drugs: ACT (artemisinin combination therapies), 41–42, 45, 47; artemisinin, 36, 41; chloroquine, 36, 41; limited research (early 1980s) on, 36. *See also* malaria epidemic

anti-TB drug market: MRs' (medical respresentatives') perceptions of private prescribers in the, 264–69; MRs' views

as an early warning system, 18–20; in global health, 16–18; how it demystifies global health projects, 26; lived realities and "target populations" and, 19, 248; marketing practices and, 258; as a methodological tool of inquiry, 11; of Mozambique public sector and ART, 175–78; the public health landscape and, 133–39; salvage, 210–36

European AIDS Society, 96

European AIDS Treatment Group, 96

Evans-Pritchard, E. E., 208, 215

evidence-based medicine (EBM): accountability measured by "audit" of, 58, 76–77; controversy over merger of public health and, 64–67; creation of experimental metric for health care created by, 55; as default language for health intervention issues, 7–8, 25–26; examining the issues related to, 14; IIS on impact of health insurance schemes on child health, 67–72; LAM's story on pioneering problem-solving innovations, 356–62; NGO-industrial complex and audit culture issues of, 76–79; origins and rise of, 55–58; producing and privatizing profits in global public health use of, 72–76; shift of priorities of public health caregiving due to, 55; taken as the gold standard, 55–56; TAR Health Bureau-US project derailed by, 79–83; translational research orientation to study, 348, 355–62. See also biomedical science

evidence-based public health (EBPH): controversy over merger of public health and EBM in, 64–67; producing and privatizing profits in, 72–76; RCT-model research driven by, 59–64. See also global public health

explanatory models, 256

Farber, Amy, 356–58, 359, 360, 361–62

Farmer, Paul, 9, 252, 256

Fassin, Didier, 27, 28–29, 109, 215, 355, 363, 364

Feachem, Richard, 38, 45

Federal of Pharmaceutical Manufacturers Associations, 37

Federation of Medical Representatives Association of India (FMRAI), 261

Feierman, S., 148

Fidler, David, 335–36

fiscal concerns: accountability measured by EBM audit culture, 58; Chile's labor system and economic uncertainty, 277, 287–92; economic trickle-down theories, 251, 338–41, 355–56; EMB audit culture and NGO-industrial complex, 76–79; of evidence-based medicine in global public health, 72–76; Ghana Guinea Worm Eradication Program and Northern Ghanan farmer, 219; Island Insurance Study (IIS) cost-effectiveness and, 270–71; market-driven research methodology, 74–75. See also poverty

Fischer, Michael M. J., 347

Folkman, Judah, 352, 354, 360

food security issues, 177–79

Fortun, Kim, 370

Fortun, Michael, 370

forward-looking orientation: building public health civil society through, 348, 371–73; dialogue as beginning the, 371

Foucault, Michel, 114, 116, 313, 338

Foul Water, Fiery Serpent (film), 232

"4-H Club," 94

Frank, Volker, 287

Gandhi, Mahatma, 115

Gates, Bill, 48

Gates Foundation: EBM standards and accountability followed by, 58; focusing on innovative approaches to resource constraints, 179; global eradication of malaria called for by, 48–50; global health funding by, 6, 367

Geissler, Wenzel, 213–14, 219

Genetic Alliance, 356

genomics: benefits of information on, 371; Open Source Drug Discovery Project (OSDD's) completion of tuberculosis genome, 369–70; as tool for emergent ecological consciousness, 368–69

German Leprosy and TB Relief Association (GLRA), 255

Ghana guinea worm: brief history in West Africa, 210–15; controversy over ABATE chemical bringing back the, 208, 226–27, 228–29; *Cyclops* crustaceans ("water fleas") beginning life cycle of, 210–11; *Dracunculus insignis* (guinea worm) infecting dogs, 235;

health interventions (*cont'd*)
    security shaping modern, 6; interpreting the entire intervention scene, 214–15, 217–18; Island Insurance Study (IIS), 67–72; movement toward cost-effective and scalable, 8; as research, 65–66; Ugandan therapeutic clientship as, 134, 140–67, 365–66. *See also* ART programs; global health; magic-bullet approaches
heart disease: as chronic disease, 302, 303, 304; metabolic syndrome factor in, 321
Herzfeld, Michael, 76
HIPAA (US Health Insurance Portability and Accountability Act), 356, 362
Hirschfield, Lawrence, 110
Hirschman, Albert O., 14, 16
Hispanics: chronic disparities and public health genetics, 318–22; women targeted as at-risk population, 320–21
HIV/AIDS: AIDS "exceptionalism," 94, 98; CDC's first report (1981) on, 93–94. *See also* CD4 counts
HIV/AIDS epidemic: compassion for AIDS orphans and depoliticitization of, 127; emergence of children in the, 112–13; examining South African politics of childhood in context of, 27–29; food security issues related to, 177–79; framed in terms of innocent and deserving children, 119–20; framed in terms of "sexual promiscuity," 119; ignorance and fear reactions during beginning of, 92; Museveni's National Resistance Movement mobilization around, 143; "right to know" versus "know your rights" related to, 101–3; universal access to AIDS therapies, 332; viral-associated cancers and, 185. *See also* AIDS orphanhood
HIV/AIDS research: concerns over quasi-experimental models of evaluation in, 82–83; Global Fund's approach and funding percentage of, 44
HIV/AIDS transmission: ABC approach to preventing, 104, 105; debate over criminalizing, 95–97; how injustices can facilitate, 103; mother-to-child, 112, 116–20, 168, 176; "people-centered" approach to, 103–7
HIV/AIDS treatment: calls for structural-rights interventions and, 103; diversity

of international settings for, 7; examining privileged domain of knowledge in, 26–27; human rights language used to advocate for, 91–92; Iran's WHO Best Practices program for, 364; "people-centered" approach to, 103–7; PEPFAR and, 168; projectified care approach used in Uganda, 6, 140–45; "right to know" approach to, 91–92; therapeutic clientship used to receive, 134, 140–67; universal access to, 332; violation of human rights as barrier to, 103–7. *See also* ARVs (antiretroviral drugs)
HIV-related discrimination: Nkosi Johnson as face of, 114; "sexual promiscuity" as justifying, 119
HIV status: concept of "citizenship" in Ugandans with, 164; limited rights of African women with, 97, 100; right to know others,' 93–97; right to know your own HIV serostatus, 97–101
HIV testing: China's legal treatment of drug users and, 99–100; informed consent prior to, 99; issues related to mandatory, 97; Mozambique incorporation into primary health care, 170–71; right to know status of others,' 93–97; WHO's emphasis on, 98
Hopkins, Donald, 216
"horizontal" disease-specific control programs, 46
"How Not to Roll Back Malaria" (*New York Times* editorial), 46–47
humanitarianism: evidence-based standards of evaluation and, 60; health interventions shaped by, 6; paradoxes of, 210; political role of moral sentiments and, 132; trade-offs between market-driven and NGO, 367
human rights: advocating HIV treatment through language of, 91–92; criticism of "Western" values determining, 99; HIV treatment compromised by violation of, 103–7; Partners In Health approach to, 87; "people-centered" approach to, 103–7; shifts in moral culture and, 362–67. *See also* Brazilian constitutional right to health; global health politics; "right to know"; social justice approach
Human Rights Watch: documenting increasing African cancer rates, 184; opposing HIV-related restrictions to entry

judicialization of socioeconomic rights
health litigation, 334–38; continuity of
care through medical technology access
and, 341–44; crucial issues raised by
pharmaceuticalization of health care
and, 328–34; far-reaching impact in
post-apartheid South Africa, 336; role of
market forces in, 328–29. *See also* global
health politics

Kaler, Amy, 157
Kenyan study on worm infections, 17–18
Khoury, Muin, 316–17, 317
Kim, Jim Yong, 98
Kleinman, Arthur, 256, 257
Knight, Kelly, 83–84
knowledge: global health policy function
of, 26–27; as privileged domain in HIV/
AIDS treatment, 26–27; "right to know"
aspect of, 26–27; structural rights
related to, 27
Kochi Arata, 47, 49–50
Kremer, Michael, 17–18
Kuhn, Thomas, 83–84

labor: Chilean informal "indefinite contracts" system of, 277, 287–88; Chilean
piecework sewing in *la rueda,* 288–89;
Pinochet regime's reform of the Labor
Code, 287–88
LAM (lymphangioleiomyomatosis):
description of, 356; "empirical lantern"
story of, 356; LTA devoted to fighting,
356–61, 362; Novartis-sponsored RCT
on, 359–62; pioneering problem-solving
innovations to fight, 356–62
LAM Treatment Alliance (LTA), 356–61,
362
Lancet (journal): article criticizing Roll
Back Malaria program, 46; editorial
celebrating malaria eradication goal, 49;
"Epitaph for Global Malaria Eradica-
tion?" editorial, 34; Global Mental
Health: 1 Year On series of, 279–80;
Molyneux's article on guinea worm
eradication, 232; "Movement for Global
Mental Health" campaign launched by,
280; "Treating Depression in Primary
Care in Low-Income Women in San-
tiago, Chile: A Randomised Controlled
Trial," 282
Lancet Oncology journal, 183

Latour, Bruno, 256
laughter: autopalliation through, 200–202;
Botswana cultural artifact regarding
pain and, 198–200
League of Nations Health Organization,
118, 350
Lee Jong-wook, 47
Lévi-Strauss, Claude, 218
Lhasa Health Bureau, 80
lifestyle diseases: diabetes labeled as, 351;
genetic predisposition to, 317–18; obesity framed as, 303, 304, 305, 310–11,
314–15
Lissouba, Pascal, 36
Liverpool School of Tropical Medicine, 40
Livingston, Julie, 136, 182, 364, 366
long-lasting insecticidal nets (LLINs), 47
"looping effects," 256
LTFU (lost to follow–up) risk: Mozambique
ART programs and, 175–76; pregnant
women and, 135–36
Lupin Ltd. (India): rise as leading producer
of anti-TB drugs, 257–59; as TB Alliance
stakeholder, 254; "tracking pharmaceuticals" project on anti-TB drug market
role of, 257–75. *See also* "Champions of
the Chest"

Madagascar malaria epidemic (1988), 31
magic: ethnographic accounts on witch
doctor healing with, 218; public health
magic-bullet competing with local, 223–
29; Ugandan witch doctor, 140, 141
magic-bullet approaches: ABATE chemical
formula to kill guinea worm larvae as,
208, 226–27, 228–29; competing with
local witch doctor magic, 223–29; cultural barriers to using devices distributed
by, 223–25; description of, 3–4, 223;
guinea worm water filters perceived as,
221, 225–26; launched against malaria
(mid-1950s), 30, 349–50; Roll Back
Malaria (RBM) positioning itself as, 24,
48. *See also* health interventions
Malaria: According to the New Researches
(Celli), 349
malaria containment programs: Brundtland's WHO leadership impact on,
38–39; Global Fund's funding of, 44;
Global Malaria Control Strategy (1992)
on, 36–37; insecticide-treated mosquito
nets (ITNs) strategy of, 40, 44, 45;

neoliberalism: audit cultures of, 76–77; labor regimes of, 287; reemergence of, 38, 50; state and, 330; structural adjustment and, 167; patienthood in, 134; privatization of health in, 71–72; public-private partnerships and, 39

Nepal: anti-TB drug market in, 256–75; examining the TB programs in, 256; Lupin's increasing dominance of anti-TB drugs in, 259; unethical marketing practices of MRs in, 268

nevirapine, 112

New Orleans program, 25

"new variant famine," 177–79

New York City's condom distribution, 104

New York Times: "How Not to Roll Back Malaria" editorial in, 46–47; Kenyan worm infections story by, 17; on local resistance to guinea-worm eradication efforts in Nigeria, 214; reporting Seretide (inhaler) as bestselling drug, 306

"NGO industrial complex," 25

NGOs (non-governmental organizations): being pressured to work with local public sector, 180–81, 223–29, 364–67; EBM's profits and the NGO-industrial complex and audit culture, 76–79; Global Fund's CCM requirement of, 43–44; increasing demands for accountability of, 77; international health proliferation of, 77–78; most of PEPFAR funding channeled to, 166–67; "NGO Code of Conduct for Health System Strengthening" proposed for, 179–80; storage of health workers due to higher wages paid by, 135; TAR Health Bureau project partnership with, 79–83; therapeutic clientship role of, 134; trade-offs of humanitarian intervention by, 367. *See also* civil society; PEPFAR (US President's Emergency Plan for AIDS Relief)

Nguyen Vinh-Kim, 151

Nigeria: "Eradicating Guinea Worm Without Wells: Unrealized Hopes of the Water Decade" report on, 221; "resistance in the population" to eradication of guinea worm in, 214–15, 217

Nkosi's Havens (homes for HIV-positive mothers and children), 114

noncompliance: asthma medication, 305–6; Barbados framing asthma as problem

of inhaler, 306, 309; cultural factors to consider in, 214–15, 217; economic costs to Barbados of asthma, 313–14; economic costs to Trinidad, 314. *See also* compliance

The Normal and the Pathological (Canguilhem), 218

Novartis, 359

Novartis India, 254

obesity: American shame approach to, 310; biomedical asceticism approach to problem of, 310–11; as chronic disease problem, 303, 304, 305; economic costs to Trinidad of noncompliance cause of, 314–15

"open-source anarchy," 251, 336

ORG-INS (India), 263

orphans: AIDS orphanhood of, 27–29, 111–13, 125–28; historic Western concerns over, 124–25; "philanthropic abduction" creating, 125; UNICEF estimates on worldwide number of, 125. *See also* children

OSDD (Open Source Drug Discovery Project) [India], 369–70

Packard, Randall, 349

pain: Botswana's oncology ward and logics of, 183–85; as fundamental social experience in Botswana's cancer ward, 202–3; as individually held experience that "shatters language," 184; reasons for marginalization of in African clinical medicine, 188–91; relationship between laughter and, 198–202

pain management: in Botswana's cancer ward, 187–91; by silencing patient complaints in Botswana's cancer ward, 191–97

palliative care: African palliative care movement, 188; Botswana patients' use of laughter as form of autopalliation, 200–202; developing guidelines in Botswana, 188; shared history of cancer and, 190–91

Pan American Health Organization, 31

pandemics, 369

para-aminosalicylic acid (PAS), 258

parasites: failed DDT-centered (1950s to 1960s) to eradicate malaria, 23, 32–34,350; Ghana guinea worm,

parasites (*cont'd*)
138–39, 207–36; Kenyan study on worm infections, 17–18; malaria carried by Anopheles mosquitoes, 350; *S. sanctipauli* blackflies causing river blindness, 223–24, 227

Park, Sung-John, 164

Partners In Health: human-rights approach by, 87; social justice approach of, 10

patents: Brazilian constitutional right to health implications for, 326–29; Brazilian patient-litigants challenging, 325–28, 332–38; "golden rice" issue, 354; PXE International providing challenges to "ownership" of disease and, 356; WTO membership requiring India rewrite their patent laws, 353. *See also* pharmaceutical corporations

patient advocacy movement, 323

patient-citizen-consumers, 338, 355

patient empowerment movement, 311, 323

patients: concerns over erasure of caregiving relationship to, 86; "empirical lantern" for understanding the, 14, 17; global health stuck in access mindset instead of value to, 8–9; growing public health focus on future of, 322–23; litigating, 326–27; rare disease trials and, 327, 339, 341, 359; silencing pain complaints by Botswana's cancer ward, 191–97; Ugandan therapeutic clientship engaged in by, 134, 140–67. *See also* ART programs; compliance; ethnographic case studies; subjects

patron-client systems: exchange between unequal parties in, 154–58; personalistic African, 151; Ugandan therapeutic clientship form of, 134, 140–67

Patton, Michael Quinn, 82–83

"people-centered approach": game-changing impact of the, 105–6; to HIV and transmission and treatment, 103–7; NGO Code of Conduct and, 179–80; to strengthening public services, 176

People's Republic of Congo, 36

PEPFAR (US President's Emergency Plan for AIDS Relief): complex political economy of, 167–68; examining the global health role of, 6, 135; HAI as designated partner for central Mozambique with, 167–68, 169–71, 176, 180–81; impact of funding NGOs over public sector by,

166–67, 171, 367; policy on supporting many different ART programs, 143, 152; role in postwar Mozambique's AIDS epidemic, 171–75; SAPs (structural adjustment programs) constraints on funding by, 167, 365; Ugandan Mukuju Health Center ART program funded by, 142, 365. *See also* NGOs (non-governmental organizations)

Persistent Organic Pollutants Treaty (2001), 42

Personal Genome Project (PGP), 368

Petersen, Hector, 115

Petryna, Adriana, 1, 29, 80, 85, 87, 243, 250, 251, 355, 363, 364, 366, 370, 371, 372

Pfeiffer, James, 135, 136, 166, 364, 366, 370

Pfizer India, 258, 274

pharmaceutical company drug donation programs, 6

pharmaceutical contract research organizations (CROs), 59–60

pharmaceutical corporations: Eli Lilly, 254; Lupin Ltd., 245, 254, 257–75; Novartis, 359; Novartis India, 254; TB treatment through PPMs (Public-Private Mixes), 244–45, 253–54; trade-offs of humanitarian intervention by, 367. *See also* patents

pharmaceuticalization of health care: crucial issues raised by judicialization of socioeconomic rights and, 328–34; examining the challenges of, 15; extension of diagnostic categories linked to, 315–16. *See also* health care

pharmaceutical market: Brazil as eighth largest, 249; how Chile's National Program for the Diagnosis and Treatment of Depression was shaped by, 277–99; Indian and Nepal's anti-TB drug, 245, 254–72; unequal drug pricing worldwide issue of, 331. *See also* medications

pharmaceutical researchers: Arterolane developed through cross-national collaboration, 353; international health work role of, 59–60; use of RCT model to unite international health programs and bench science of, 60–64; Synriam synthetic for treating malaria, 352–53; troubling uptake of high-tech treatments and, 339; working on orphan disease

randomized controlled trials (cont'd)
and, 339. *See also* biomedical science;
pharmaceutical researchers; subjects
rape: mythical association with black
males, 123; South African crisis of, 124;
South African HIV epidemic context of
child, 121–24; uncritical explanations of,
126; violence history and, 127; "virgin-
cleansing myth" driving, 123
Rasmussen, Sonja A., 317
R-cinex, 257, 269
Reagan, Ronald, 38
resiliency-training programs: to low SES
school-age children, 72–73; questionnaire instruments used in, 73–74; solution to ethical conundrum of, 73
resource constraints: Gates Foundation focus on innovative approaches to, 179; as
justifying cost-effectiveness approaches,
181
Revised National TB Control Programme
(RNTCP) [India], 255, 275
Ributin (rifbutin 150mg), 258, 261–62
rifampicin, 257, 258, 266
Rififi (film), 261
rights-based pilot projects, 6
"rights of the child" (UN, 1989), 110–11
"right to know": Chinese laws related
to HIV testing drug users and, 99–100;
comparing WHO's and UNICEF's
campaigns for, 92–93, 101–2, 106; criticism of "Western" values determining,
99; debate over balancing individual
and community rights, 96; HIV treatment and, 91–92; knowledge aspect
of, 26–27; "know your rights" versus,
101–3; others' HIV status, 93–97;
possible policy changes through, 107;
TAC's broad-based campaign on,
103; your own HIV status, 97–101,
102. *See also* global health activism;
human rights; "your right to know"
campaigns
right to health: as constitutional mandate,
327–30, 332, 371; high drug costs and,
343–44; interpretations of scope of,
101–5; litigation and judicialization of,
326, 332–37, 343; pharmaceuticalization and, 329, 363
river blindness: *S. sanctipauli* blackflies
causing, 227; study on campaign to
eradicate, 223–24

Rockefeller Foundation, 37, 349
Roll Back Malaria (RBM): British bilateral
assistance agency support of, 40; criticisms and reorganizations of, 45–48;
eight MDGs and objectives of the,
40–41; Global Fund support of, 43–44,
46; global health politics and role of,
23; Global Malaria Action Plan by, 48;
insecticide-treated mosquito nets (ITNs)
strategy of, 40, 44, 45; LLINs (long-
lasting insecticidal nets) term used by,
47; origins and partners in, 39–40; positioning itself as a magic bullet, 24, 48
"Roll Back Malaria: A Failing Global
Health Campaign" (*British Medical
Journal*), 46
Román, Oscar, 283

S. sanctipauli blackflies, 227
Sachs, Jeffrey, 39, 42
Salazar, Gabriel, 287
salvage ethnography: description and
debate over, 210; on the Guinea Worm
Eradication Program experience, 215–
36; on Guinea worm in history of West
Africa, 210–15
Samba, Ebrahim, 37
SAPs (structural adjustment programs):
innovations to overcome constraints
of, 365; origins of World Bank/IMF,
173; PEPFAR funding constraints by,
167; postwar Mozambique rebuilding
through, 174
SARS crisis, 369
Save the Children Fund, 58, 77, 118
"Save the Guinea Worm Foundation," 232
Scarry, Elaine, 184, 187
Schoolnik, Gary, 370
Science (journal), 39
Scott, James, 111
Section 27 (formerly AIDS Law Project),
103
security issues of health interventions, 6
Seidu-Korkor, Andrews, 220, 221
Shanta Biotech (Hyderabad), 354
Silent Spring (Carson), 34
smallpox campaign (1960s), 216
Smith, Charlene, 123
Snyder, Michael, 351, 357, 362
social justice approach: Brazilian constitu-
tional right to health, 326–29; decline
of civil society as transactional locus for,